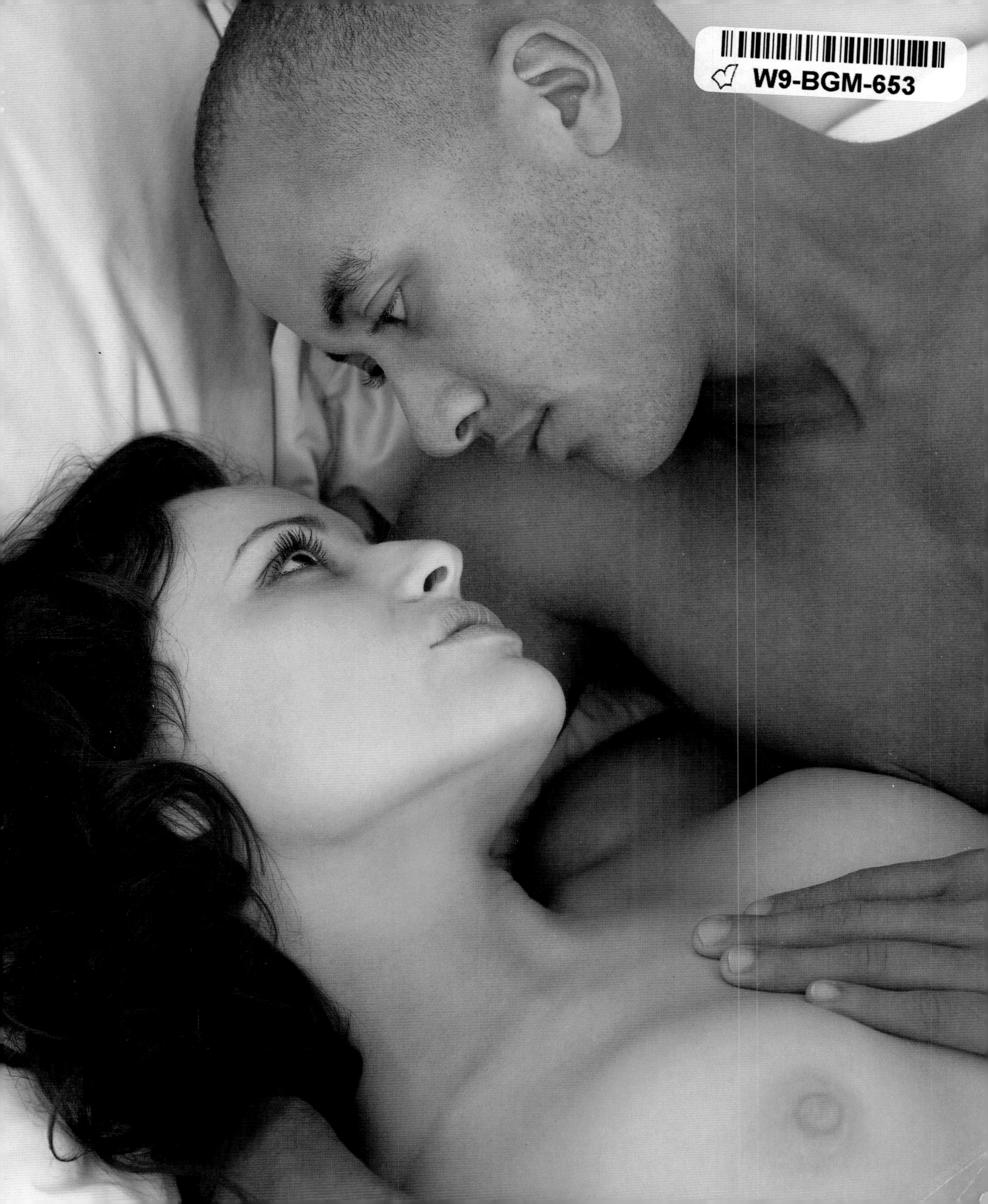

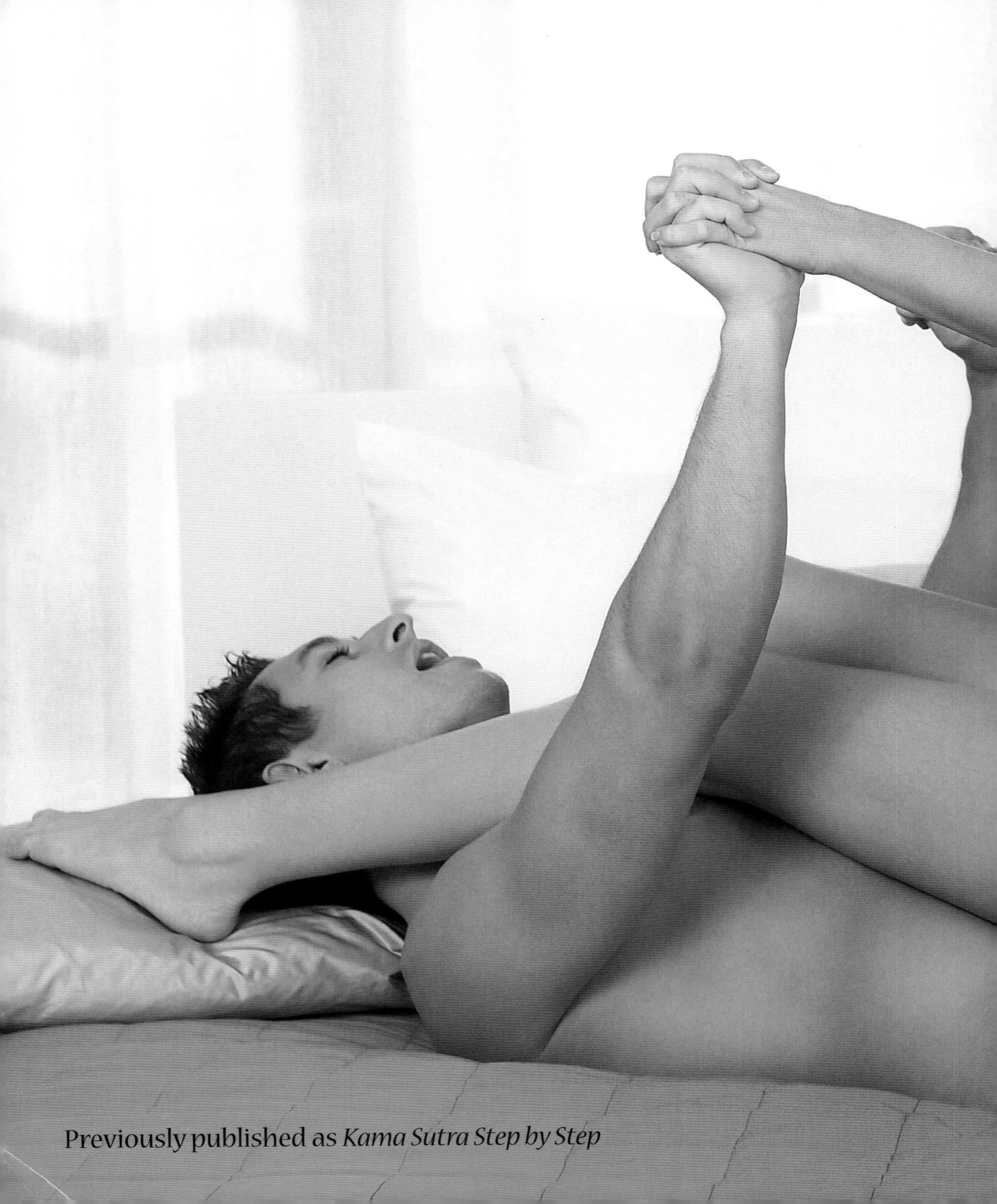

Previously published as *Kama Sutra Step by Step*

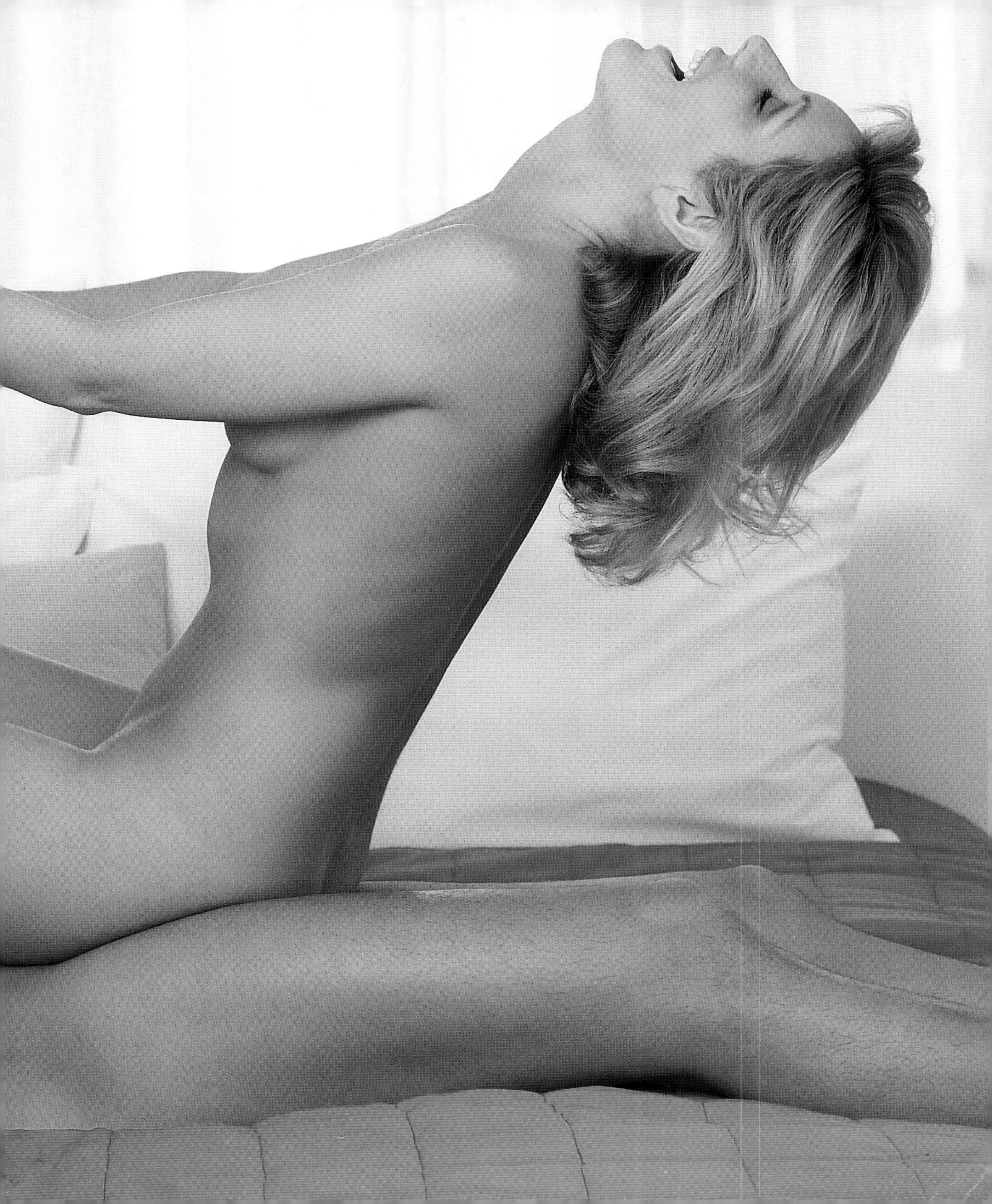

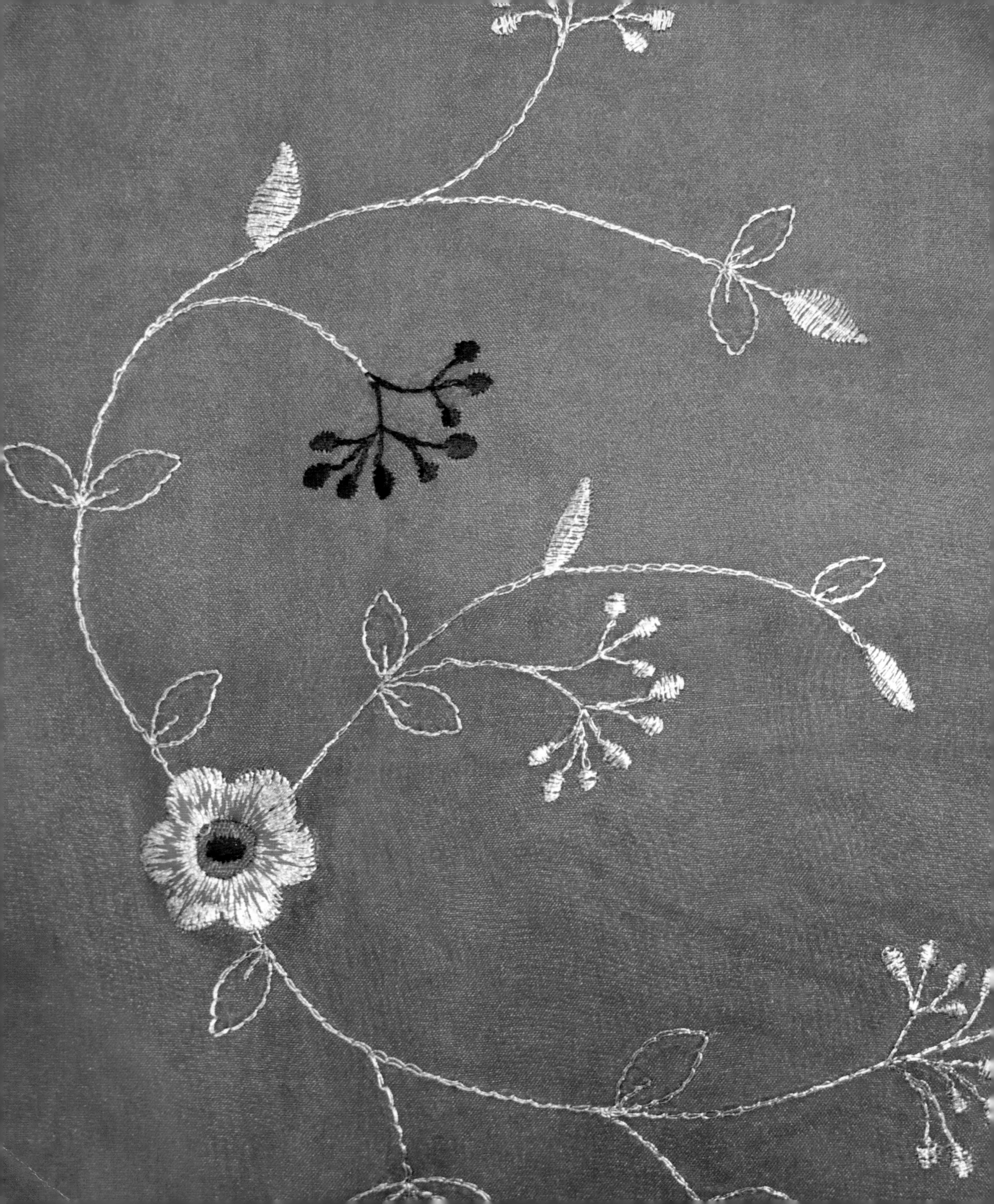

Contents

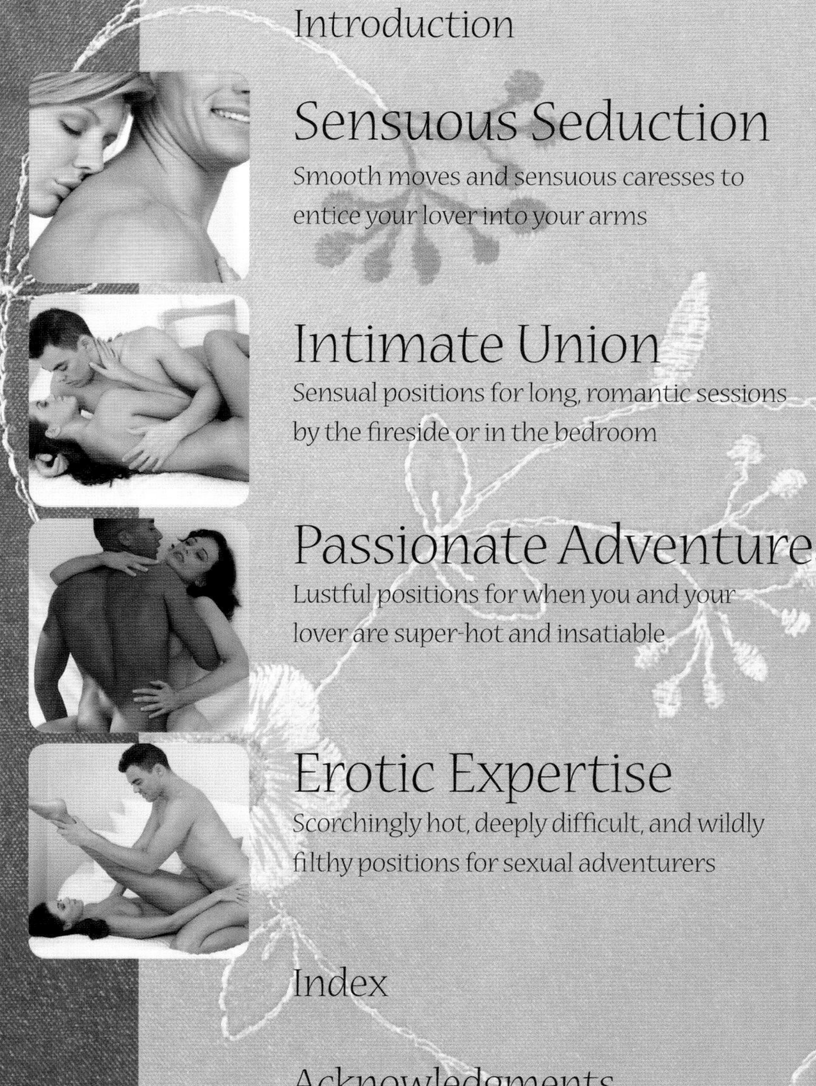

Introduction

Erotic, exotic, and acrobatic, the jaw-dropping, joint-cracking sex positions of the *Kama Sutra* have enthralled readers for centuries. But behind the sexual gymnastics, the book itself is filled with ancient sexual wisdom that will benefit any couple.

What is the *Kama Sutra*?

The original *Kama Sutra* was written in 3rd-century India by a man known as Vatsyayana Malla. It had no pictures and the text appeared in Sanskrit "sutras": short, pithy phrases that were designed to be memorized. Little is known about Vatsyayana, but he was eager to establish his squeaky-clean motives, saying that he composed the *Kama Sutra* "in chastity and in the highest meditation."

More is known about the two British men who picked up the *Kama Sutra* in the 19th century and set about getting it translated into English. Their names were Sir Richard Francis Burton and Forster Fitzgerald Arbuthnot, and their translation revived modern interest in the ancient text. Burton was an explorer, writer, and soldier. Arbuthnot was an ex-civil servant and translator. Their mission was to bring the erotic wisdom of the East to Victorian England; no easy task given the repressive attitudes of the time.

As Burton and Fitzgerald were aware, the *Kama Sutra* was not the only sex manual to come out of Asia over the centuries. The *Ananga Ranga* is another Indian love text, written in the 15th century by Kalyana Malla. It was intended to "prevent lives and loves being wasted" due to ignorance of the divine pleasures of the arts of love. *The Perfumed Garden* came from 16th-century Tunis and was written by Sheik Nefzawi, to encourage sexual satisfaction, and hence fidelity, in the married couples of the kingdom. Positions from both titles appear in this book, along with some from *The Tao*, a series of ancient Chinese pillow books.

The generally more open and relaxed sexual climate of the 1960s meant that the *Kama Sutra* could finally come out of hiding, and people have been happily bending themselves into its sexual knots ever since.

The unseen *Kama Sutra*

Despite its worldwide reputation for exotic and saucy sex positions, the *Kama Sutra* isn't all about sex. It consists of seven books, only one of which discusses sex in detail.

The other six books have nothing to do with the nitty-gritty of sex. Instead, they describe how men and women should behave in sexual and romantic relationships. Vatsyayana

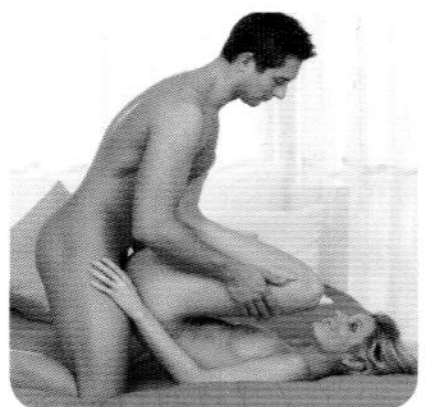
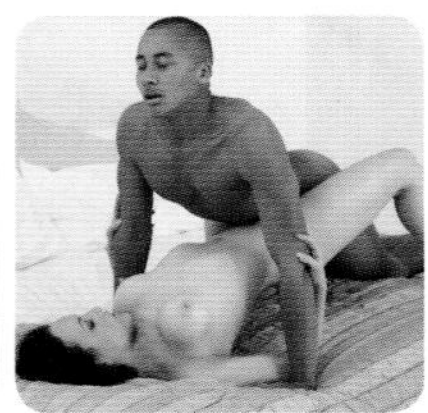
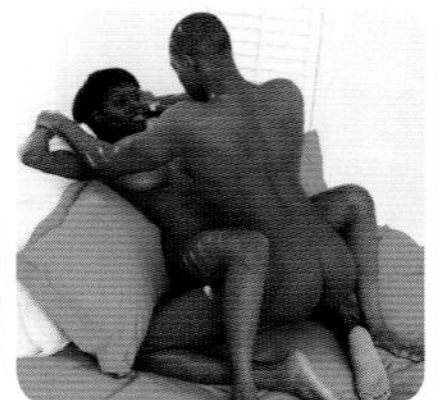
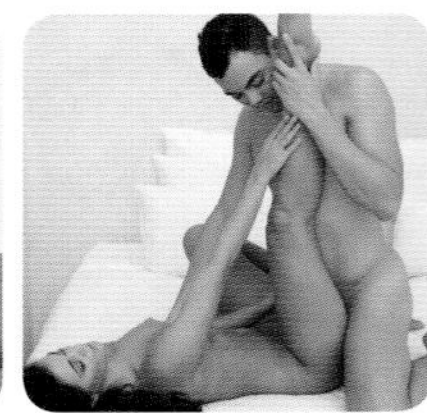
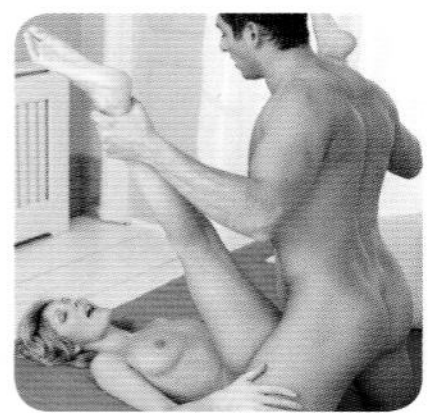
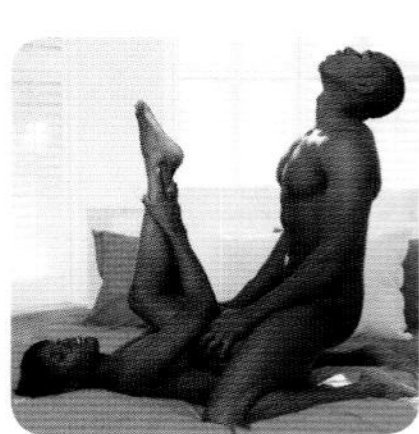

"Kama is the enjoyment of appropriate objects by the five senses of hearing, feeling, seeing, tasting, and smelling, assisted by the mind together with the soul." KAMA SUTRA

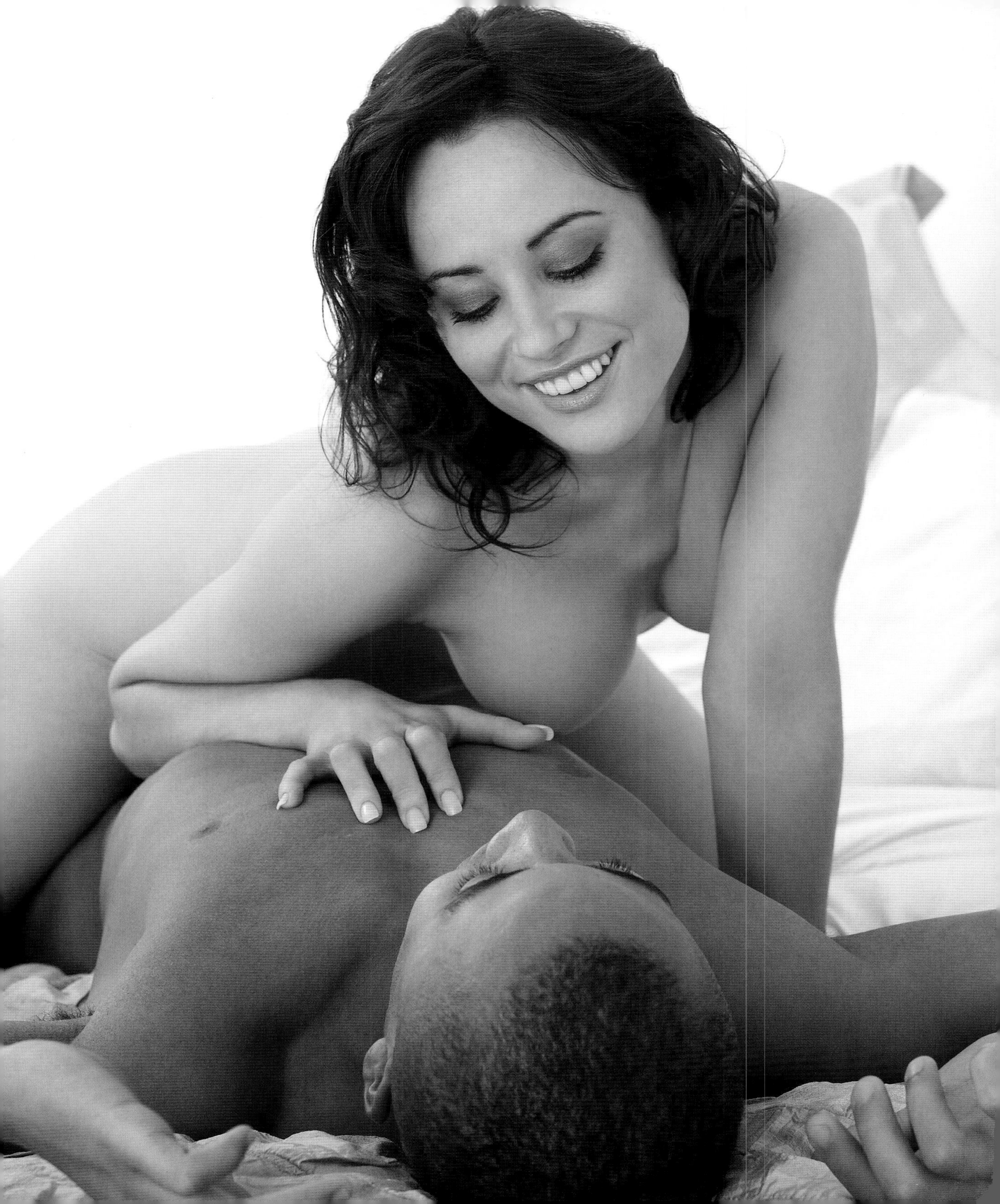

dispenses lengthy advice to men on how they should attract a woman, especially a virgin (the whole of book three), and how to manage her once she's been snared. Women are furnished with instructions on their correct conduct as wives, courtesans, members of the harem, and romantic gossipers and go-betweens.

Simply being good in bed wasn't enough in Vatsyayana's eyes. Along with the *Kama Sutra*, 64 other fine arts should be studied. These include: preparing wines, fruit juices, and other drinks; teaching parrots and mynah birds to talk; knowledge of omens; carpentry; sleight of hand; improvising poetry; dancing; cutting leaves into shapes; and rubbing, massaging, and hairdressing. If you want to be an accomplished lover, ancient Indian-style, the *Kama Sutra* book one contains the full instructions.

Whether it's luring a virgin into bed or visiting a harem, very few sexual deeds and misdeeds are frowned upon in the *Kama Sutra*. It's even OK for a man to steal another man's wife. More than OK in fact; Vatsyayana lists the reasons a married woman might resist a suitor (understandable ones such as love for her husband, regard for her children, or contempt for the suitor…), then offers men instructions on how to quash each one of these reasons. Here's how a man should snare a married woman:

"He gazes at her constantly… When she is looking at him he should speak to his friends about her… Then within her hearing, and without looking at her at all, he talks about the Kama Sutra*."*

Vatsyayana also gives the thumbs-up to husbands having multiple wives, mistresses, and concubines. But, as always in the *Kama Sutra*, lovers must abide by the rule book:

"Whatever love-play one woman favors, or whatever peculiarity her body may have, or whatever reproach she lets slip during pillow talk—he must not tell that to the other women."

Toys, props, and potions

The *Kama Sutra* isn't averse to a little artificial help in the quest for great sex. For men who can't satisfy their lovers, Vatsyayana recommends the aid of a dildo made of gold, silver, copper, iron, ivory, or buffalo horn. Alternatively, a man can attach a well-greased cucumber, lotus stalk, or bamboo stalk to his hips and use that as a penis substitute during intercourse with his (presumably long-suffering) wife. And if a man wants to increase the size of his member, he need only rub it with insect bristles, massage it with oil for 10 nights, and wait for it to swell. Oh yes, then lie face-down on a bed and dangle his penis through a hole cut especially for the purpose.

Potions can also help you to procure a lover. Vatsyayana recommends ointments and powders (even eye make-up) made from hogweed, clarified butter, wild ginger, and blue lotus leaves to help the cause. These "erotic esoterica" are listed at the end of the *Kama Sutra* as an appendix of back-up techniques to be used when all else fails. As Vatsyayana says: "A person who has not obtained the object of their desires may have recourse to these secret recipes."

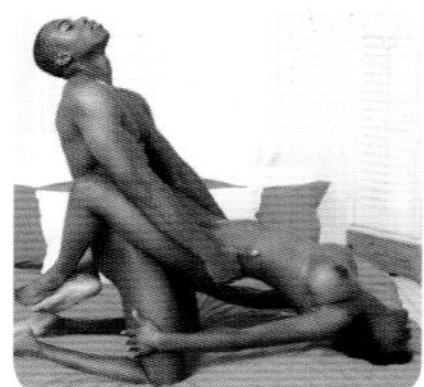
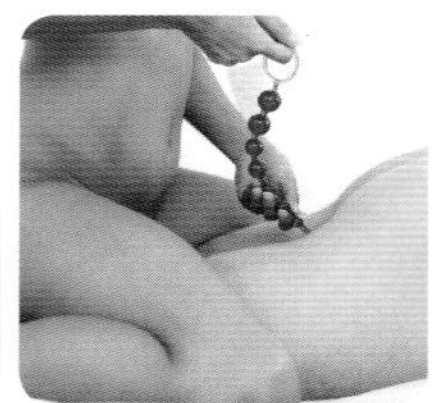
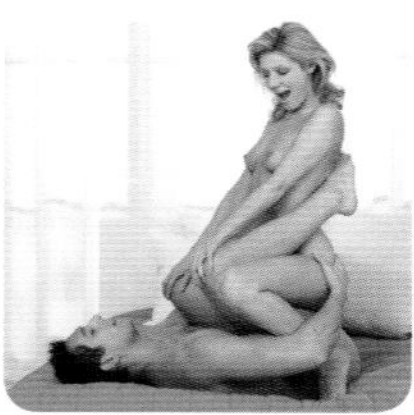
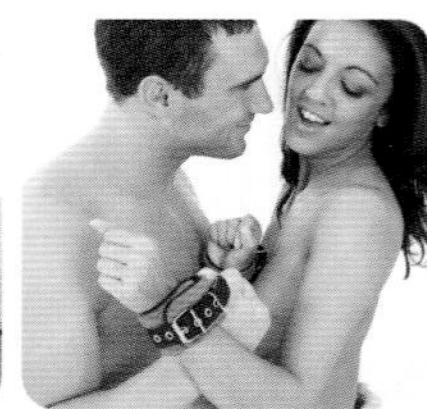
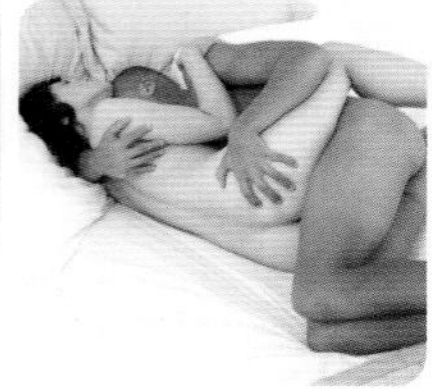
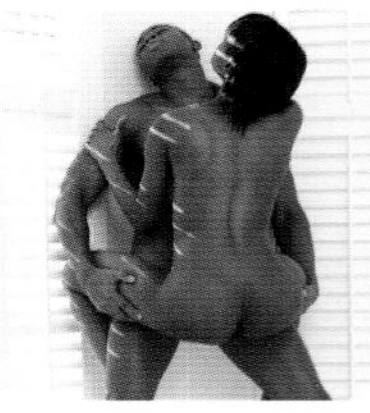

"Sexual intercourse being a thing dependent on man and woman requires the application of proper means…" KAMA SUTRA

Thankfully, modern sex toys are rather more advanced than the marital aids of 3rd-century India. Contemporary versions are body-friendly, multitasking, and precision-targeted to thrill your erotic hot spots. (And they are unlikely to make your penis swell.) It is now possible to stimulate your lover exactly where they like for as long as they like, or to deliver vibrations direct to their genitals just by texting their cell phone. And toys and props are no longer seen as remedies for bad sex; they're there to enhance our abilities rather than compensate for lack of them.

Sprinkled throughout the following chapters are tips and suggestions about how to incorporate sex toys and props into your love life, to maximize your between-the-sheets pleasure. Use them to take your arousal a notch higher and to give your lover a titillating surprise.

The *Kama Sutra* in your bed

So without further ado, it is time to discover the book that lifts, spins, twists, and flips everything you knew about sex positions. It not only gives you the sheer range of Eastern love postures, but shows you how you can actually try them for yourselves. If you don't know how to split the bamboo or play the transverse lute, you soon will.

Each sex position is broken down into stages, to help you untangle the knots of limbs. Sexy photographs guide you through every leg lift, skin caress, thigh squeeze, and pelvic thrust. Explicit instructions explain exactly what to do, ensuring that you and your lover are never left dangling from the ceiling light thinking, "What next?" And if there's a prop or technique that will enhance your pleasure in a particular pose, it's highlighted for your attention.

Both the erotic temperature and the level of difficulty goes up a notch in each chapter, so if you're feeling smoochy, sensual, and in the mood for something easy, start in chapters 1 or 2. But if you're sizzling and up for a challenge, thrust straight ahead to chapters 3 and 4.

The techniques and positions on the following pages are all sourced from the Eastern erotic texts the *Kama Sutra*, the *Ananga Ranga*, *The Perfumed Garden*, and *The Tao*. You can pick and mix them to create a wild marathon of sex positions that leaves you hot and gasping. Alternatively, you can take one or two and linger over them with luscious intensity; treat yourself to a tantra-style session in which you get into position and stay there for the duration. Keep yourselves at an erotic simmer with lots of sexy eye contact, deep synchronized breathing, and internal squeezes from your pelvic-floor muscles.

So put your best sheets on the bed, slip off each other's clothes, and launch your lust by selecting your first position. Then go forth and tangle your limbs.

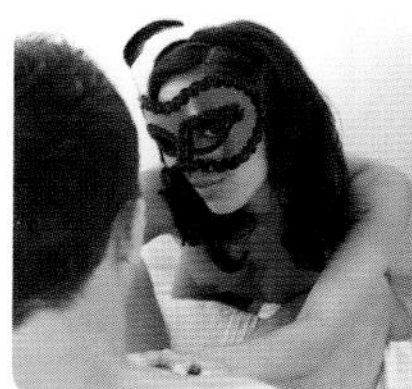
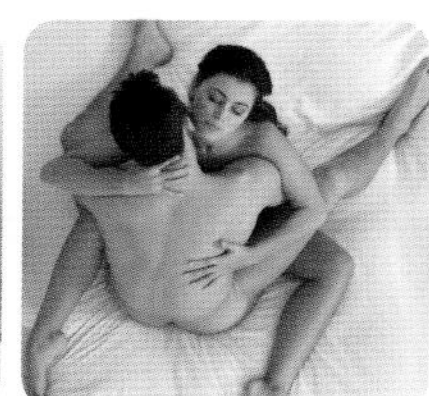
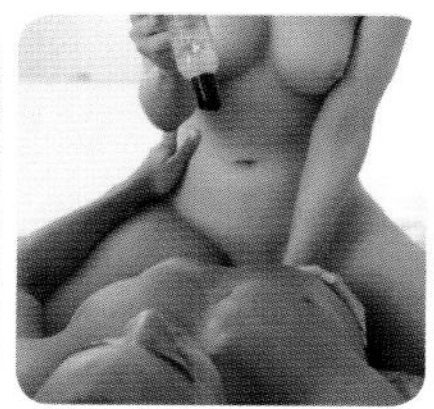
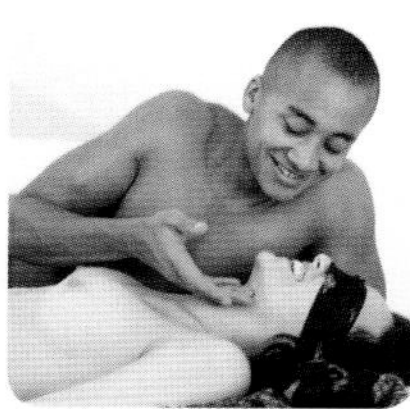
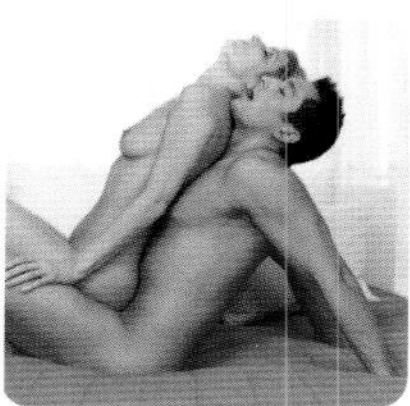
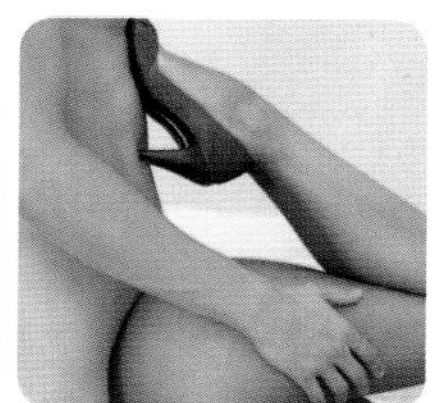

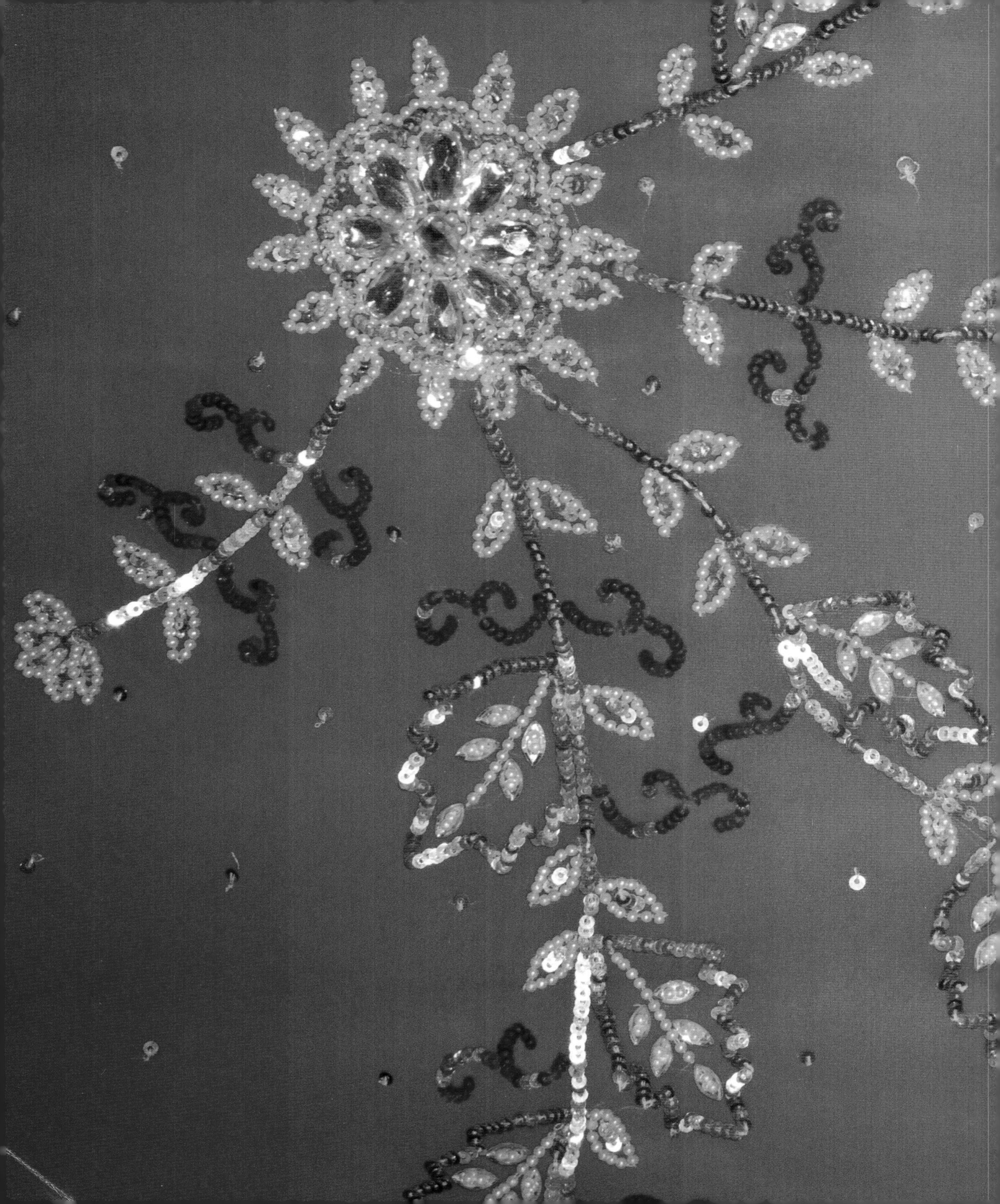

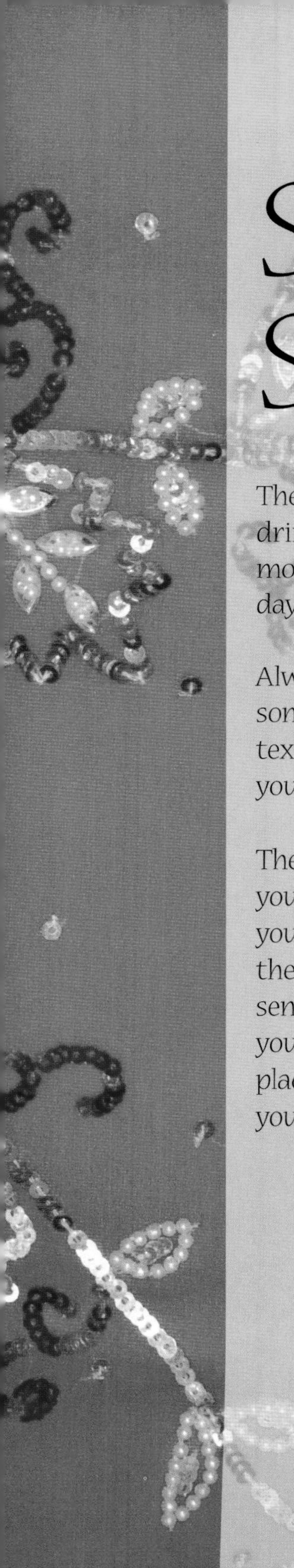

Sensuous Seduction

The curtains are closed, the candlelight is flickering, the drinks are chilling… all you need now are some smooth moves to entice your lover away from the rigors of the day and into your melting embrace.

Always bear in mind that no seduction is complete without some serious kissing, *Kama Sutra*-style. However, the ancient texts insist that, once you've aroused your lover with a kiss, you must be prepared to follow up with other seductive skills.

The following pages show you how to seduce in style. Pick your technique and apply it with all the seductive mastery you can muster. If you choose to undress your lover, peel off the layers in a way that borders on reverential. If you opt for a sensual embrace, make it time-stoppingly intense. If you treat your partner to some oral loving, show them that there's no place in the world you'd rather be. Whatever you do, devote yourself, mind and body, to the moment.

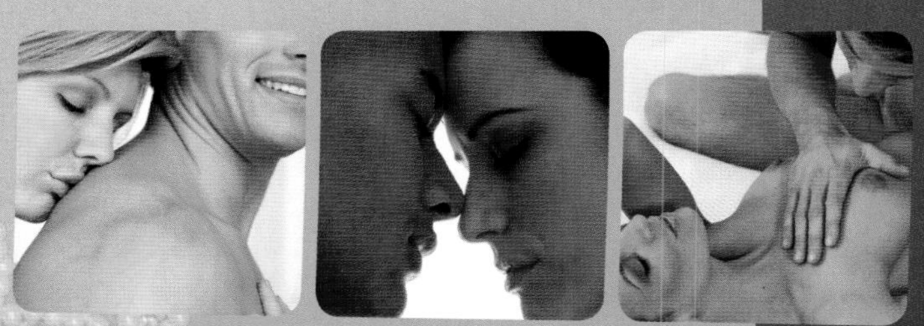

Seduction

Seduction can happen in the wink of an eye or the sending of a wickedly explicit text message. It can also be a more lengthy, lingering affair, in which you can make use of the techniques shown here. Either way, take your lead from the *Kama Sutra* and make seduction your top priority.

The must-have-it mood

It's easy to pounce on your lover when you're in the mood. The challenge comes when they're NOT in the mood. Maybe they've just come home from work, maybe they've got stuff on their mind… Your job is to turn them around and get them into a must-have-it mood. And to do this you need some hot seduction techniques under your belt. Try any of the following to drive your lover wild with desire:

Call your lover when you're just minutes away from meeting them. Tickle their sense of anticipation by telling them that you're so horny that you want to have sex straight away. Tell them to prepare accordingly. Or, if you want to appeal to your lover's sense of fun, try seducing them with sheer playfulness. Challenge them to a pillow fight or dress up in their underwear and demand that they undress you.

Turn the tables

If you're always the one to seduce and initiate in your sex life, try shaking things up with some reverse psychology. Tell your partner that you're going on a sex "detox" for a few days. Hint that you could be persuaded to break your fast if the right kind of temptation came along. You'll see a whole new side of them as they struggle to get you into bed.

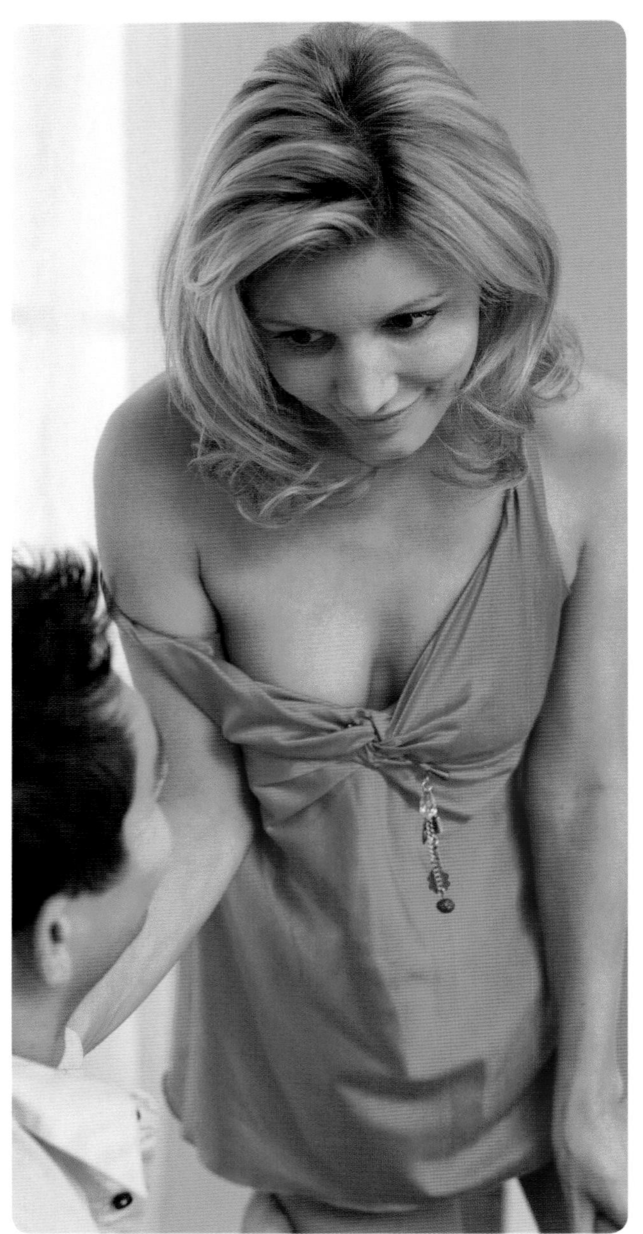

The power of the mind

If you can fill your lover's head with lust and lechery, you may find that their body is raring to go before you even touch them. Try asking your lover to describe in detail a sexy act they'd like to perform on you.

"He should seat her on his left side and, holding her hair, and touching also the end and knot of her garment, he should gently embrace her with his right arm." KAMA SUTRA

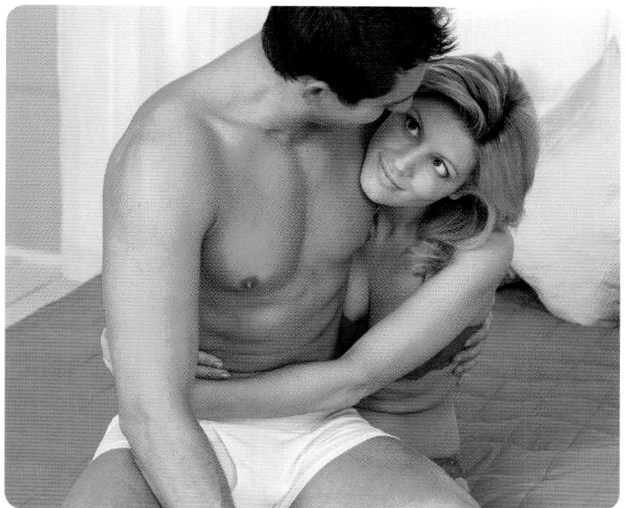

Erotic suggestion

Follow Vatsyayana's advice and indulge in some sexy chat to get things going: "... talk suggestively of things that would be considered coarse, or not to be mentioned in society."

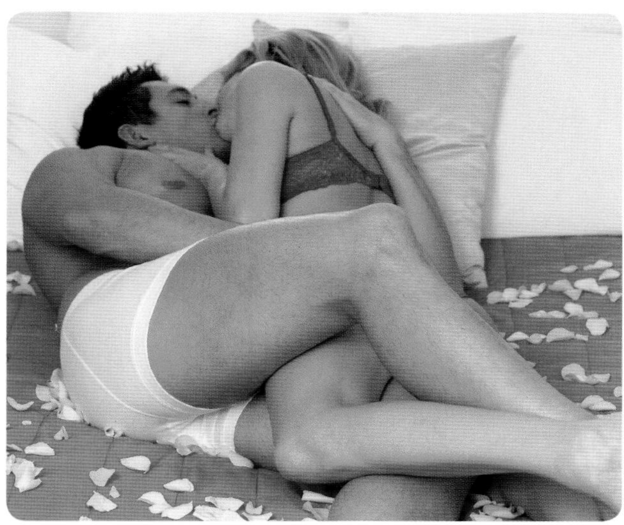

Flirting with finesse

Show your sexy intentions by decorating the bed with flower petals. Then drag your partner into the bedroom for some good old-fashioned flirting and fondling, so they know exactly what you have in mind.

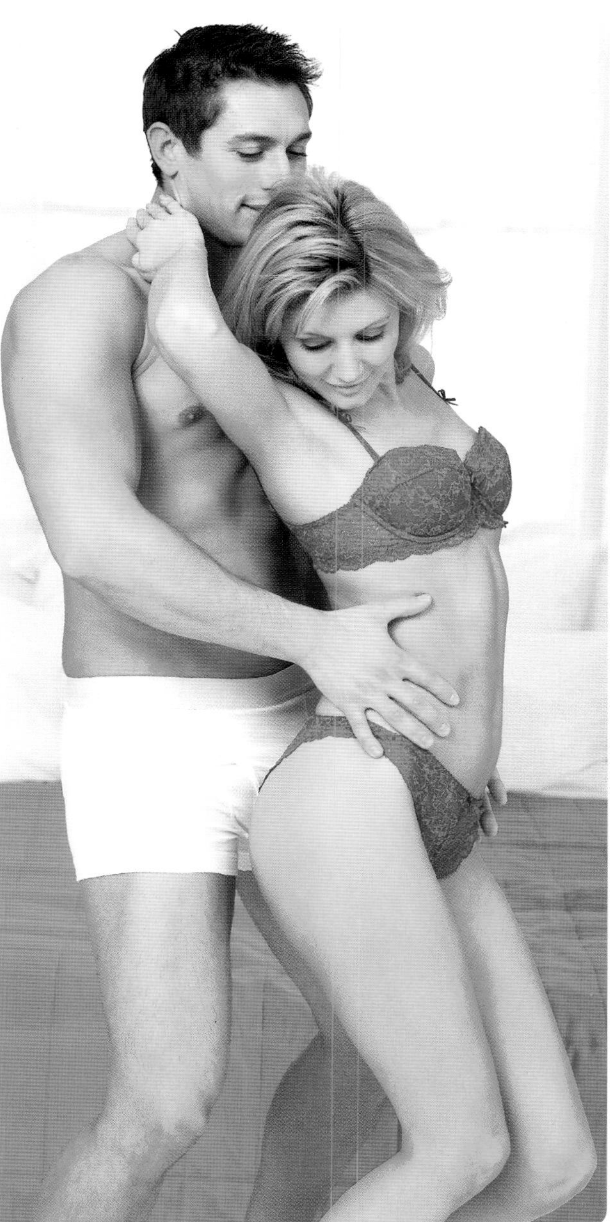

Setting the mood

You can also set the mood dial to seductive by doing something arousing together, such as slow and sexy dancing. Start off clothed and help each other slowly undress as the dance heats up.

Embraces

An erotic embrace can take the sexual mood from tepid to torrid in the bat of an eyelash. Little compares to the experience of standing with your body in a tight clinch against your lover's. It allows you to put all the stresses and strains of the world behind you, and to enter the realm of your senses.

External enjoyments

The ancient erotic texts are united on the subject of embraces: they are essential preliminaries to the act of love. The *Ananga Ranga* refers to them as "external enjoyments" that "should always precede internal enjoyments." Their job is to "develop the desire… These affect the senses and divert the mind from coyness and coldness."

Embraces are so important that they are listed for every occasion. Some of the embraces that the *Kama Sutra* recommends, such as The Twining of a Creeper, should be "performed at the time of greeting a lover," and are intended as sensual expressions of affection. Others, such as The Embrace of Milk and Water, are intended to get you hot under the collar.

Reaping the rewards

The message is pretty simple: spend lots of time embracing in the build-up to sex. Hugs, strokes, snogs, and cuddles ramp up the sexual tension so that sex becomes more explosive when you get down to it. And don't save embraces just for sex; make them part of everyday life so that any moment can be sensual. Hug hello, lie entwined while you're watching a movie, and say goodbye with a sexy full-body embrace.

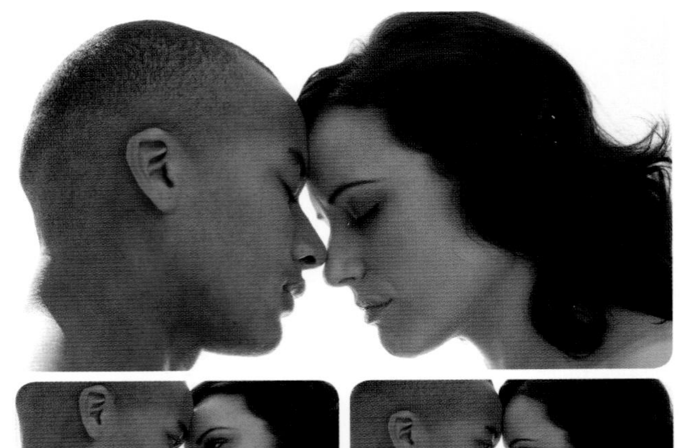

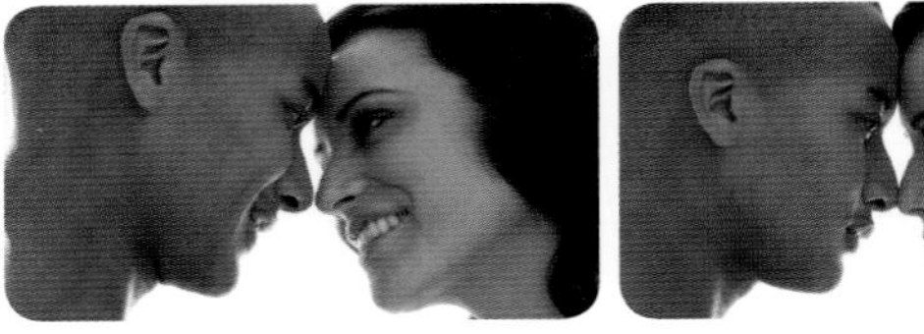

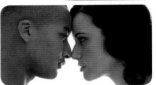

Embrace of the forehead

You lean towards each other so that your foreheads are pressed together. Be still for a moment to feel your partner's breath caressing your face, and enjoy the intimacy of close union.

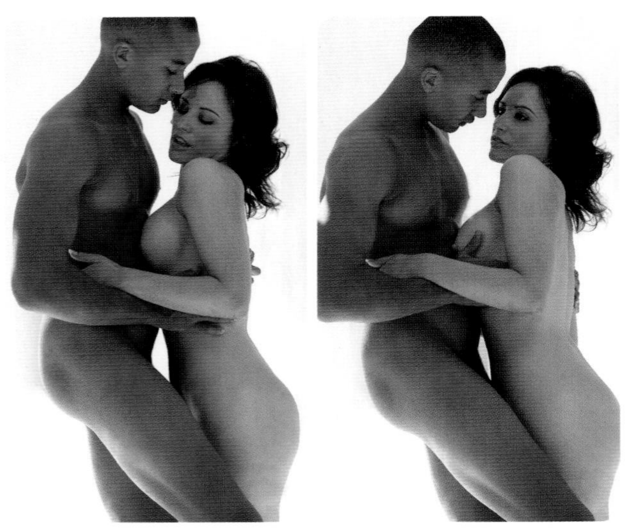

The piercing embrace

She presses her breasts against his body in a passionate I-want-you-right-now gesture he won't be able to resist. He cups her breasts in his hands and strokes them gently.

"Embracing is of such a nature that men who ask questions about it, or who hear about it, or who talk about it, acquire thereby a desire for enjoyment." KAMA SUTRA

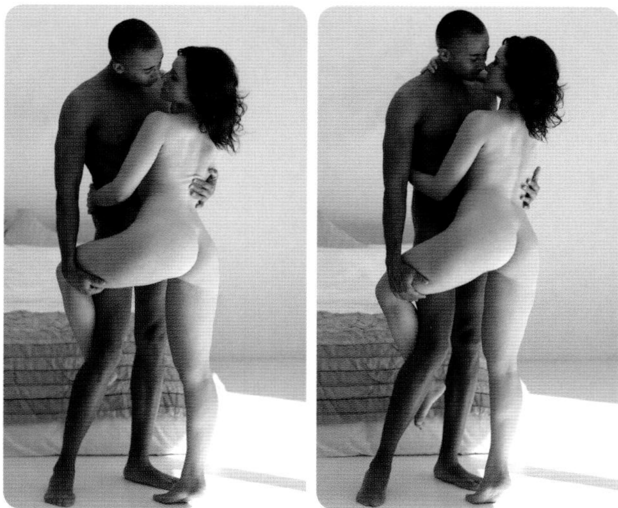

The twining of the creeper

She clings to his body with all her limbs "as a creeper twines round a tree." She bends his head towards her face so that she can gaze at him lovingly before kissing him softly and sensuously.

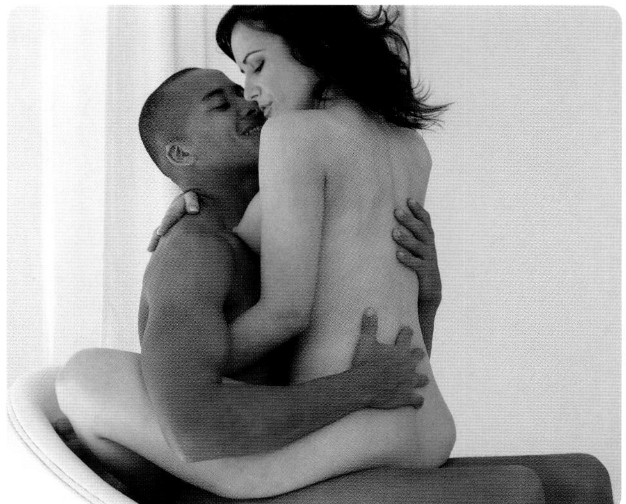

The embrace of milk and water

She sits on his lap and wraps herself tightly around him. He holds her close in his arms. The fact that your genitals are in such close proximity is a real turn-on. Imagine you're trying to "enter into each other's bodies."

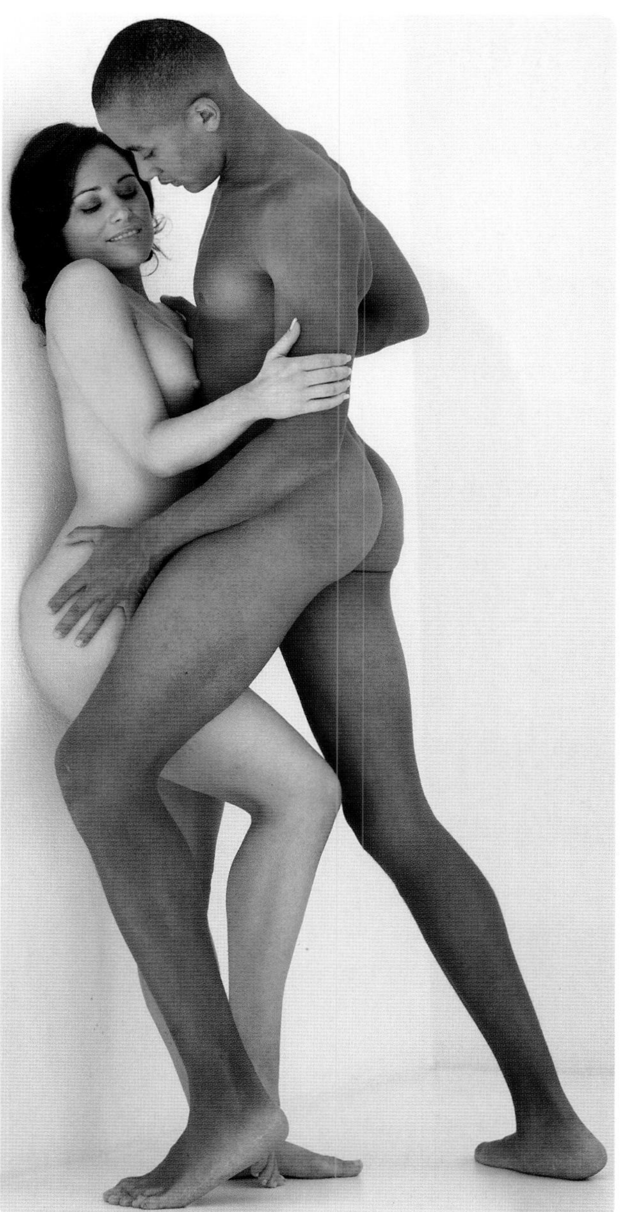

The pressing embrace

Overcome by lust, he presses her against a wall and moves in to cover her body with his. Try grinding your hips together to get the sexual tension going; you probably won't be able to control yourselves.

Kisses

Kisses are carefully stage-managed in the *Kama Sutra*. There's no going in all tongues blazing; you gather momentum slowly: a brush of a lip here and a slip of a tongue there. Only certain parts of the body should be kissed: forehead, eyes, cheeks, throat, chest, breasts, and the interior of the mouth.

The perfect kiss

There are a few simple rules laid down in the ancient texts to ensure that every kiss inspires adoration rather than revulsion in your partner. Many of them hold true today.

The first is to make sure that you taste gorgeous. The *Kama Sutra* recommends eating betel leaves "together with other things that fragrance the mouth". You should feel breath-confident, however, with the contemporary equivalent: brushing, flossing, and mouthwash.

The second is to use your teeth as well as your lips and tongue. According to *The Perfumed Garden*, nibbling a woman's lips produces a particular type of saliva that is "sweet and exquisite".

Finally, all the texts agree that, if kissing makes you both dizzy with desire, you should follow it up with sex. As *The Perfumed Garden* says: "Kisses are useless if unaccompanied by the introduction of a penis... you should abstain if you are not able to copulate or you will light a fire that only sterile separation can quench."

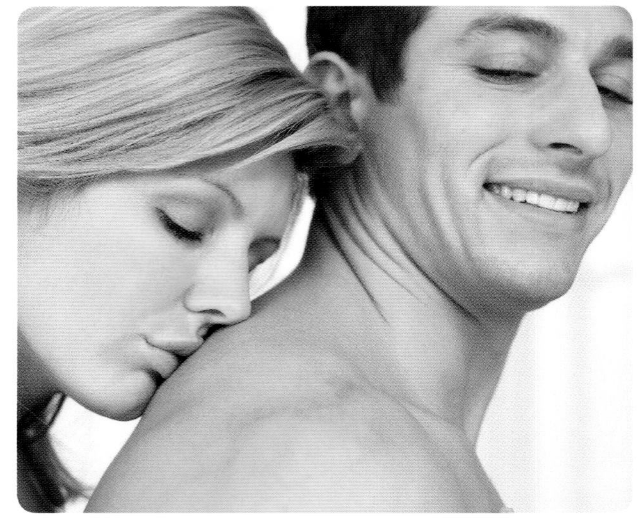

The kiss that turns away

She kisses him softly but insistently when he's looking away from her. Her aim is to turn his attention away from whatever he's doing, and focus it all on her and her desires.

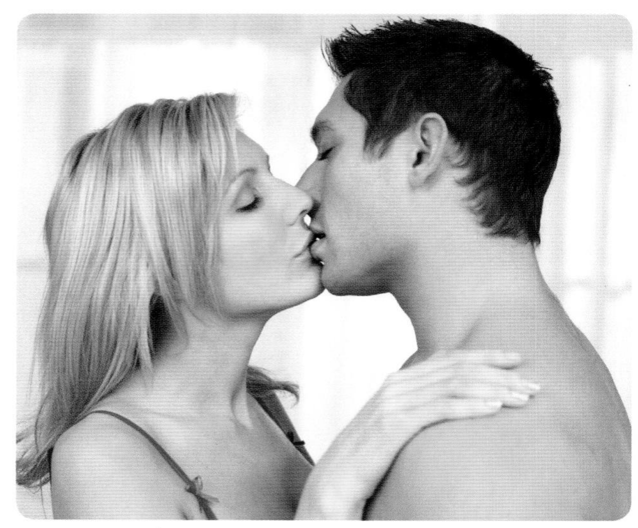

The straight kiss

She presses her lips gently against his as you both relish that first tingle of contact. Caress each other with your breath as you barely touch each other. Keep the mood sensual and teasing: no tongues yet.

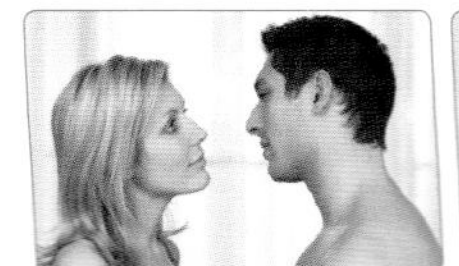
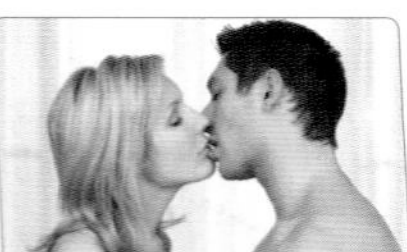
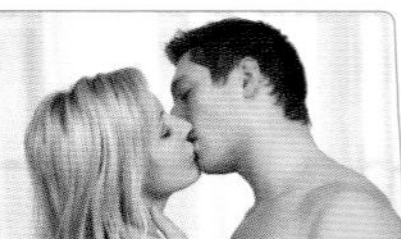
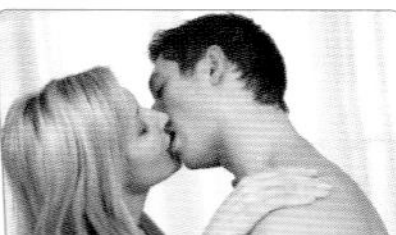
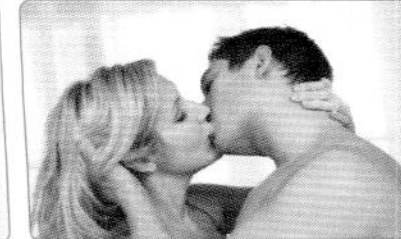

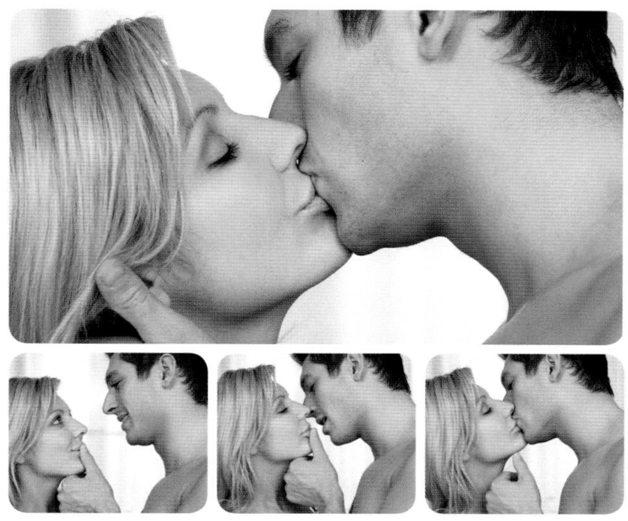

The greatly pressed kiss

In a moment of cheeky intimacy, he looks her in the eye, draws back a little, and pinches her lower lip between his thumb and finger. He then follows up by pressing his lips tightly against hers.

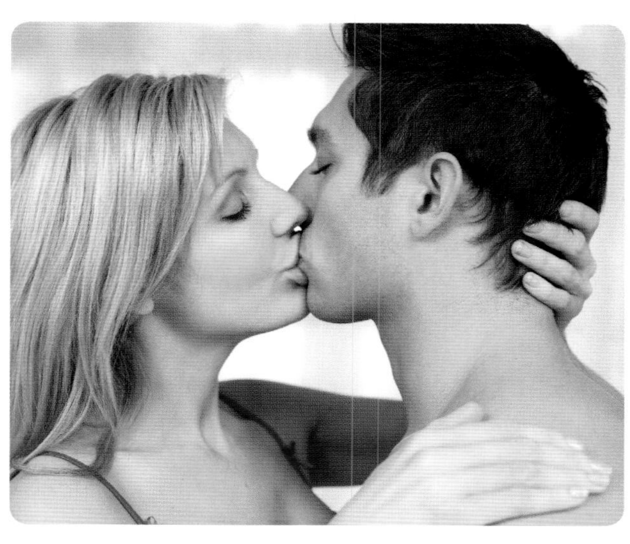

The clasping kiss

She holds his head in her hands and takes both his lips between hers, sucking them and caressing them with her tongue. She then puts her tongue in his mouth and twines it around his.

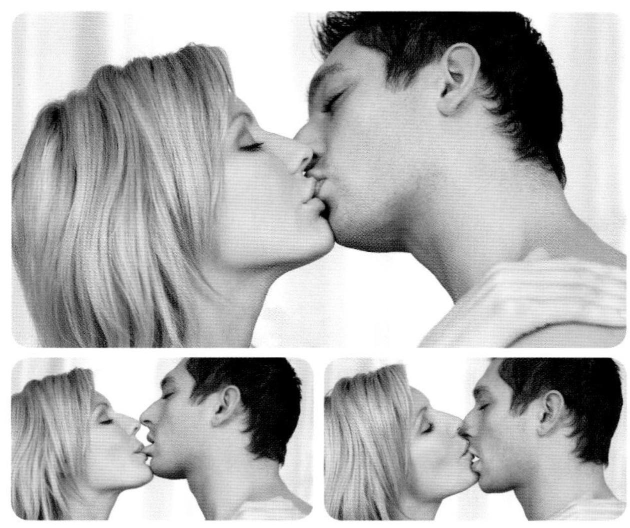

The kiss of the upper lip

He encloses her upper lip between his, and she kisses his lower lip. Let the tip of your tongue tantalizingly brush your lover's lip (but keep the tongue touches light and occasional).

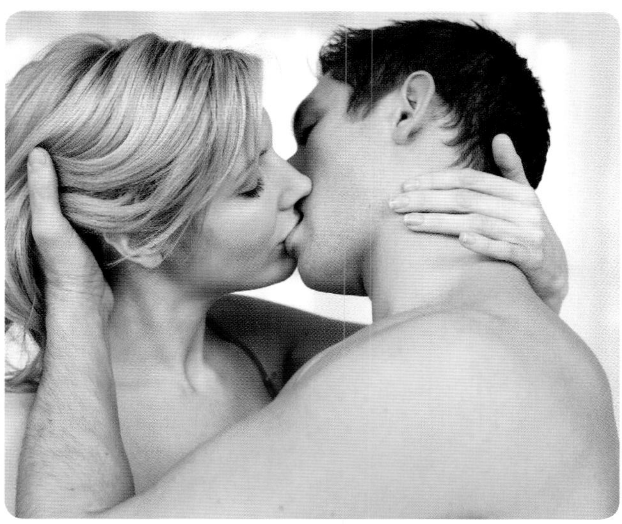

The bent kiss

Finally, when the lure of a tongue-twining kiss becomes irresistible, he presses his lips against hers, and she angles her head to the side. You both close your eyes, part your lips, and go for it.

"Whatever things may be done by one of the lovers to the other, the same should be returned." KAMA SUTRA

Massage strokes

Stroking and rubbing were vital pre-sex warm-ups in the East. Women, especially, were thought to be in need of a man's strokes and caresses to get them in the mood. Try a few of these massage techniques to prove that men are just as susceptible to seductive strokes as women.

Melting massage

Make your pre-sex massage sensual rather than clinical with lots of warm scented oil. Pour some into your hands, rub them together, then let your palms glide smoothly over your lover's skin. Or gently warm the oil on a radiator, and drizzle it straight on. Dedicate entire massage sessions to his or her pleasure. Pure bliss means being able to relax in the knowledge that you won't have to get up in a minute and return the favor. And be creative. Your hands are just one massage tool at your disposal. Others include your hair, your fingernails, your feet, even your breath. Make your lover shiver and tingle with pleasure.

One word of warning: don't press on joints or bones, or your partner is more likely to wince than melt. If you massage your lover's back, caress the muscles on either side of the spine, but avoid pressing the spine directly.

Turning up the heat

Increase the eroticism of your massage as you sense your lover becoming more relaxed and pliable. For example, as you stroke the belly, you can let your hand brush ever closer to their genitals. Or you can enhance a leg massage with some barely-there kisses on the inner thighs.

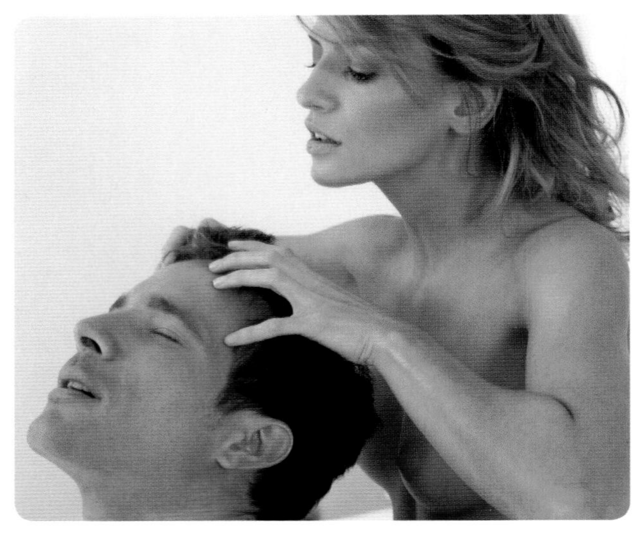

Scalp circling

She presses the pads of her fingers against his temples and moves them in slow, firm circles. She moves her fingers all over his scalp, circling as she goes, as though gently washing his hair.

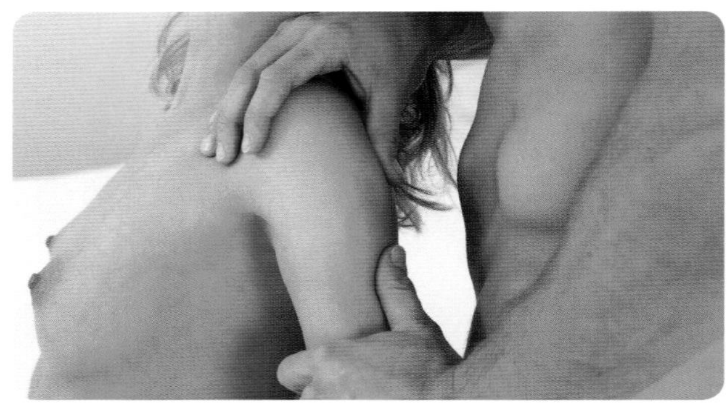

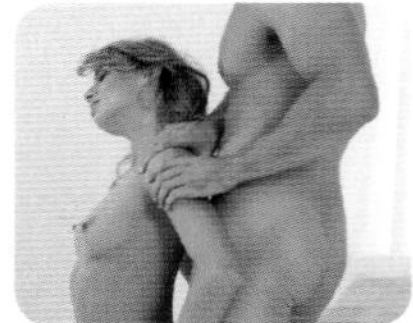

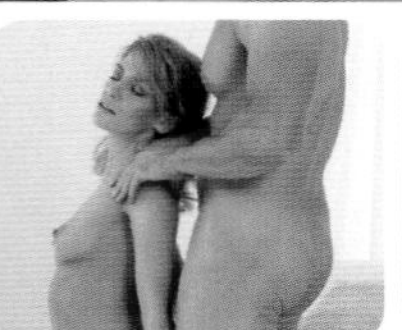

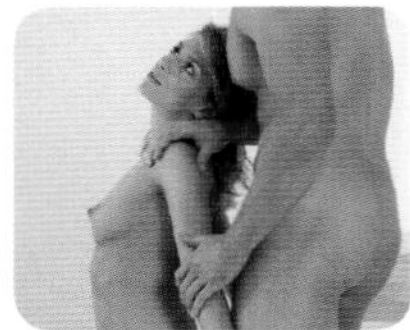

Shoulder rub

He presses his thumbs into the muscles at the back of her shoulder and his fingers into the dip just above her collarbone. He then works his hands in slow, circular kneading movements.

"Woman is like a fruit that will yield its fragrance only when rubbed by the hands." THE PERFUMED GARDEN

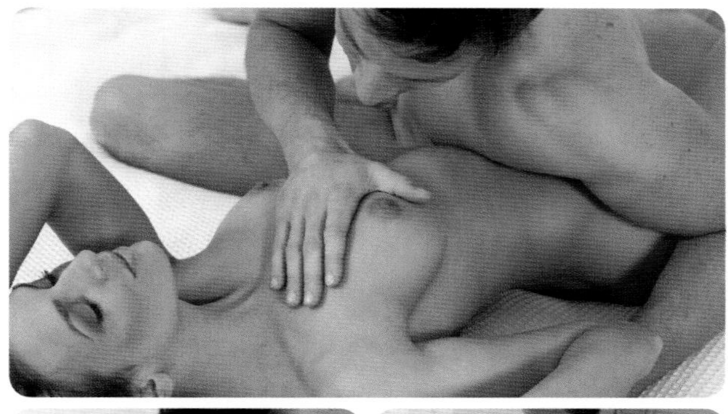

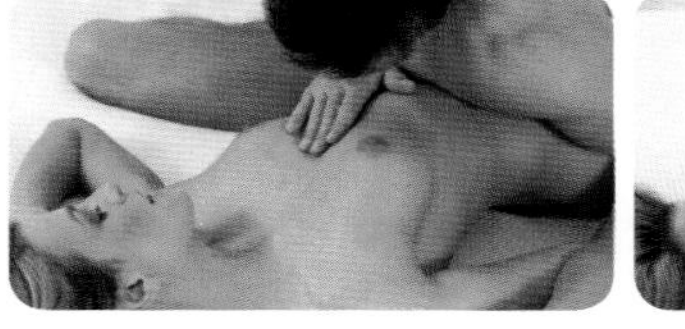

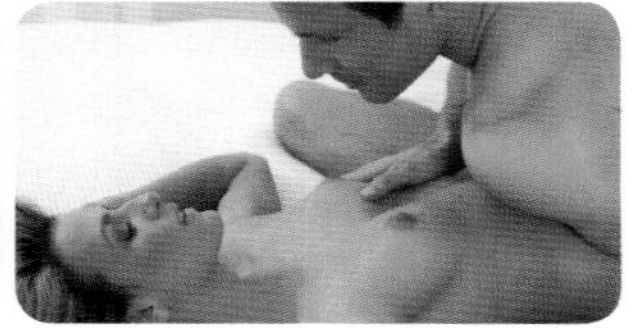

Breast strokes

Keeping his hands flat, he slides his palms across her body and over the curves of her breasts. He uses his thumb and index finger in a scissor action over her nipples, squeezing lightly as he goes.

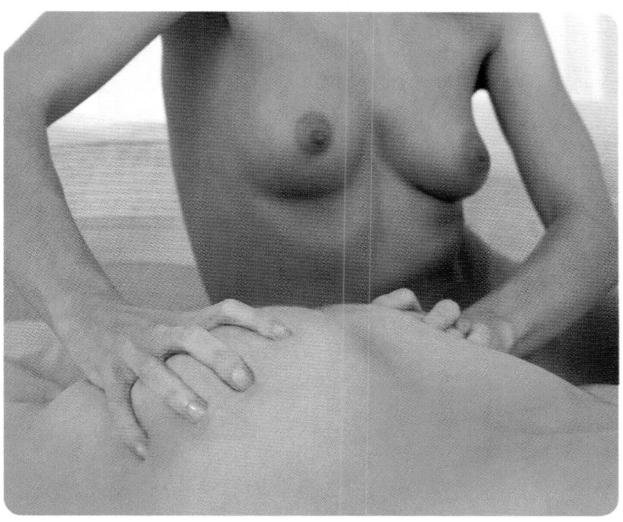

Bum kneading

She leans forward so that her upper body weight is on her hands. She then kneads and presses his muscles using the tips of her fingers, the heels of her hands, and the flat part of her fists.

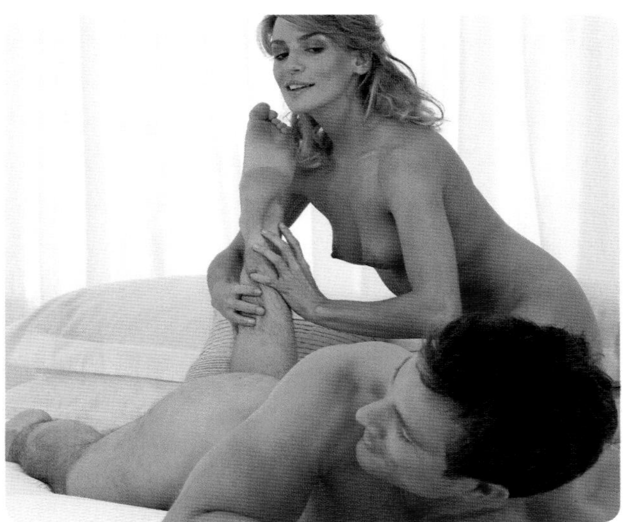

Calf pressure

She works on his large calf muscles by sliding her fingers up and down in opposing directions, circling her thumbs, and raking her fingertips across in a clawing motion.

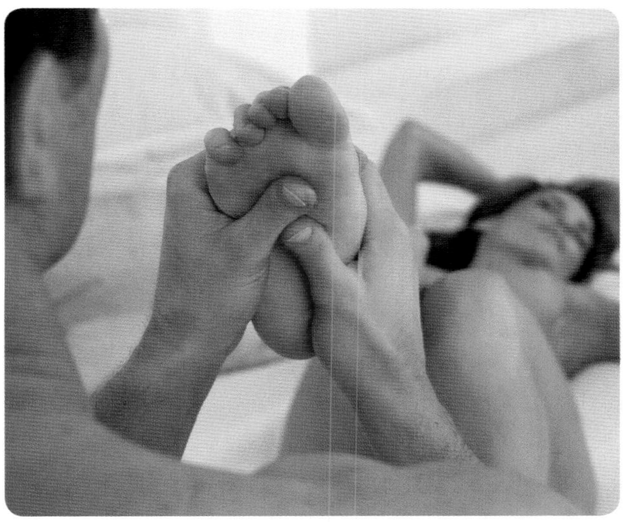

Foot warmers

He gives her a friendly foot squeeze with his thumbs on her sole and his fingers on the top of her foot. He then glides his thumbs along the bottom of her foot and pinches and squeezes each of her toes.

Undressing each other

In the *Kama Sutra* every sexual act from kissing to scratching is performed with careful and reverent ceremony, and disrobing is no exception. So if you're in the habit of ripping off each other's clothes in a sex-hungry frenzy, take a leaf out of Vatsyayana's book: turn undressing into an erotic ritual.

Naked pleasure

Instead of viewing taking each other's clothes off as the boring-but-necessary bit, treat it as part of foreplay. Imagine you're taking the wrapping off the sexiest gift-wrapped present ever. Every time you expose a new bit of your lover's body, feast upon it with your lips, tongue, teeth, hands, and eyes. As you smooth her stocking down her thigh or his pants over his hips, exploit the opportunity to brush local hot spots with your fingertips. Slow things down, and uncover each bit of your lover's body with a sense of awe.

Tips for being stripped

Concentrate on the subtle yet sublime sensation of your clothes being peeled or pulled away from your skin. If your lover gets stuck on a button or fastening, don't try to help; surrender to their control. Wear sexy or sensual fabrics that your lover will delight in touching: for example, silk, lace, leather, or latex. And embrace the erotic power of zips by wearing thigh-high zip-up boots; dresses with zips that run from neck to hem; or zippable corsets, catsuits, basques, or pouches (for him).

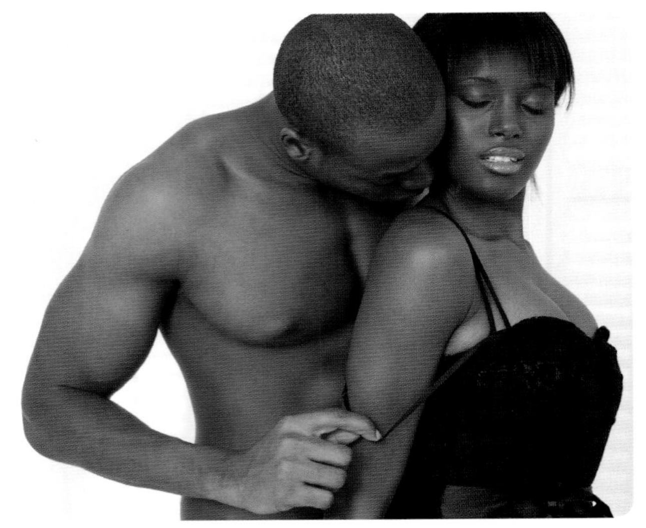

1 **Undressing her: Off the shoulder**
He gives her goose bumps as he nuzzles and licks the back of her neck. At the same time, he slides her dress off her shoulder to expose its smooth curve.

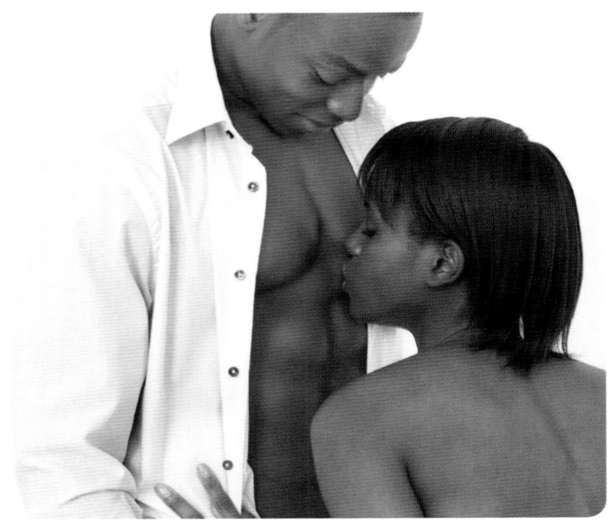

1 **Undressing him: Baring his chest**
She undoes his shirt buttons with sexy slowness, leaning in to caress his chest with her lips after each button, lighting his fire and making him think of things to come.

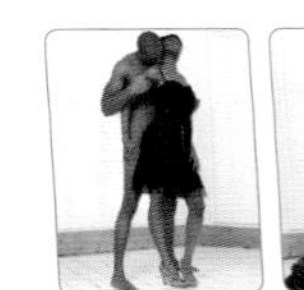
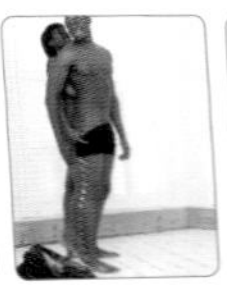
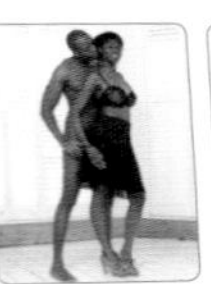
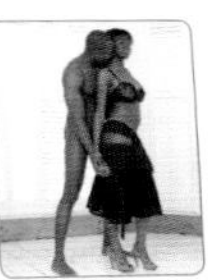
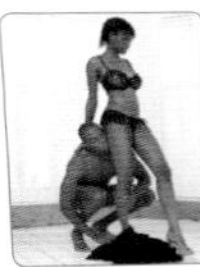
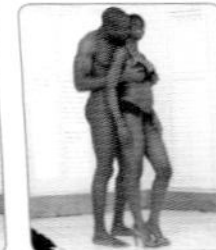
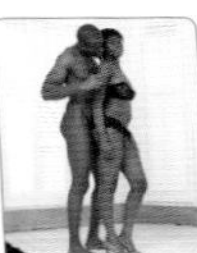
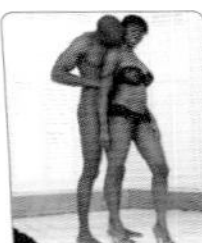
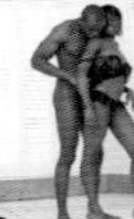

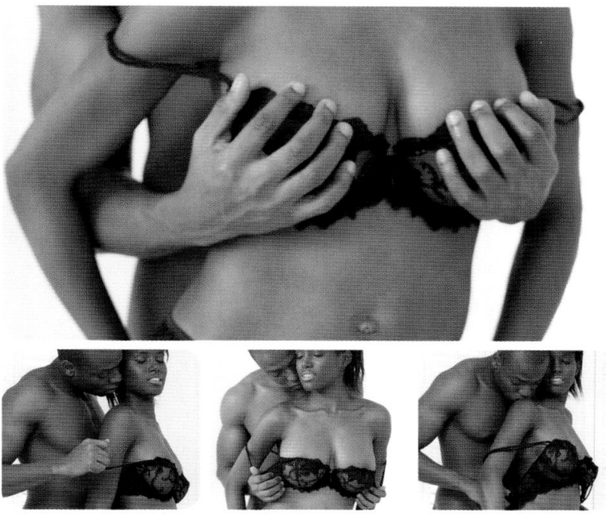

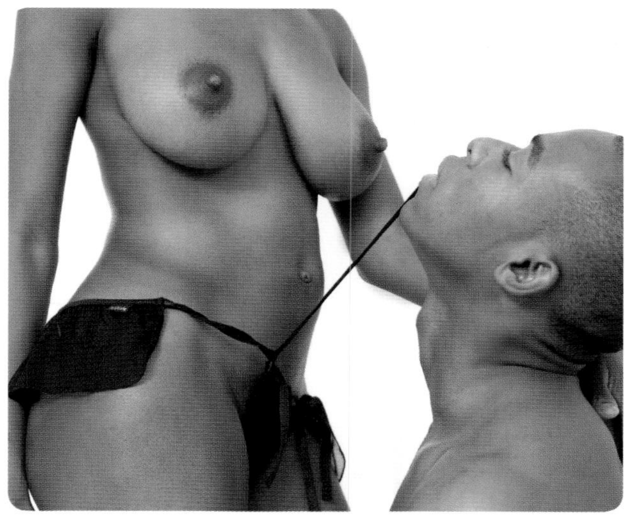

2 Undressing her: Slow unveiling

Having undone her bra, he cups her breasts through the fabric, lightly searching for her nipples with his fingertips, then tweaking and pinching them. He then slides the bra down over her shoulders.

3 Undressing her: Reveal all

He kneels submissively at her feet before taking the fabric of her panties between his teeth. He then edges her panties slowly down her thighs; even better if she is wearing drawstring underwear.

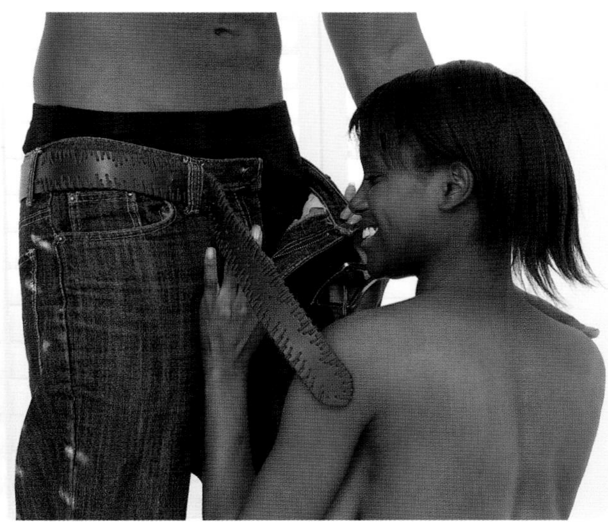

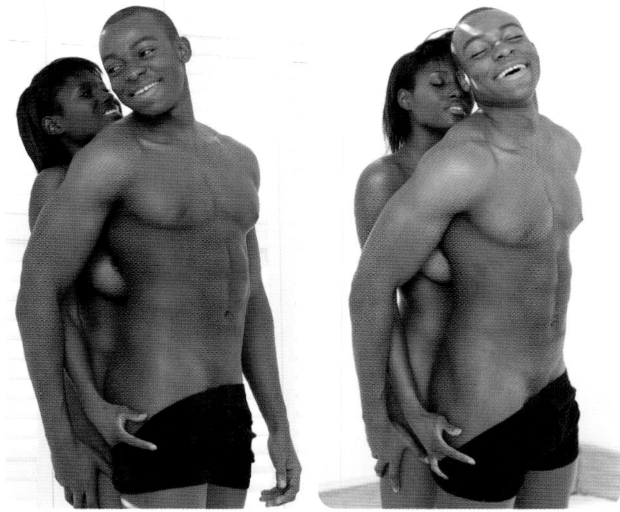

2 Undressing him: On the fly

She gazes cheekily up at him from a kneeling position as she undoes his flies and eases his trousers over his waist, her lips tantalizingly close to his crotch.

3 Undressing him: Grand finale

She slides her hands provocatively under the rim of his pants for a quick bum caress, then with a playful smile she smoothes his pants slowly over his hips...

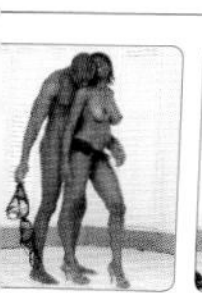

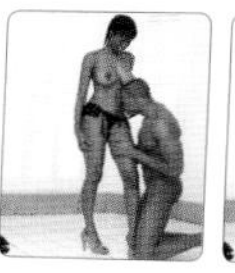

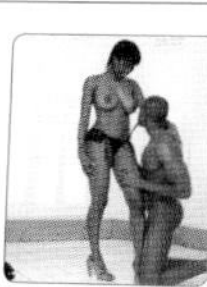

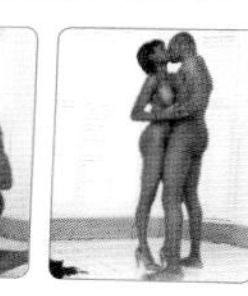

"Her petticoats are raised... and her hair is thrown into a dishevelled state, symbolizing passion." ANANGA RANGA

Biting, scratching, and striking

According to the *Kama Sutra*, marking your lover with teeth and nails is a sign of intense passion. If your partner is likely to be upset or offended rather than aroused, don't even consider this stuff. But if you're both into it, the "blows of love" can make spicy additions to your seduction repertoire.

Making your mark

Test-drive your lover's enthusiasm by incorporating the odd spank or scratch into a massage or sex. Try some nips, spanks, or scratches in places where they can be covered up by clothes. A publicly visible love bite may send your lover screaming, but, as the *Kama Sutra* says, seeing marks on *hidden* places brings back memories of love and passion.

Keeping it playful

No-holds-barred sex is one thing; waking up black and blue is another. Some people wear bites, scratches, and other sex injuries with erotic pride; others cringe with embarrassment. Check which group your lover falls into before letting rip.

Take off rings and bracelets before a spanking session. And find out how hard your lover likes their bottom spanked on a 1–5 scale: "1" is a gentle love pat, and "5" is a whack that stings and leaves you red in both sets of cheeks. You might want to disregard the *Kama Sutra* suggestion of trimming the nails of your left hand into points (unless you're into intense pain during nail play). Instead, just follow your mum's advice, and keep your nails clean and trimmed into gentle curves.

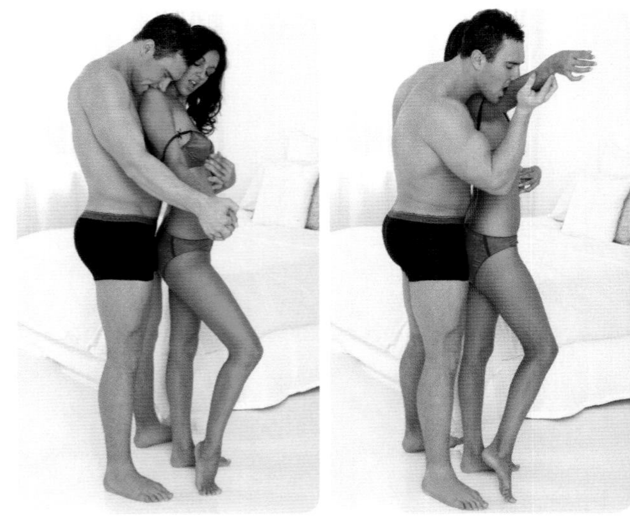

Biting of a boar

He playfully bites her shoulder and along her arm, leaving behind a series of crimson marks. The *Kama Sutra* recommends this for "persons of intense passion".

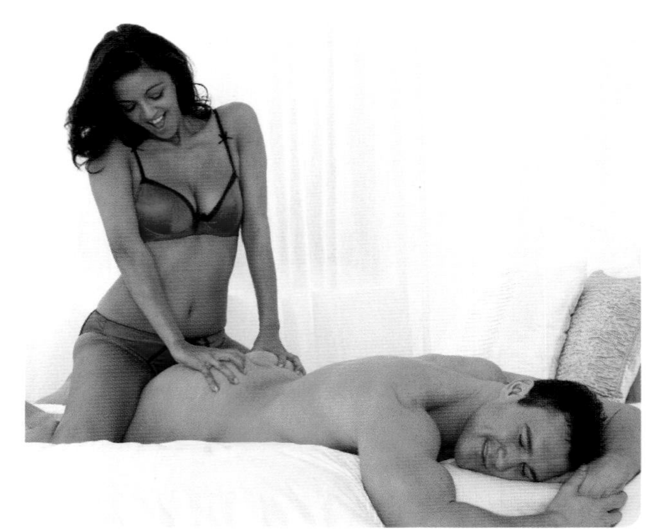

Half-moon

She presses her nails into his buttocks, and leaves half-moon shapes imprinted on his flesh. (The *Kama Sutra* also recommends making circles: two half-moons opposite each other.)

"In short, nothing tends to increase love so much as the effects of marking with the nails, and biting." KAMA SUTRA

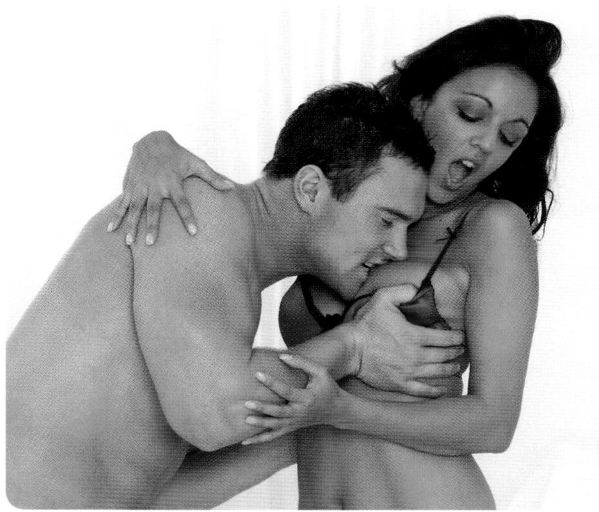

Broken cloud

He presses his mouth to her skin (anywhere on her body), sucks her flesh gently, then bites and nibbles to leave behind a mark in the shape of broken cloud.

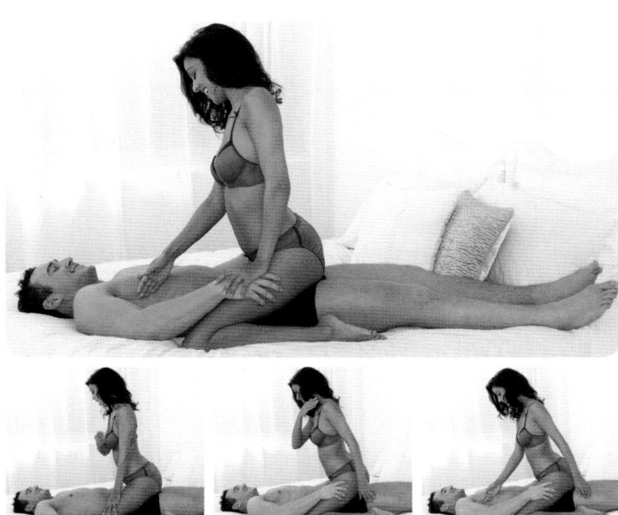

Backhand strike

She feigns anger and strikes him on the chest with the back of her hand (she can incorporate this into role-play scenarios). If he likes it, she repeats it while getting more and more "angry".

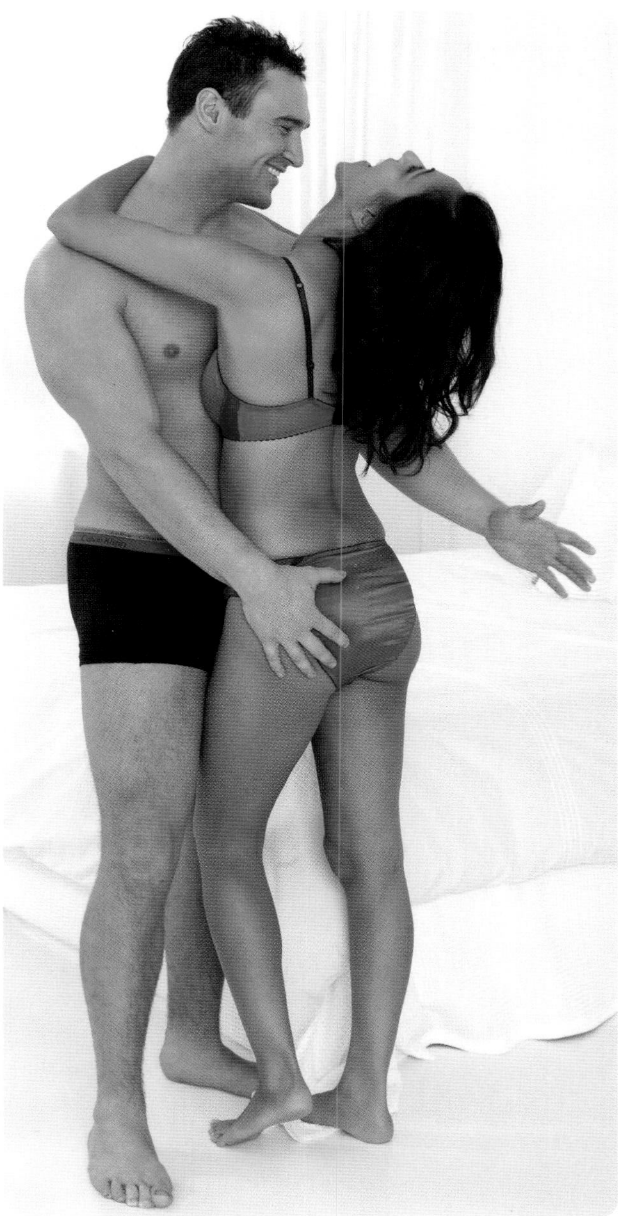

Forehand strike

He slightly cups his hand and slaps her playfully on the bum at close range. He then follows it up with a soothing buttock rub, before issuing a spank to the other cheek.

Mouth congress

Improper, against the moral code, and not for learned gentlemen was the *Kama Sutra*'s opinion of oral sex. Yet that didn't stop Vatsyayana from describing in juicy detail exactly how a eunuch or male servant should kneel between his master's legs and "suck the mango" or "swallow up".

Unsuitable practices

Fellatio in the *Kama Sutra* is purely a means for a servant to satisfy his master in between his amorous adventures. Vatsyayana preferred not to acknowledge that a chaste and beautiful woman might go down on her lover, although he does mention that "women of the harem" might occasionally indulge in a little oral to pass the time.

Oral sex to die for

If you don't have (or want) a handy eunuch or harem, you'll have to make do with each other. Although oral is a great way to warm each other up before sex, try making it your main course rather than just a starter. Knowing that your lover is committed to going the distance is a powerful aphrodisiac. When you're doing the giving, make it hot, wet, and wild. If your lover sees that you're loving it, they'll love it even more. When you're on the receiving end, show your appreciation in the form of moans, sighs, and "mmmmm"s.

Above all else, take your time. Tease before you go in for the kill. Linger on your lover's inner thighs, perineum, or pubic triangle. Spend your time kissing, tickling, nuzzling, and licking. Make sure that your lover is buzzing with lust before you apply your lips to clitoris or penis.

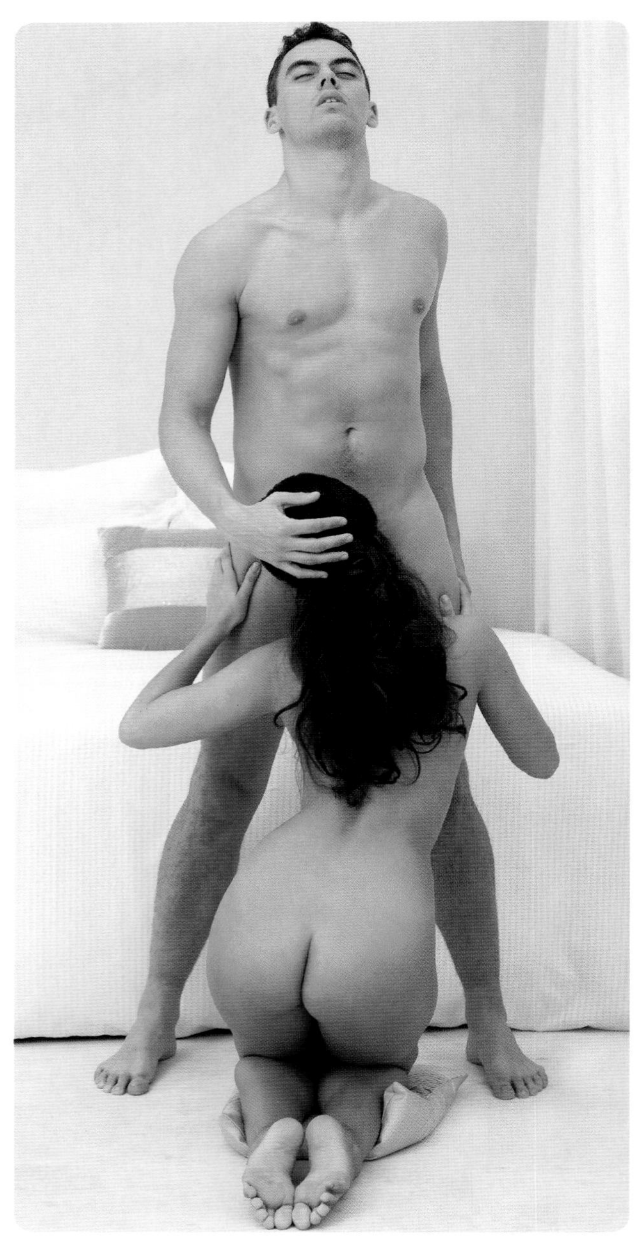

Kissing the lingam

She polishes his glans with her tongue, then she moves her mouth and fist up and down on him in unison. She then takes his whole shaft in her mouth as though she is going to swallow it (this is "swallowing up").

"Some women of the harem, when they are amorous, do the acts of the mouth on the yonis of one another, and some men do the same thing with women." KAMA SUTRA

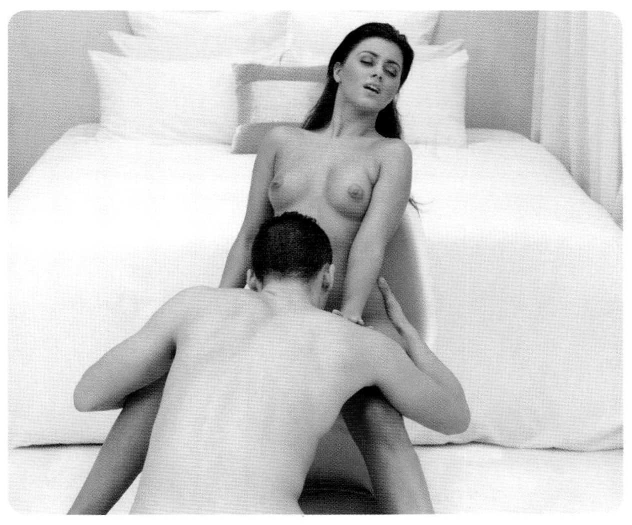

Kissing the yoni I

He sits in between her legs and puts his fingers in a scissor shape along her vulva (to expose her clitoris). He then takes the whole of her clitoral area in his mouth and gently sucks, laps, and licks.

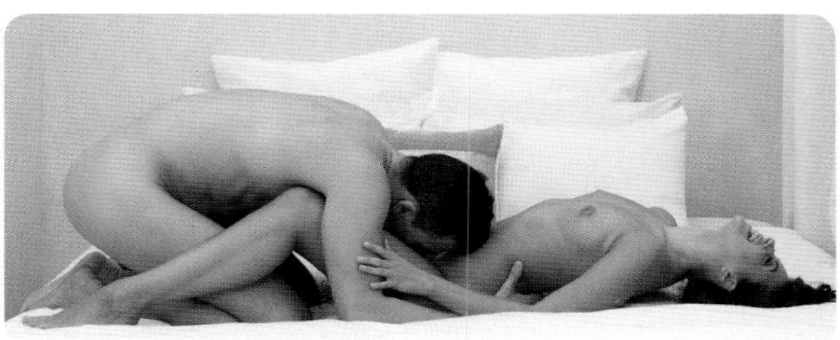

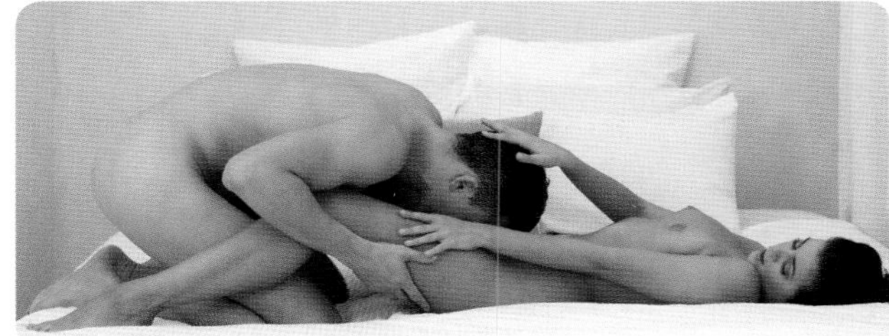

Kissing the yoni II

He kneels between her legs and swirls his tongue on her clitoris with his finger (or fingers) in her vagina rubbing or pressing her G-spot (which is on the front wall, nearest to her belly).

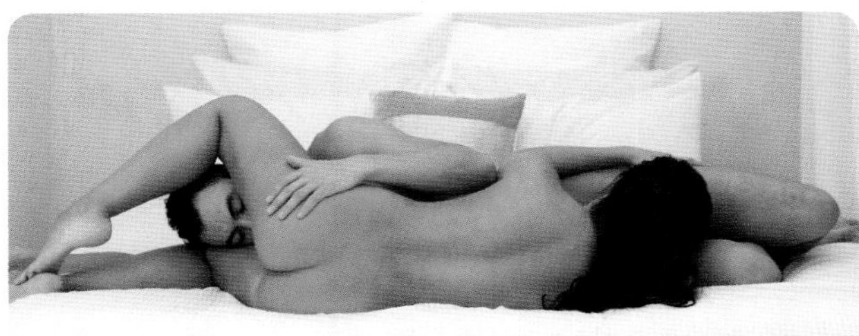

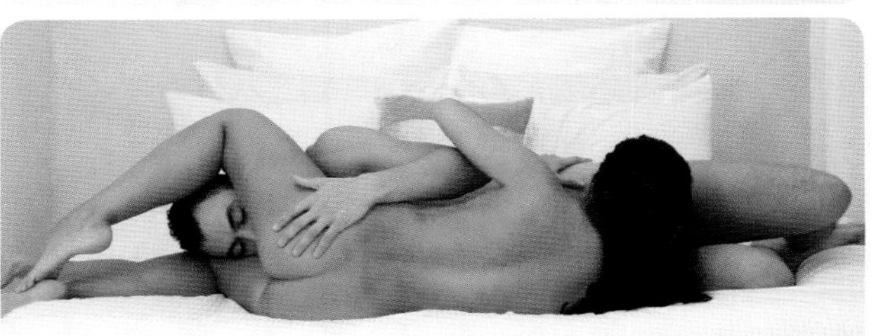

Congress of a crow I

You both lie on your sides facing each other, and start by kissing and nuzzling each other's inner thighs. You then zoom in on the genitals using a super-passionate French-kissing technique.

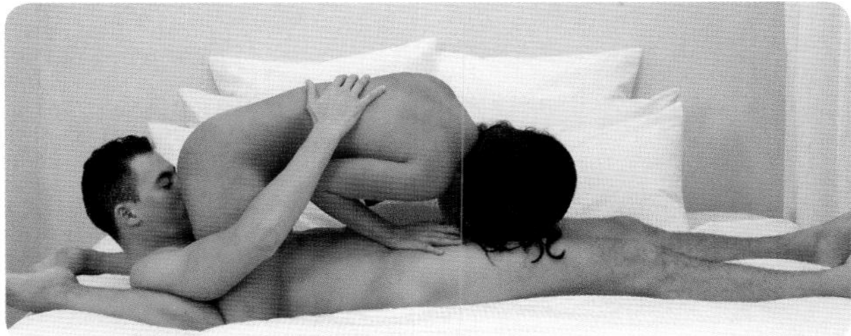

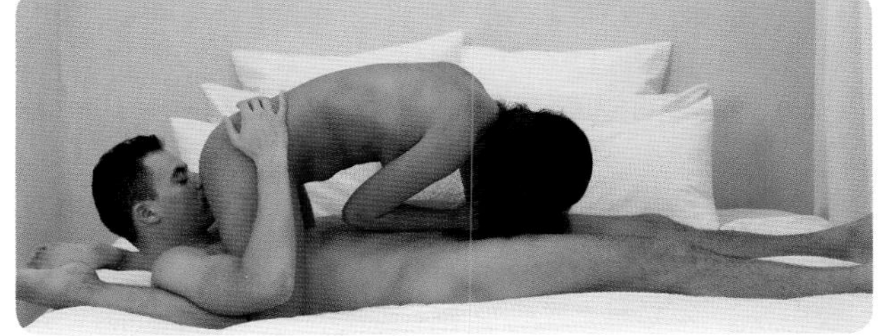

Congress of a crow II

She kneels astride his face, facing his feet, and then leans over to take him in her mouth. She bobs her head up and down on him while he flicks his tongue against her from below.

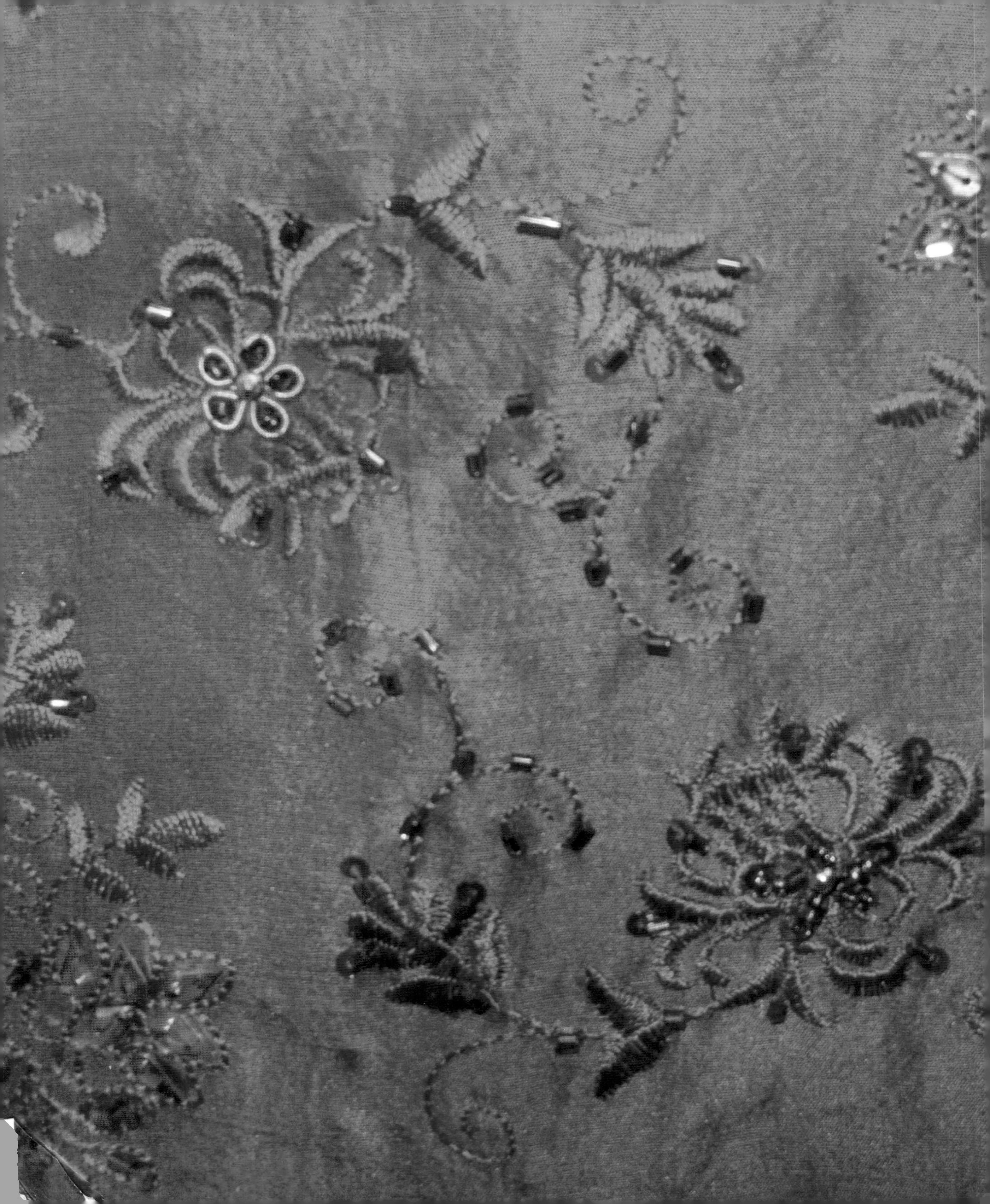

Intimate Union

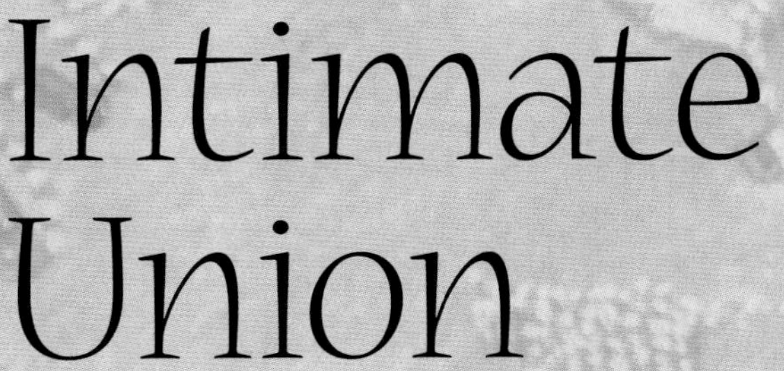

The following sex positions are made for sensual sessions in front of a log fire, love-ins in a four-poster bed, or making out in a summer meadow... or the good old-fashioned bedroom. They are chosen with romance, intimacy, and soul-melding in mind. Think tantric rather than torrid.

Here you can sample the nose-to-nose cuteness of Butterflies in Flight, the gloriously intimate Singing Monkey, and the delights of the provocatively named Cat and Mouse Sharing a Hole. But don't rely on the position alone to keep up that romantic intensity; continue with the smoldering eye contact and fingertip caresses.

In the same way that you'd choose the right wine to go with a delicious meal, choose the right sex strokes to go with the position. For example, deep thrusting might work wonderfully in The Stopperage, but be uncomfortable in Coitus from Behind. You can extend your repertoire of sex strokes by learning some ancient thrusting techniques in The Movements of Sex.

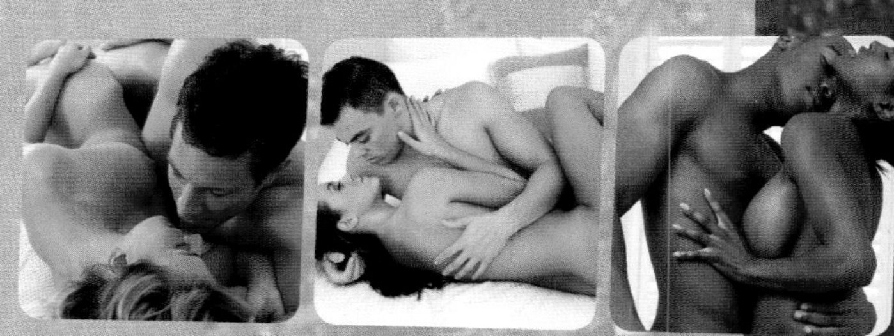

Widely opened position

☆☆☆☆ Kama sensation rating

The woman has an unusual amount of room to express her lust in this variation on the ordinary man-on-top position. Because his hips are high in the air rather than pinning her to the bed, she's free to thrust, grind, and wiggle as much as she wants.

Why it works

– You take turns to take the lead: she thrusts upward when it's her turn in charge; he thrusts downward when it's his.

– When she's the one making the moves, he experiences a sensational downward pull on his shaft.

– You can tailor the position to your mood. You can slam your bodies against each other in wild abandon or make small, gentle movements in moments of soulful intimacy.

– He doesn't put any weight on her, which is useful if she's pregnant.

Turn on...

... Try moving at the same time in a rhythm that pleasures you both: he moves down while she moves up. If you get it right, your genitals will collide in the middle with explosive results.

Turn off...

... Don't continue if this one's not doing it for you. The disadvantage of this position is that you're connecting midair with no solid surface against which to brace yourselves. If you find yourselves understimulated, lower back down to the bed.

1 The invitation

She lies back and beckons him toward her. She bends her knees and parts her legs. He kneels before her.

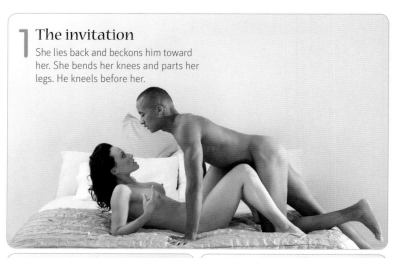

2 Slow entry

He slides on top and slowly enters her, while taking his weight on his forearms. She pulls him inside her with her hands on his buttocks.

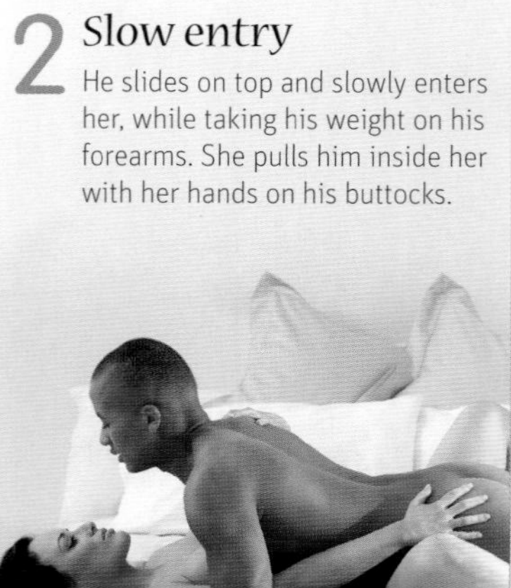

3 Press up

He pushes up on his hands into a half push-up position. He keeps his pelvis tightly pressed to hers.

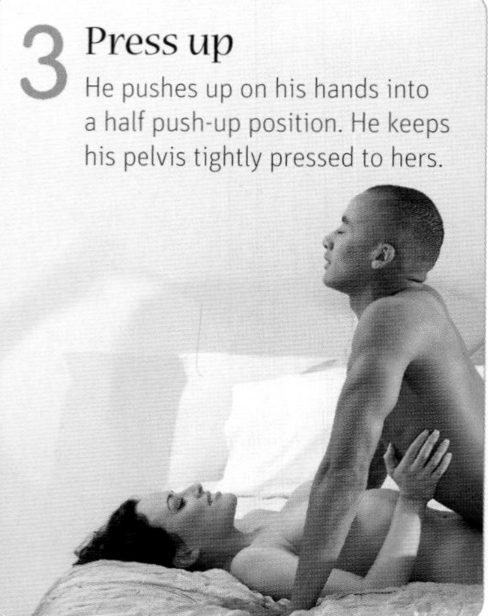

"With her head thrown down and her pelvis raised up she is wide open to him." KAMA SUTRA

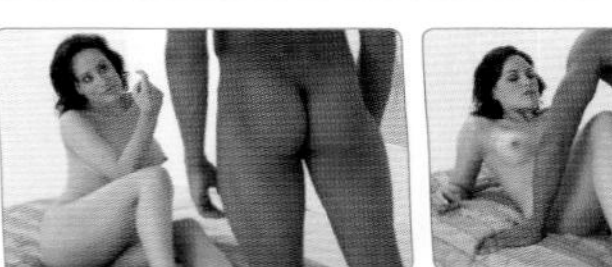

4 Liftoff

She raises her hips off the bed in a smooth, voluptuous movement, taking her weight on her feet and shoulders. He lets her movement push him up.

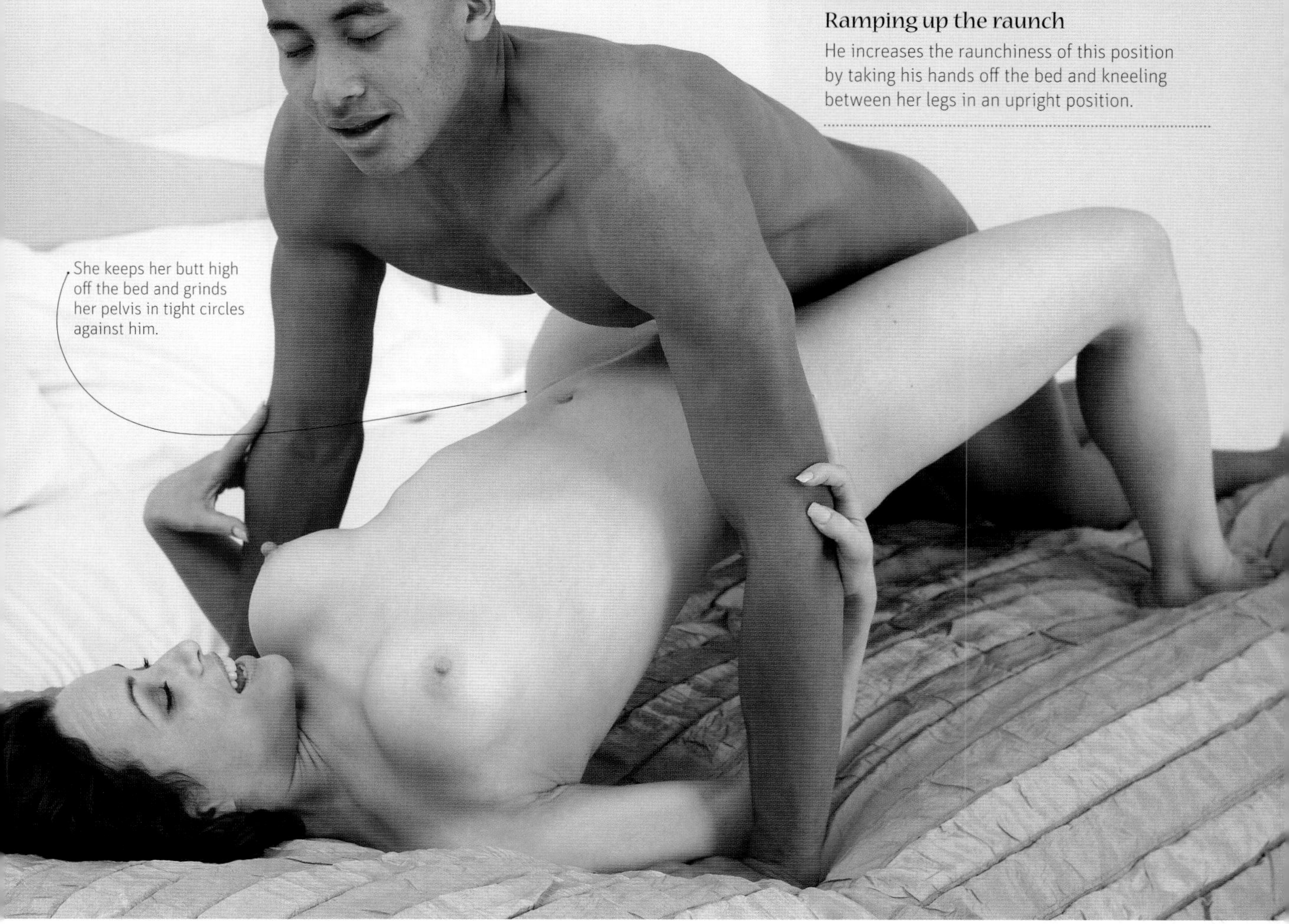

She keeps her butt high off the bed and grinds her pelvis in tight circles against him.

Taking it further

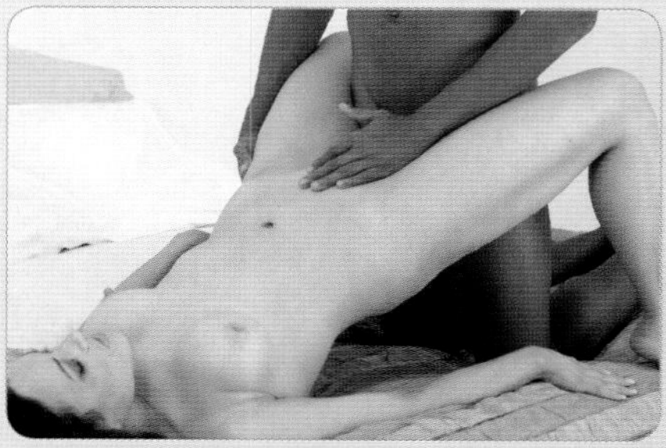

Ramping up the raunch

He increases the raunchiness of this position by taking his hands off the bed and kneeling between her legs in an upright position.

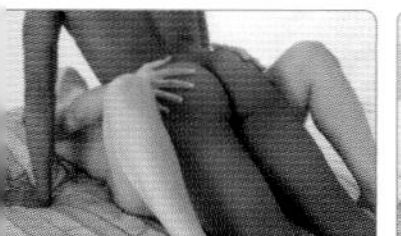
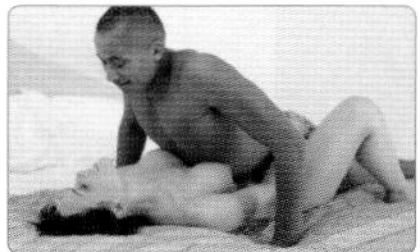
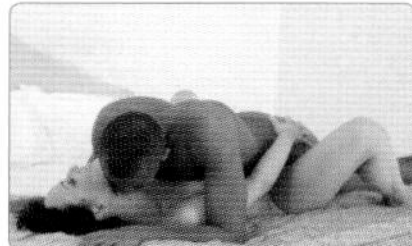
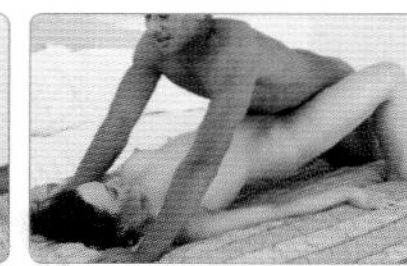
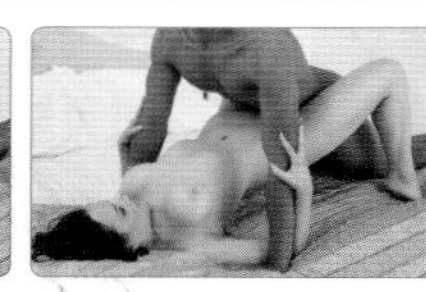

The crab embrace

☆☆☆☆ Kama sensation rating

Few positions beat this one for smoochy, intimate sex when you want to be as close as it's possible to be. Make it your opening move to a romantic reunion, use it as a way to get back in touch after an argument, or do it just because you love each other.

Why it works

- With her upper leg raised high on his hip, it's easy for him to penetrate her.
- Kissing is inevitable, whether you want to press your lips lightly together or immerse yourselves passionately in a tongue-twining, time-stopping session.
- You can combine sex with cuddling for the ultimate in sensual skin-on-skin contact.
- You're so close and intimate that you can whisper sweet nothings to each other.
- Massage fans can stroke, knead, press, and rake each other's backs.

1 Side by side

Lie on your sides with your bodies in alignment and your faces close enough to feel each other's breath.

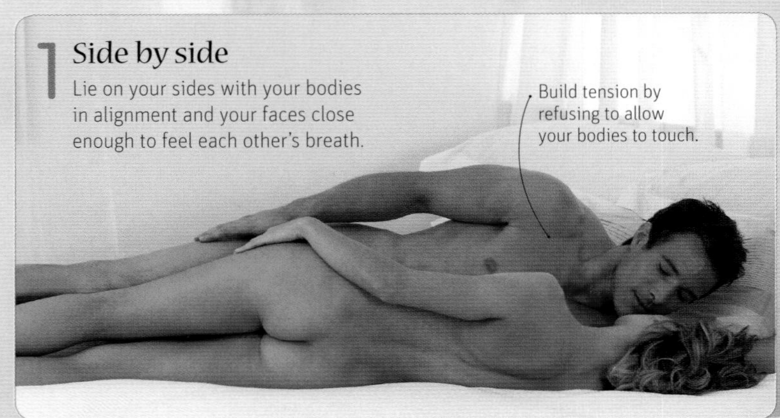

Build tension by refusing to allow your bodies to touch.

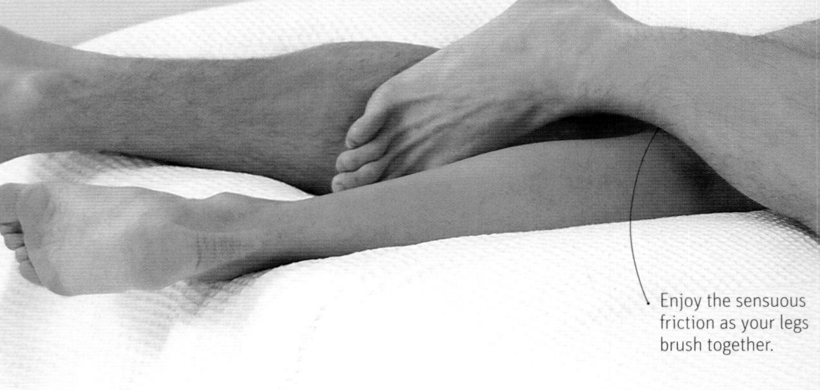

Enjoy the sensuous friction as your legs brush together.

Turn on...

... Find a steady rhythm of movement. Experiment to see what works for both of you. She can try a back-and-forth rocking motion. He can try shallow thrusting. You can take it in turns to lead, or just try moving together rhythmically.

Turn off...

... Don't worry if you can't come. You might find that you're too close to move at the pace and rhythm you need to get you off. If so, choose a raunchier position for your grand finale.

"The lust, desire, and passion of women is satisfied by sexual union." KAMA SUTRA

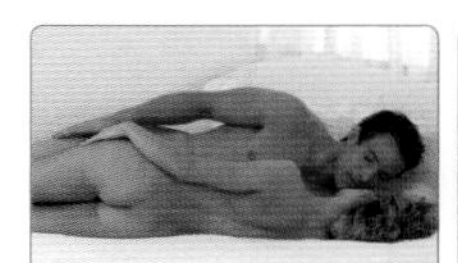

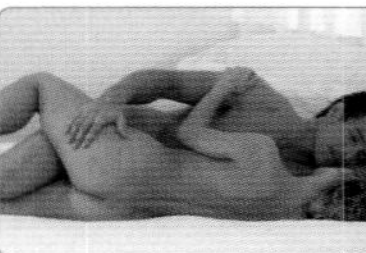

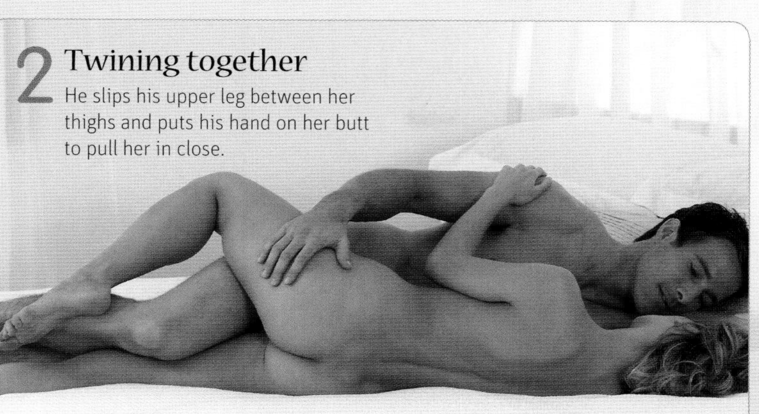

2 Twining together

He slips his upper leg between her thighs and puts his hand on her butt to pull her in close.

Taking it further

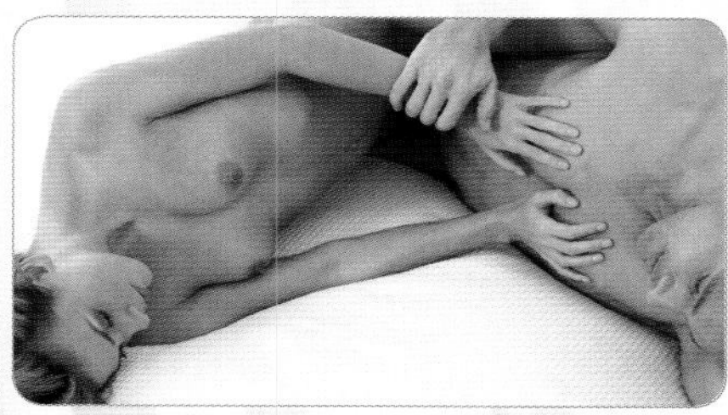

Staying in touch

If you want more freedom of movement, she can lean away from him while staying connected. Her body joins his at a right angle.

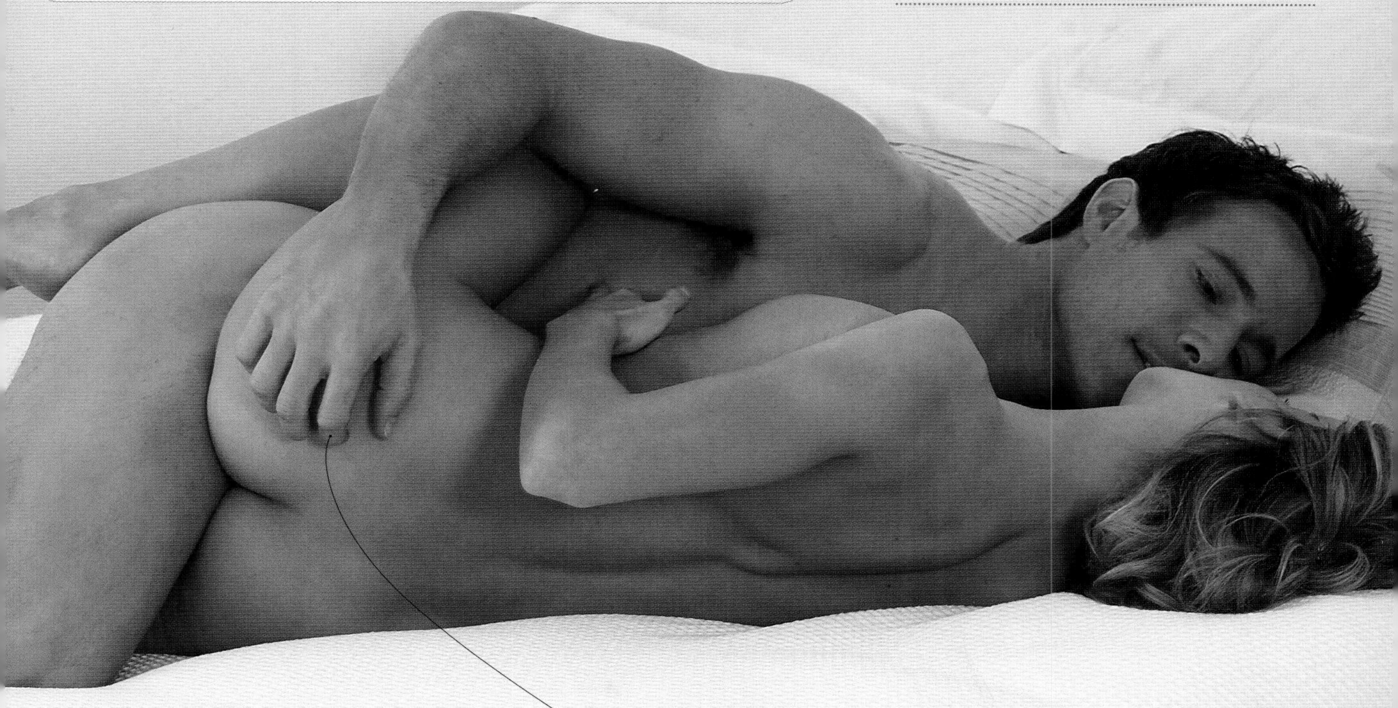

He strokes her buttocks with his fingertips.

3 Thigh clasp

She bends her upper leg and slides her thigh up along his waist. As he penetrates her, she uses her heel to pull him in.

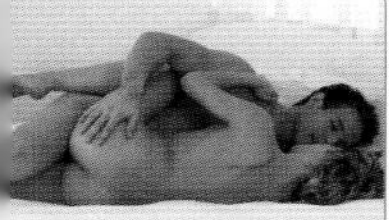
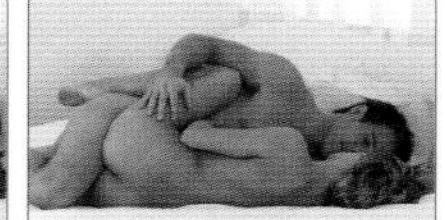
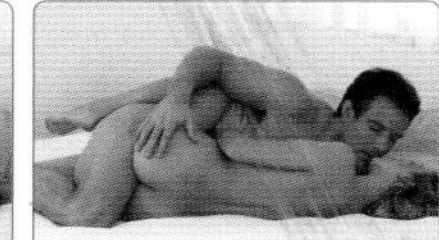
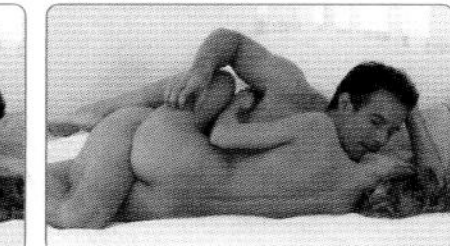
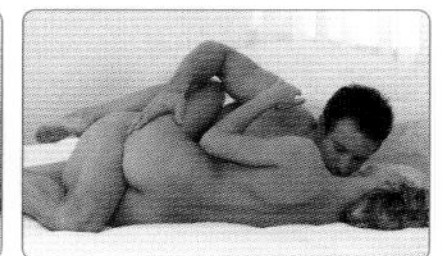

Two fishes and Swallows in love

☆☆ Kama sensation rating

Try this pair of positions when you want a teasing build-up to sex. Penetration is difficult in Two Fishes, so you can use it to ramp up the sexual tension. Then, when you're so tense you can't take it any more, she can roll on to her back and open her legs wide in greeting.

Why they work

– Two Fishes is a great position for lots of skin-stroking, ass-groping, and deep-kissing foreplay. It gives you both ample time to warm up and get your juices flowing.

– He can kick-start her arousal by slipping his hand around to caress her labia and clitoris.

– Swallows in Love (a.k.a. the missionary position) is a no-frills man-on-top position in which you're both free to concentrate on the in–out movement of his penis.

– She can grab his butt to influence the rhythm, pace, and depth of his thrusts, and rock her pelvis in time to his movements.

Turn on…

… Experiment by relaxing your entire body, including your vaginal and pelvic floor muscles. It's unusual to lie completely flat and relaxed during sex; see what sensations you experience.

Turn off…

… Don't relax to the point of inertia; he needs occasional feedback to know that you're having a good time. Show your appreciation vocally or by grinding against him as he thrusts.

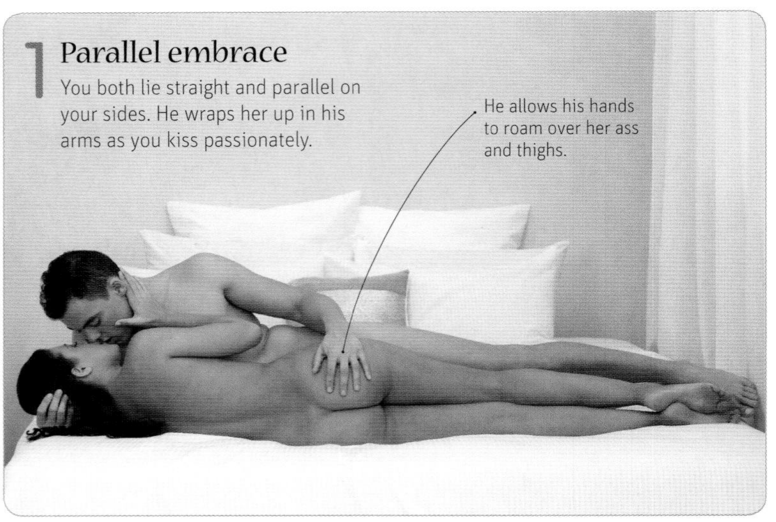
He allows his hands to roam over her ass and thighs.

1 Parallel embrace
You both lie straight and parallel on your sides. He wraps her up in his arms as you kiss passionately.

2 The hook
She hooks her legs over the top of his in Two Fishes position. He thrusts against her body without entering her.

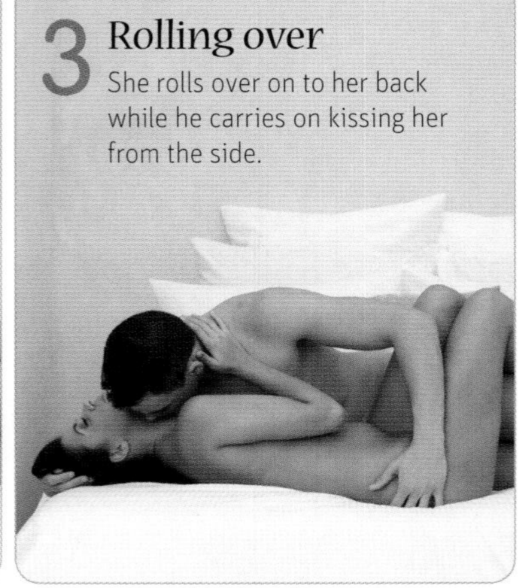

3 Rolling over
She rolls over on to her back while he carries on kissing her from the side.

"When the lingam is in the yoni and moved quickly in and out without being withdrawn, this is called 'sporting of a sparrow'." KAMA SUTRA

Taking it further

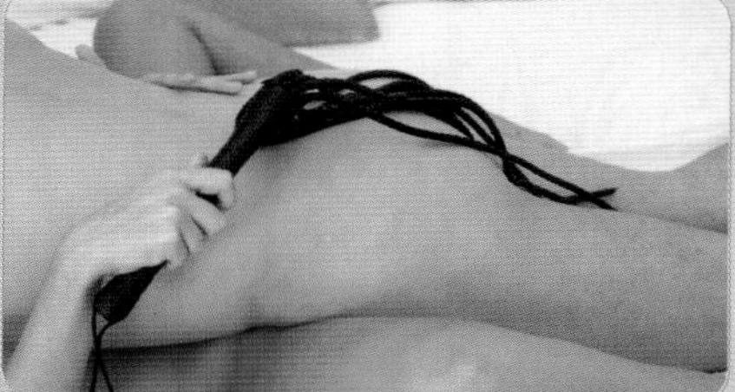

Whipping it up

If spanking is his thing, she can up the kink factor to boiling point by using a cat o'nine tails-style whip on his buttocks, instead of her hand.

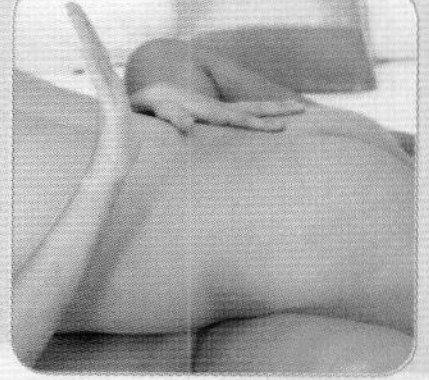

She can playfully slap his ass as he thrusts; light slaps at first, then harder if he enjoys it.

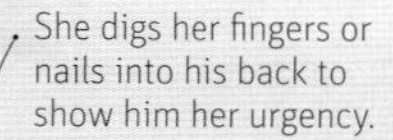

She digs her fingers or nails into his back to show him her urgency.

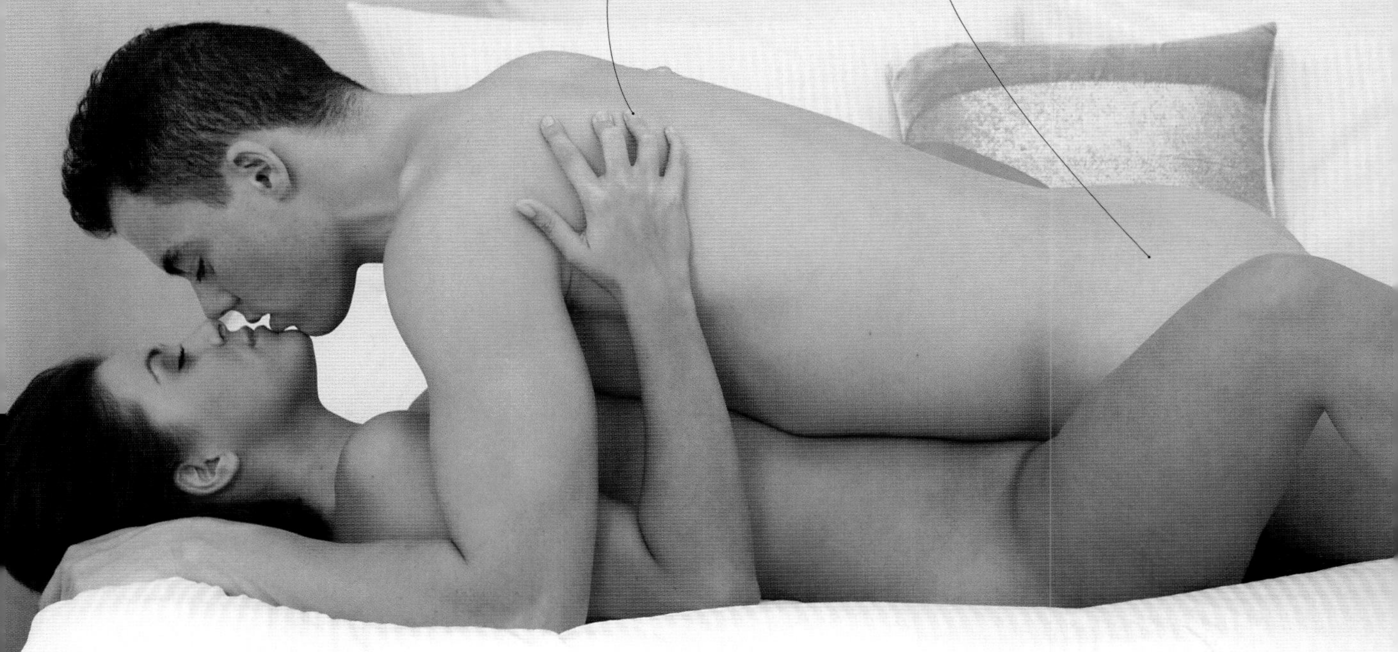

4 Man on top

He climbs on top of her, and she opens her legs to let him in. This is Swallows in Love. He takes his weight on his forearms as he thrusts freely.

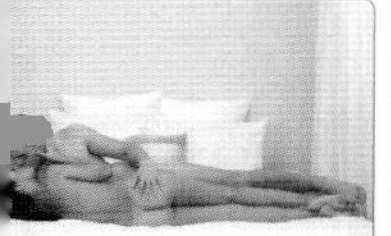
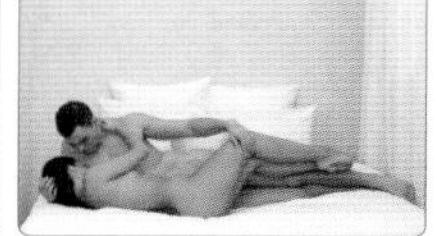
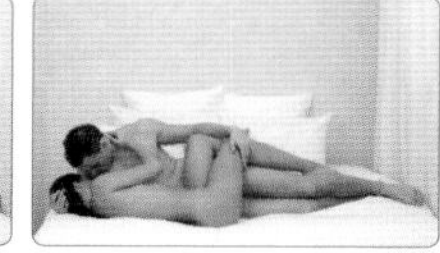
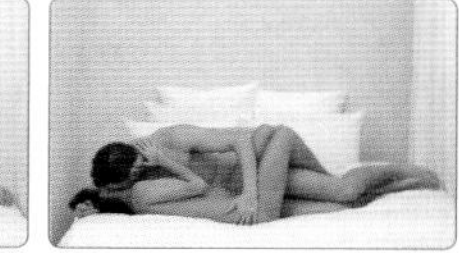
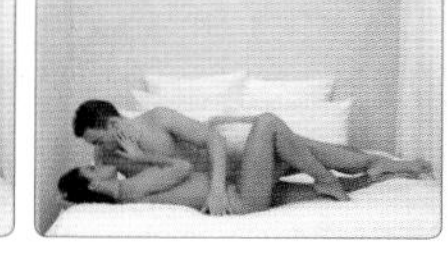
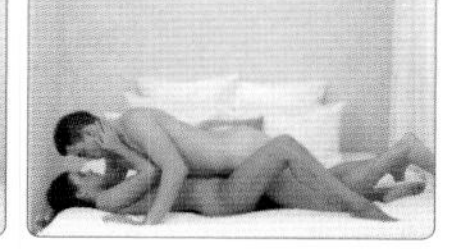

The first posture

☆☆☆☆ Kama sensation rating

This posture is aptly named because it's often the first position that lovers get into when they want good, old-fashioned man-on-top sex. It's not athletic, exotic, or artistic, but for simple, comfortable sweetness, it can't be beaten.

Why it works

- He gets the satisfaction of thrusting freely and deeply because her knees are raised.
- The shaft of his penis touches her clitoris on each thrust, giving her valuable friction where she needs it most.
- You're up close and personal, so the pleasure on your lover's face is plain to see. You can feed off each other's arousal to drive the intensity of your lovemaking sky-high.
- Her hands are free to roam all over his body to make this position supremely sensuous as well as erotic.

Turn on...

... Find a way of moving that takes her to the peak of arousal. This could be a straightforward in-and-out motion, or it could mean pressing yourself close to her body and grinding against her.

Turn off...

... Don't stop or change the pace if you sense that she's close to coming. If she's nearly there, she'll need movements that are sustained, rhythmic, and repetitive. So, if you see a look of pre-orgasmic ecstasy on her face, don't change a thing.

1 V shape

She lies back on the bed with her legs open in a V shape. He gets on all fours between her legs.

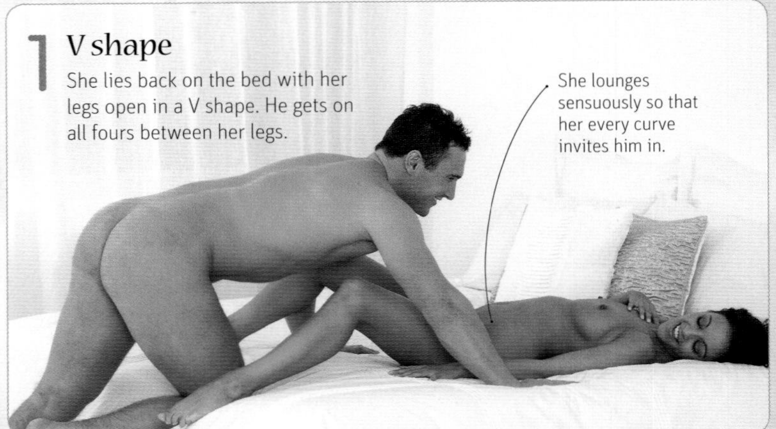

She lounges sensuously so that her every curve invites him in.

2 Face to face

He crawls up her body on all fours until his face is level with hers. He slides into a push-up position and gently penetrates her.

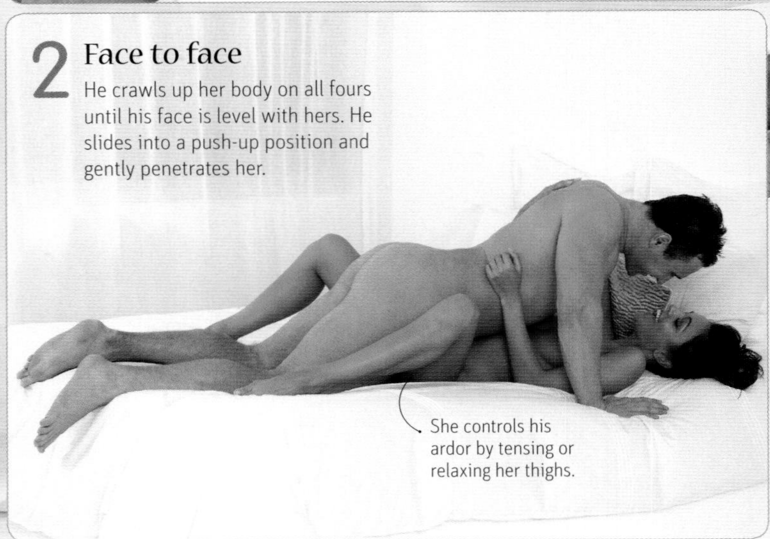

She controls his ardor by tensing or relaxing her thighs.

"An ingenious person should multiply the kinds of congress after the fashion of the different kinds of beasts and birds." KAMA SUTRA

Taking it further

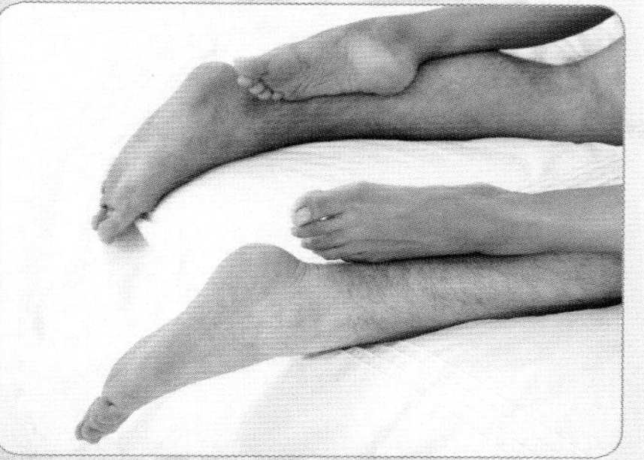

Legs entwined

She slides her feet down his legs and hooks them around his ankles. This creates a tighter genital fit and more direct stimulation to her clitoris.

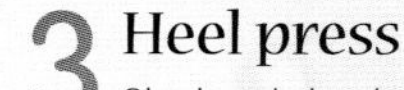

3 Heel press

She bends her knees and raises her legs so that her thighs connect with his waist and her heels press the backs of his thighs.

She uses her heels to guide the speed and tempo of his thrusts.

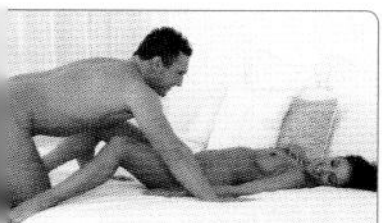
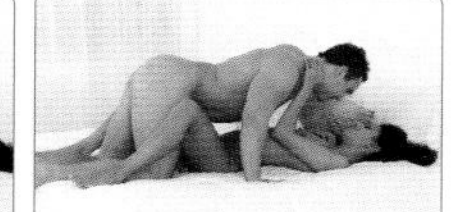
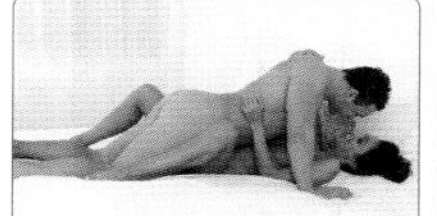
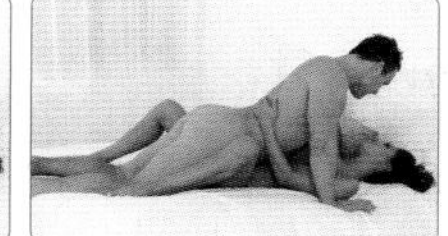
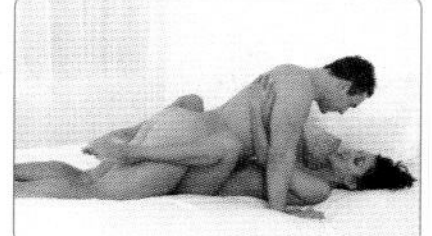
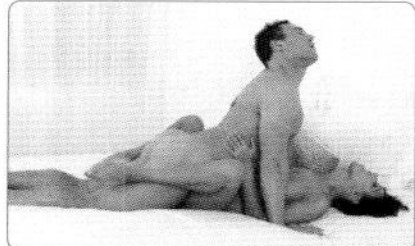

Belly to belly

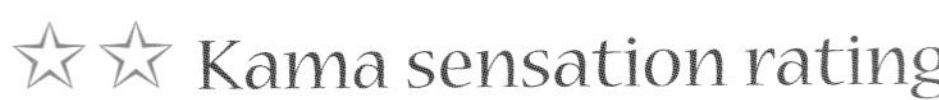

☆☆ Kama sensation rating

Sometimes sex needs to be fast and upright… Perhaps you're doing it in the shower, or maybe you're outdoors and you can't lie down. Whatever your venue, Belly to Belly is a fast-track route to penetration, without losing the intimacy of face-to-face, skin-on-skin contact.

Why it works

– You can graduate from kissing to full-blown sex in seconds. The immediacy of your lust is an aphrodisiac for both of you.

– You don't even need to undress; she just slips off her panties and lifts up her skirt. He then drops his pants, and away you go.

– His penis enters her at an unusual angle, creating plenty of stimulating friction against her clitoris and labia.

– You can make sex feel extra-dirty by telling each other your naughtiest fantasies, as you are at such close quarters.

Turn on…

… Use techniques to make her taller if there's a height difference between you. She can try wearing heels, or she can stand on the bottom step of a flight of stairs with him just below.

Turn off…

… Don't bother with this position if she's tiny and he's super-tall. No amount of squatting on his part or stretching on her part will help you to achieve penetration if you're not height compatible. Try Suspended Congress (see page 186) instead.

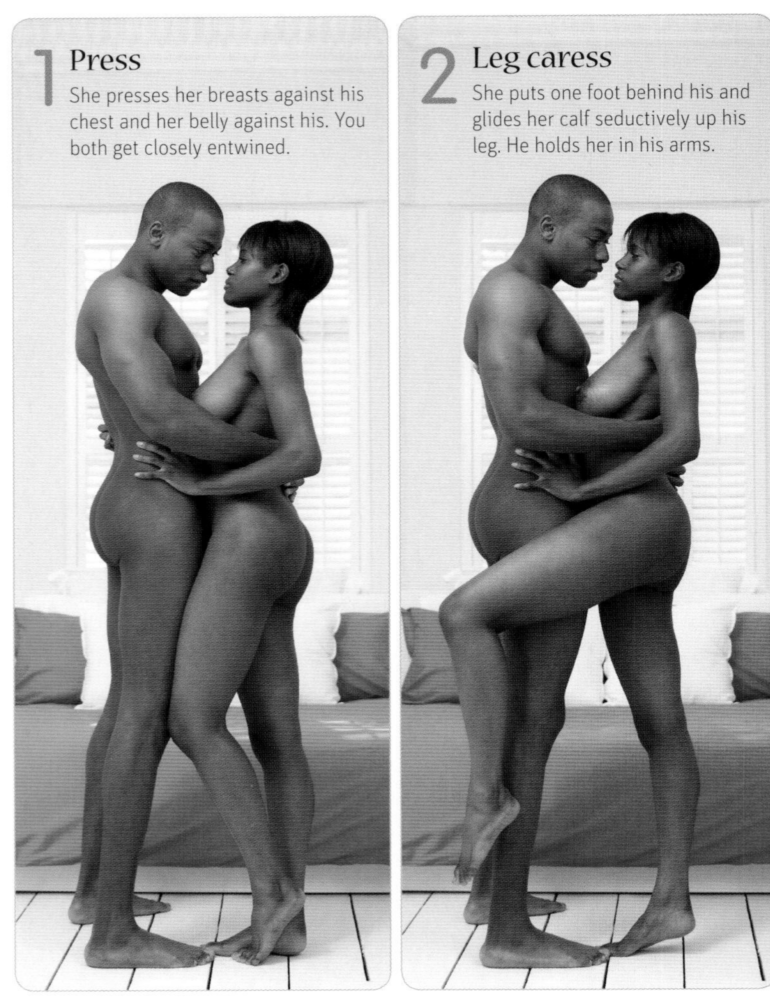

1 Press
She presses her breasts against his chest and her belly against his. You both get closely entwined.

2 Leg caress
She puts one foot behind his and glides her calf seductively up his leg. He holds her in his arms.

"One can practise the more unusual techniques in water—standing, sitting, or lying down—because it is easier that way." KAMA SUTRA

3 Leg up

She hooks her thigh around his waist so that he can guide himself into her. She puts her arms around him, and he puts a helping hand under her thigh.

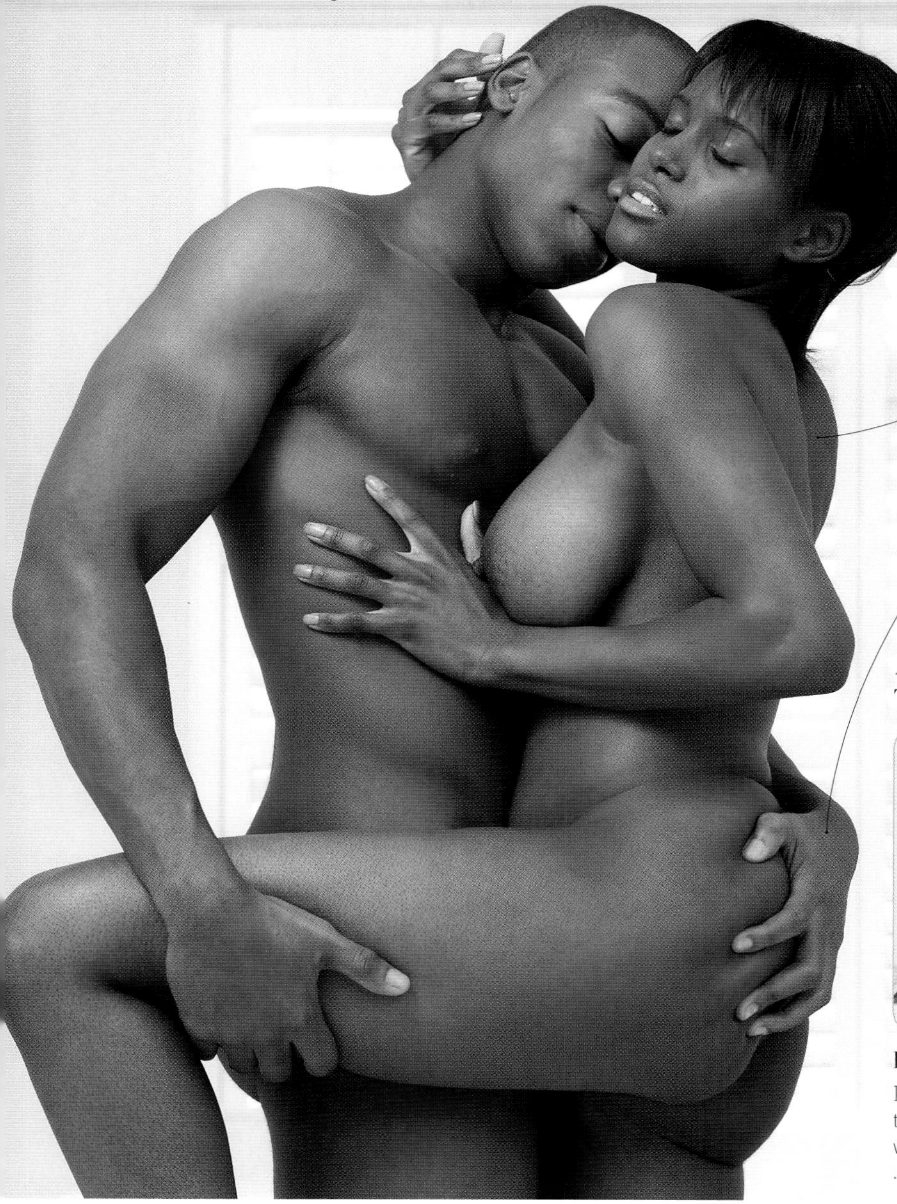

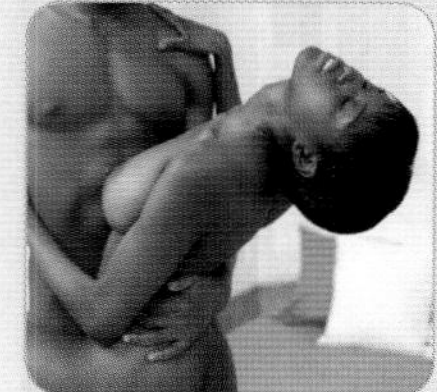

She can arch her back and push her pelvis forward to meet his thrusts.

He uses his supporting hand to give her buttock a sexy squeeze as he thrusts.

Taking it further

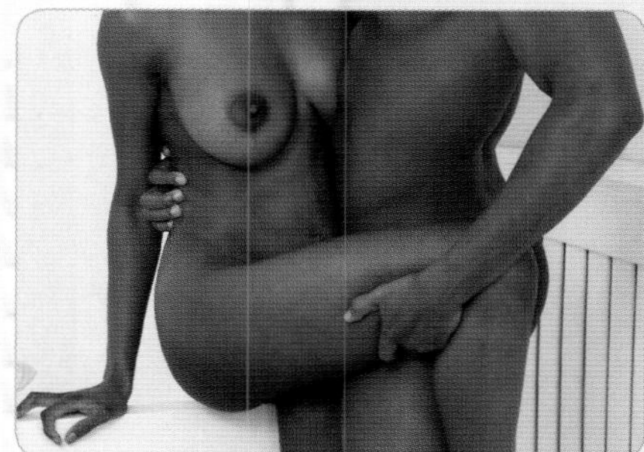

Kitchen canoodling

If there's a big height difference between the two of you, she can sit on a kitchen counter while he stands between her legs to penetrate.

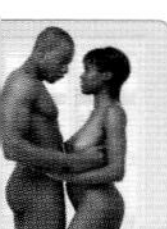
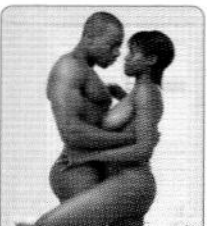
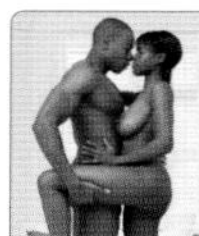
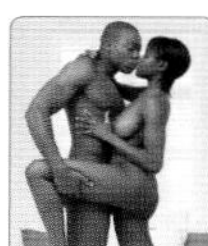
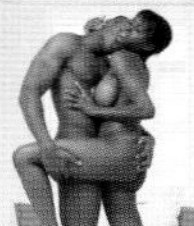

Clasping and Side-by-side clasping

☆☆☆☆ Kama sensation rating

Clasping is a hot variation of the missionary position in which she traps him with her feet around his legs. To mix things up mid-session, you roll over into a side-by-side position. And, if you want to, you can keep rolling so that she has a turn on top too.

Why they work

- If you both use a rocking motion in the Clasping position, she has a good chance of reaching orgasm. She rocks down while he rocks up (see The Movements of Sex, page 60).
- The Clasping position is one of the best positions for cuddling, hugging, nuzzling, kissing, and smooching.
- Side-by-Side Clasping changes the tempo and puts her on a more equal basis; she can push back and forth while he remains still.
- Rolling on to your sides is a good way to temper his lust and make sex last longer if Clasping is pushing his buttons too quickly.

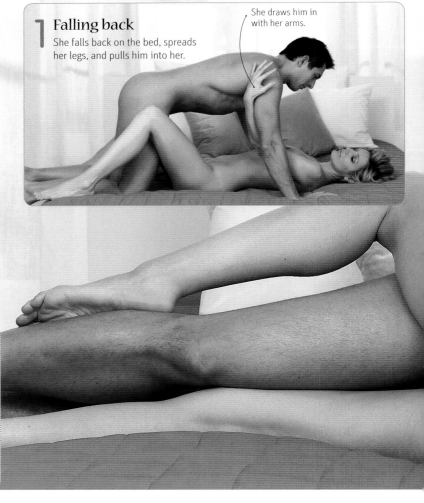

1 Falling back

She falls back on the bed, spreads her legs, and pulls him into her.

She draws him in with her arms.

Turn on...

... Hook your arms underneath her and clasp her shoulders with your hands in the Clasping position. This pulls you up her body, which means that your penis presses hard on her hot spots.

Turn off...

... Don't lean on her. Spread your weight equally between your forearms and knees so that she's not crushed, and make your thrusts light and smooth.

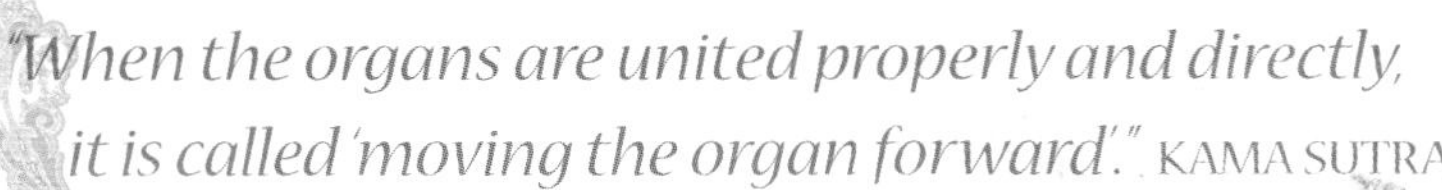

"When the organs are united properly and directly, it is called 'moving the organ forward'." KAMA SUTRA

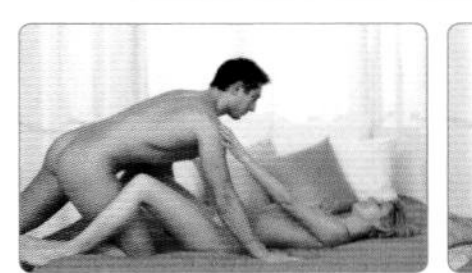

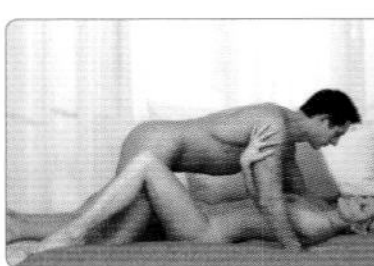

2 Clasping limbs

Once he's in, she clasps him with her hands around his body and her feet around his calves. This is the Clasping position.

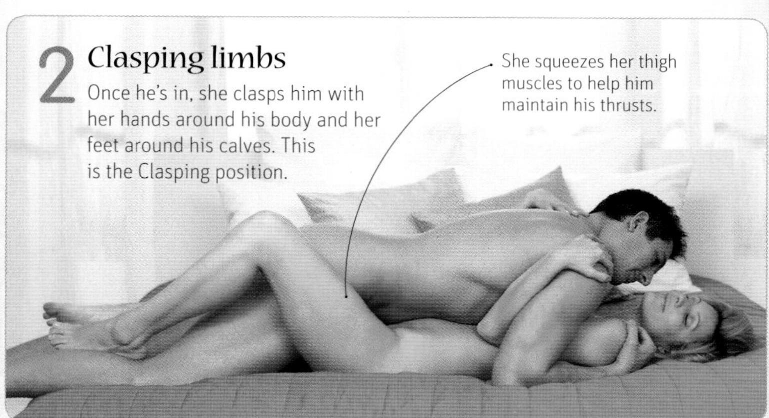

She squeezes her thigh muscles to help him maintain his thrusts.

3 Hugging and rolling

He holds her tight and rolls through 90 degrees into the Side-by-Side Clasping position. She moves her lower leg so that it is parallel with his.

Keep each other pressed close by putting your arms around each other.

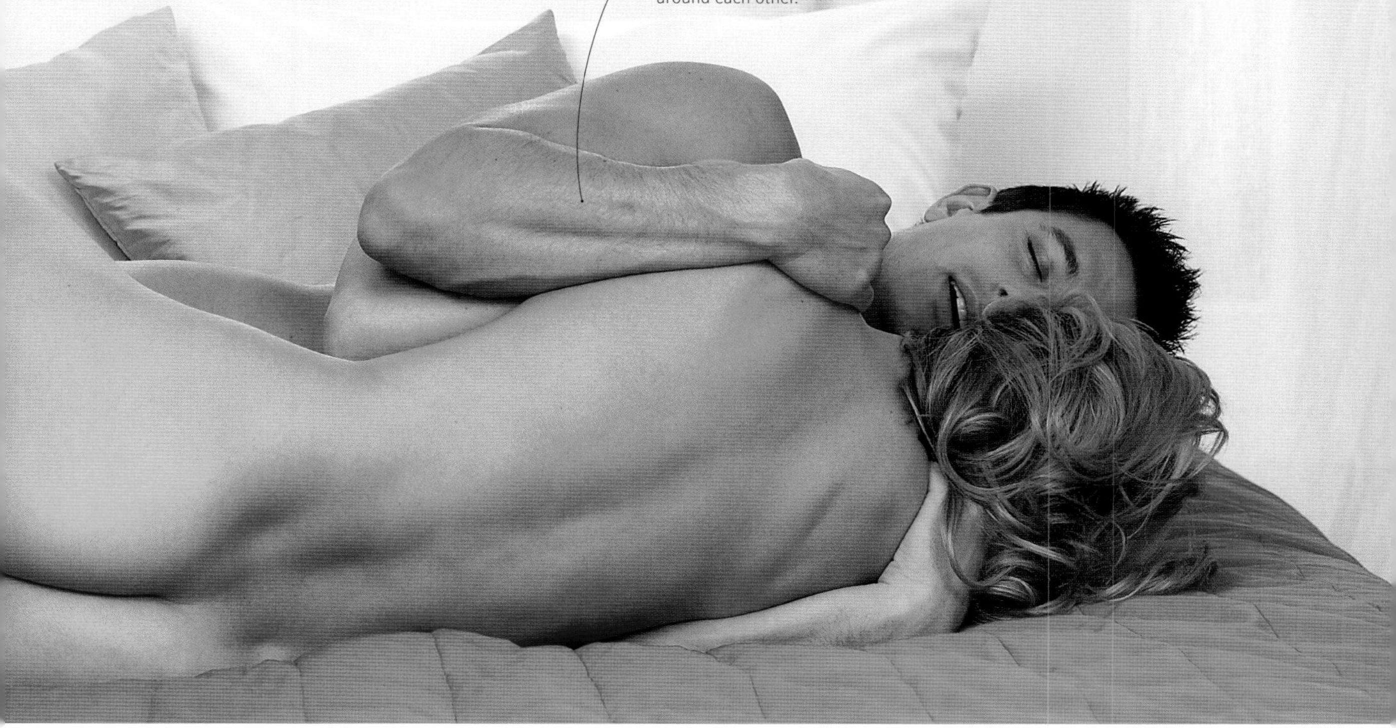

Taking it further

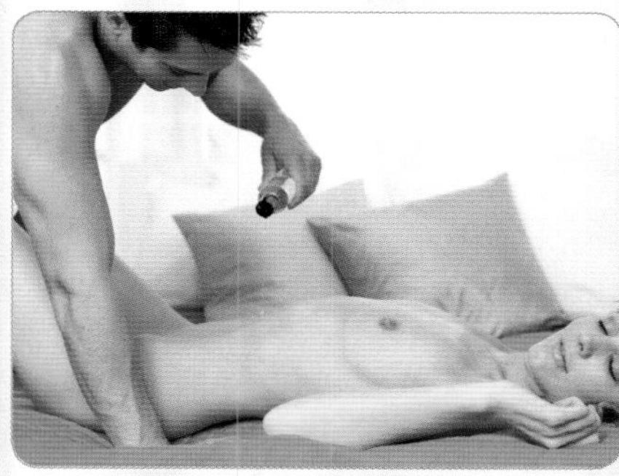

Getting slippery

Massage oil into each other's skin, then slither and slide your way through sex. A PVC sheet on the bed or floor means you can get as oily as you like.

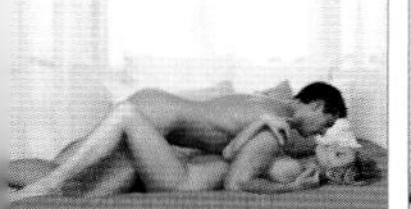
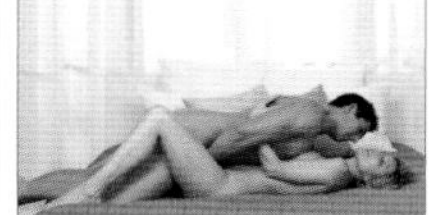
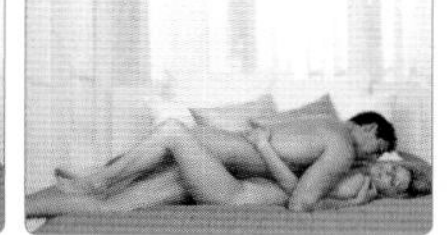
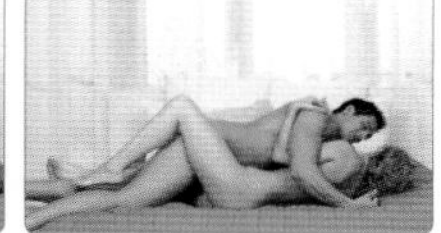
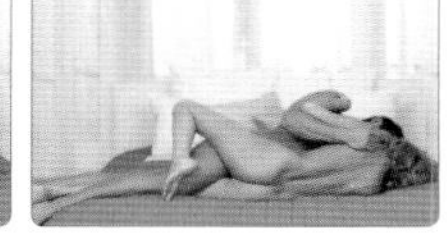
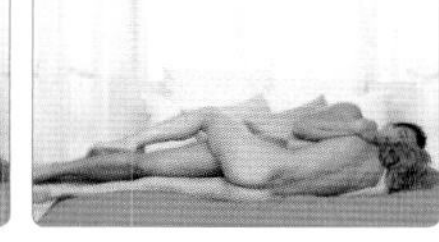

Love's fusion

☆☆ Kama sensation rating

This is the sexual equivalent of a mug of cocoa: warm, nurturing, and comforting. He takes her in his arms, and she snuggles against him as you gently rock against each other. What you miss out on in dizzying passion you'll make up for in intimacy, romance, and tenderness.

Why it works

– In this position, his penis nudges her vaginal entrance or penetrates by just a small amount. This is good for her because the outer third of the vagina is the part that's most sensitive to stimulation.

– He gets to show his caring side by taking a gentle and loving approach to sex.

– There's no performance pressure on her: she can lie back and feel cuddled and secure in his arms.

– Love's Fusion helps you to bond when you've been away from each other, or to make up after you've had an argument.

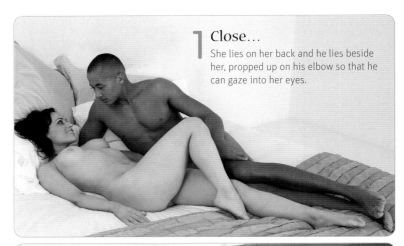

1 Close...
She lies on her back and he lies beside her, propped up on his elbow so that he can gaze into her eyes.

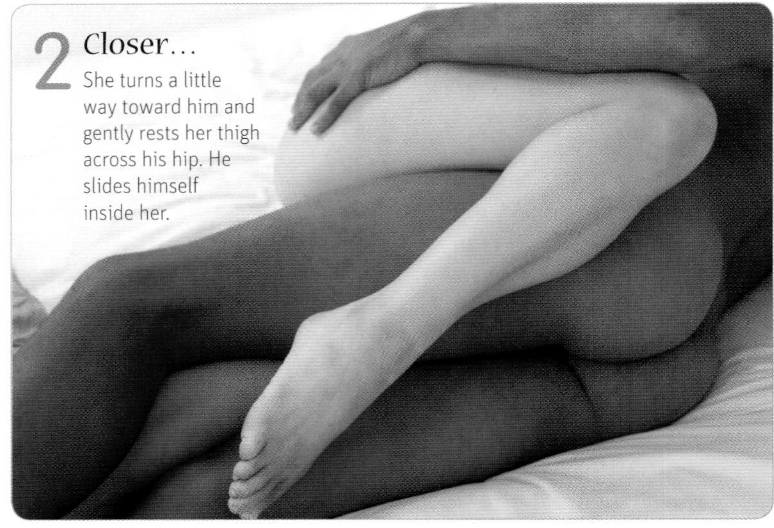

2 Closer...
She turns a little way toward him and gently rests her thigh across his hip. He slides himself inside her.

Turn on...

... Give yourselves up to romance. Whisper to each other. Stroke each other's skin. Kiss each other not just on the mouth, but all over the face and neck.

Turn off...

... Don't neglect the nether regions. This position is not high on genital stimulation for him because his penis doesn't penetrate very far. If she feels his erection losing power, she can scoot down to lend a helping hand (or mouth) to recharge him.

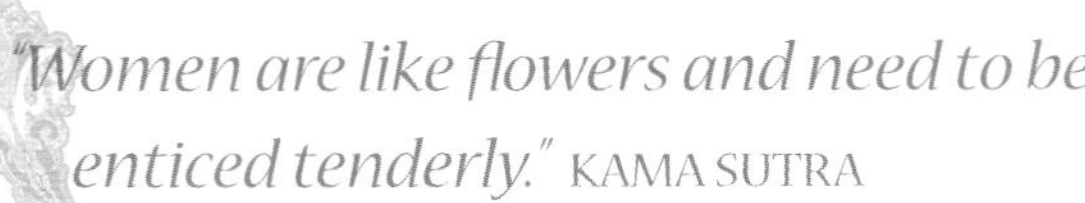

"Women are like flowers and need to be enticed tenderly." KAMA SUTRA

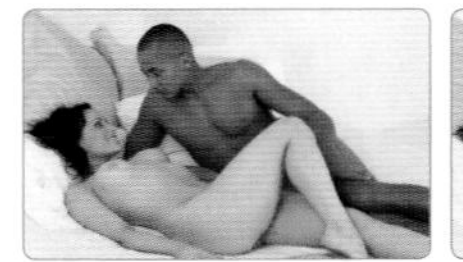

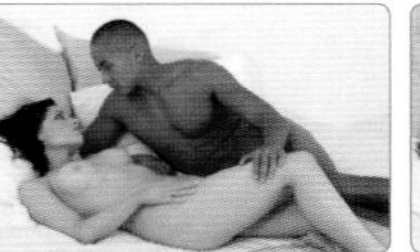

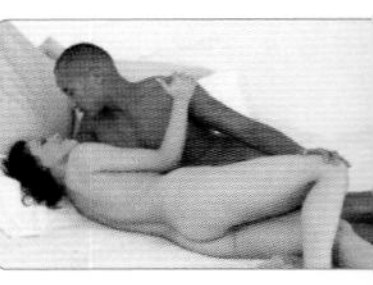

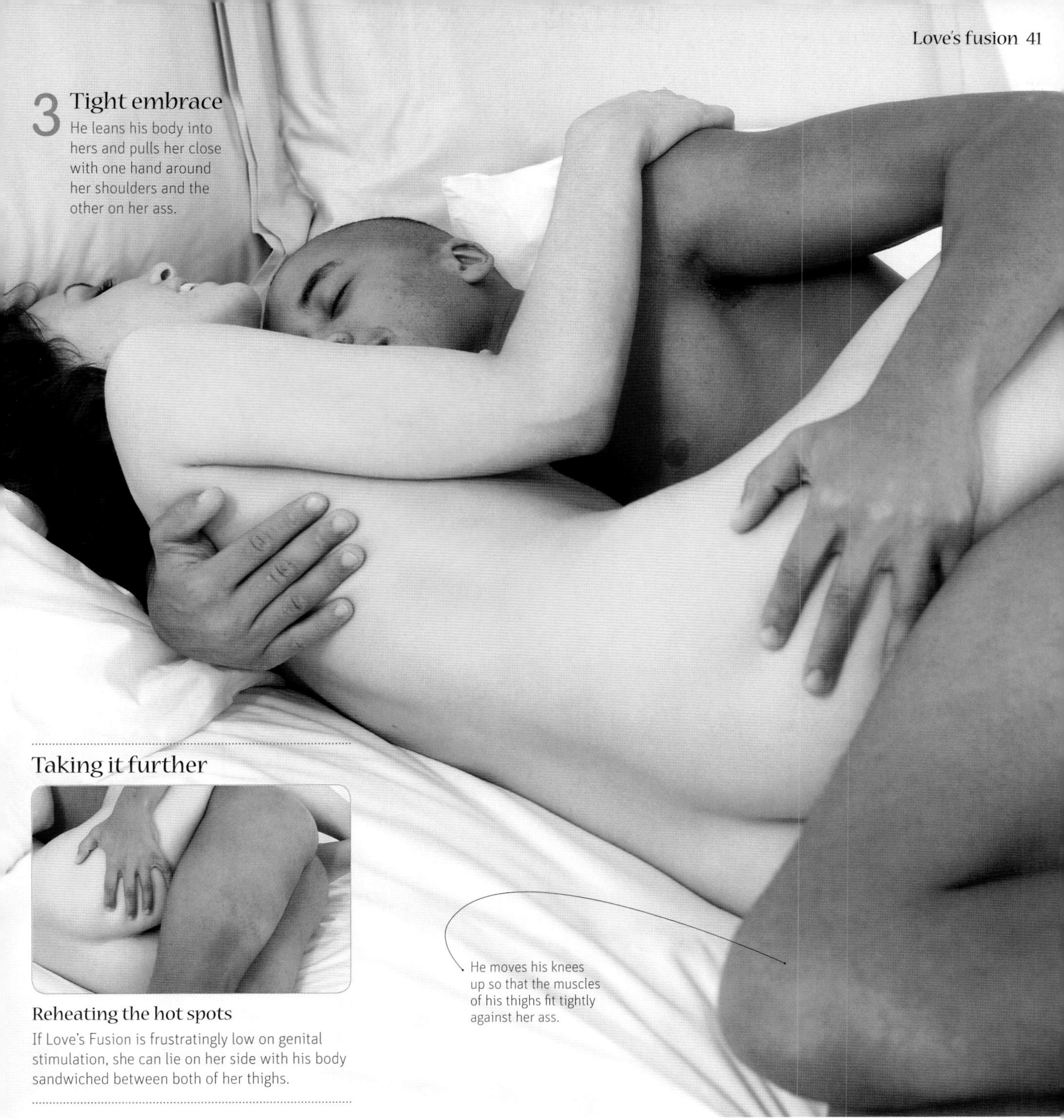

3 Tight embrace

He leans his body into hers and pulls her close with one hand around her shoulders and the other on her ass.

He moves his knees up so that the muscles of his thighs fit tightly against her ass.

Taking it further

Reheating the hot spots

If Love's Fusion is frustratingly low on genital stimulation, she can lie on her side with his body sandwiched between both of her thighs.

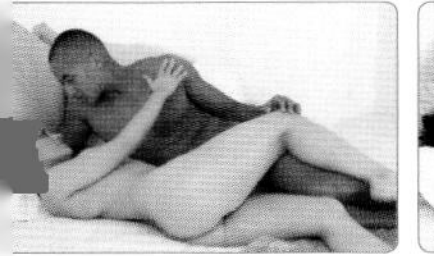
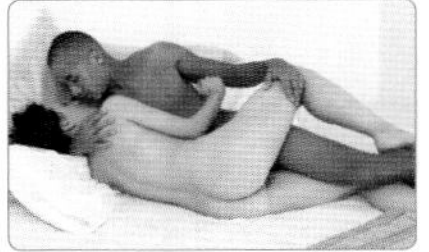
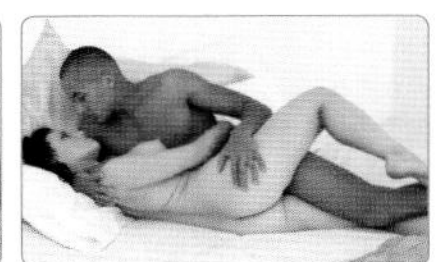
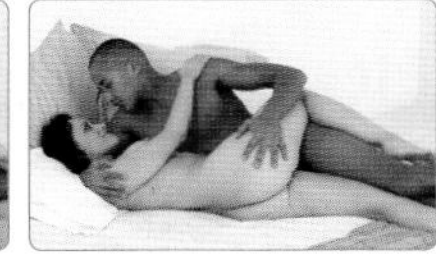
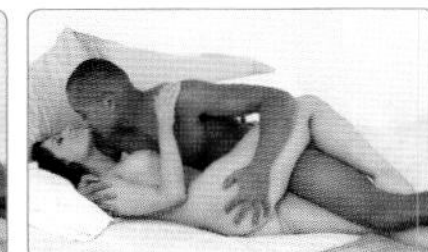
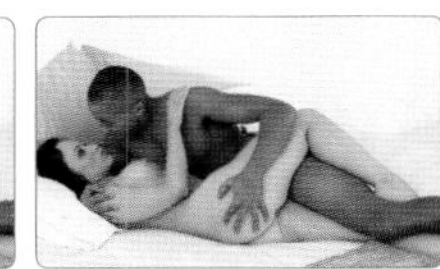

Mandarin duck

☆ Kama sensation rating

This unusual position involves some demanding leg tangles; it may not be the fastest route to penetration and orgasm, but it's fun to try if you're in a creative, experimental mood. You can always laugh and tumble your way into an easier position if it goes wrong.

Why it works

– If you get it right, the angle at which his penis enters her vagina may produce some new and intoxicating sensations.

– You both enjoy the satisfaction of trying something a little out of the ordinary.

– You can have sexy fun cooperating with each other to get into position.

– You'll be so preoccupied with figuring out which leg should go where that you'll leave all your sexual inhibitions behind.

– You're face to face, so you can enjoy each other's expressions of pleasure/amusement.

Turn on…

… Turn your phones off, lock the door, and try it when you've got a long, lazy afternoon that you can devote to spending in bed. Make it part of a sequence of positions you've never tried before.

Turn off…

… Don't berate yourself if it's not working. If his penis won't bend at the right angle, her knee won't point in the right direction, or he can't keep his balance, turn to another page and try something more satisfying and less demanding.

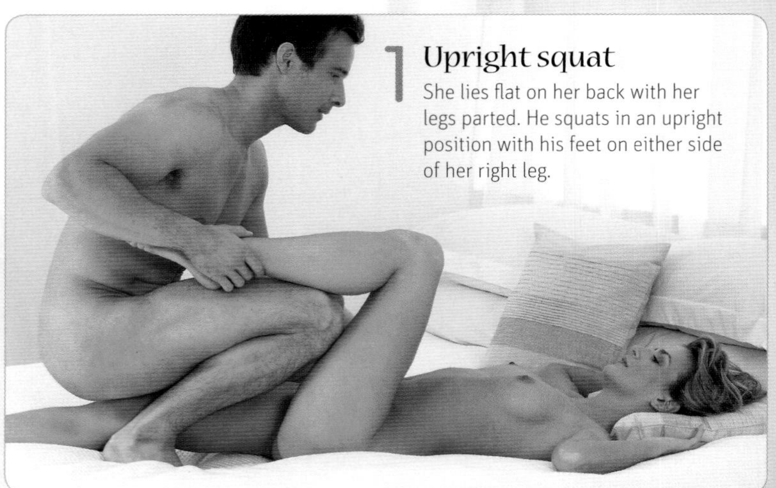

1 Upright squat
She lies flat on her back with her legs parted. He squats in an upright position with his feet on either side of her right leg.

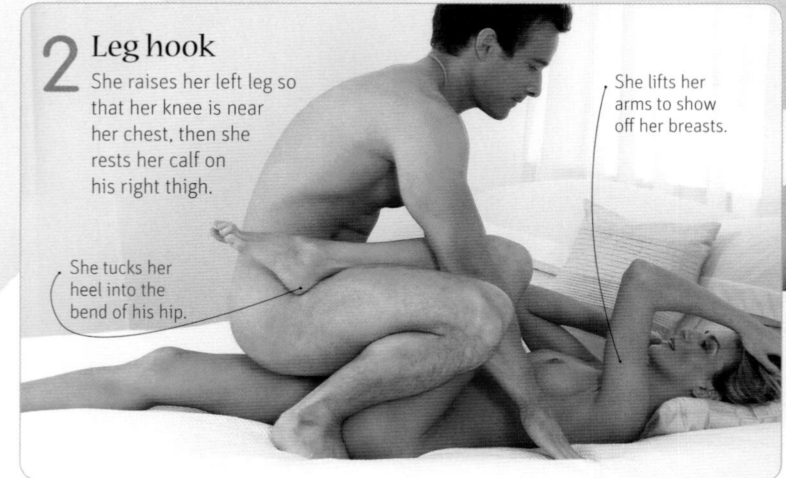
She lifts her arms to show off her breasts.
She tucks her heel into the bend of his hip.

2 Leg hook
She raises her left leg so that her knee is near her chest, then she rests her calf on his right thigh.

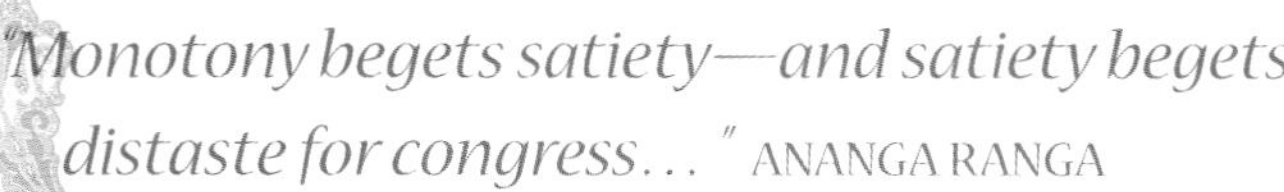

"Monotony begets satiety—and satiety begets distaste for congress…" ANANGA RANGA

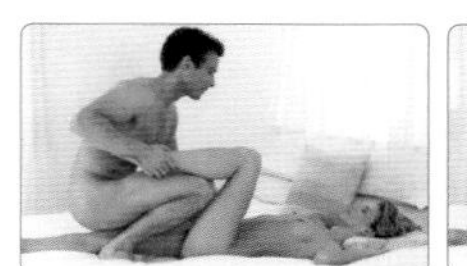

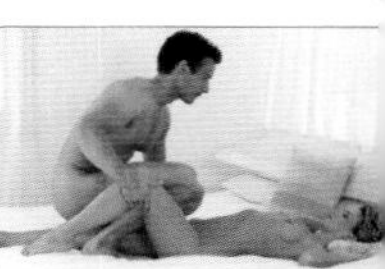

Taking it further

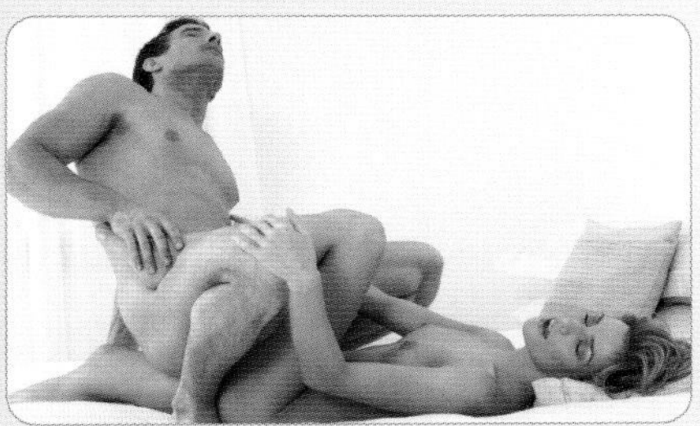

Increasing the tension

He creates a slow but sustained build-up of erotic tension by rocking gently back and forth, hopefully tipping both of you over the edge.

She helps to support him in case he loses his balance as he moves.

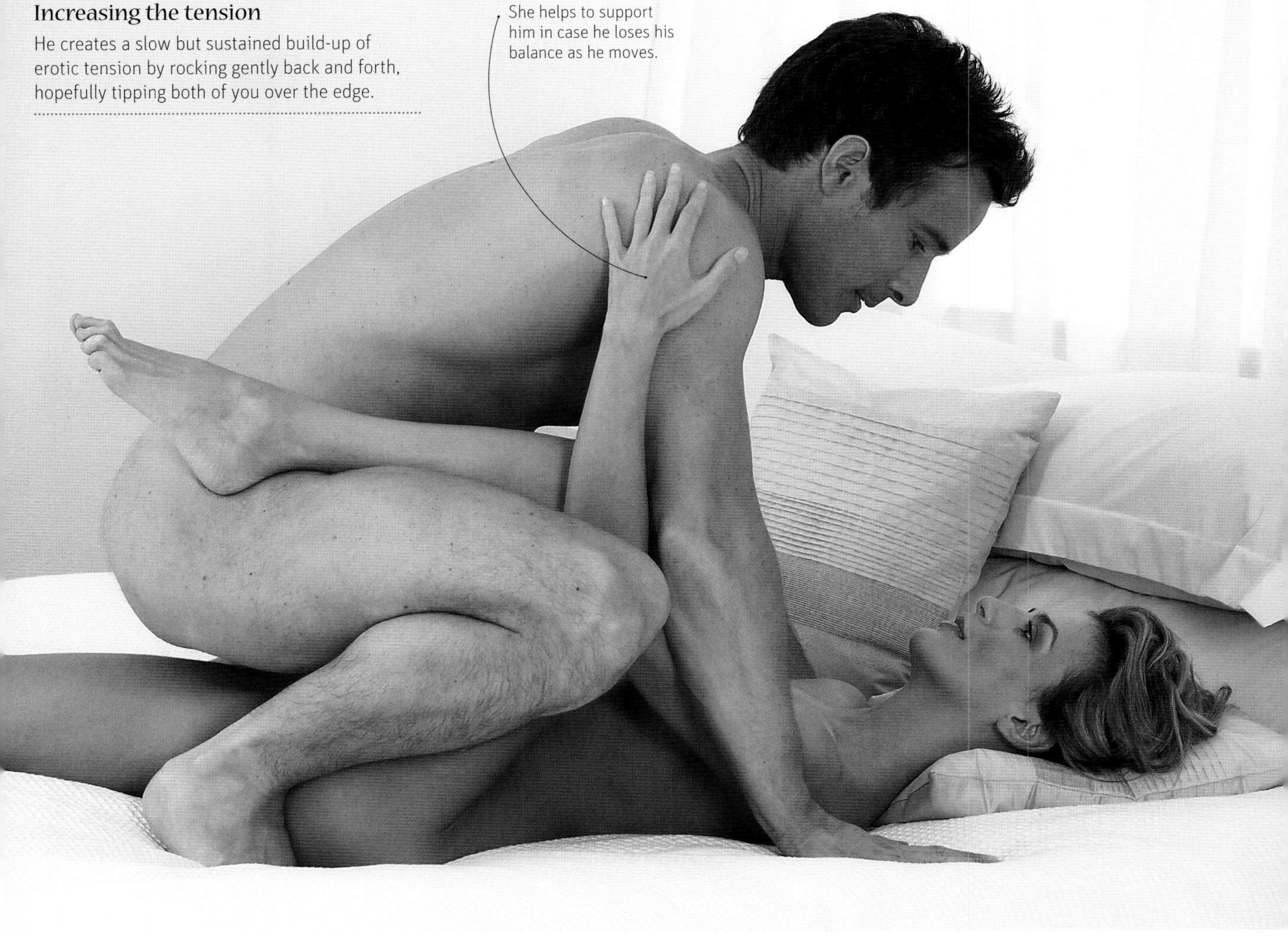

3 Supported squat

He lowers himself into a deeper squat so that he can enter her, then rests his butt gently on her thigh and supports his weight by leaning forward on his hands.

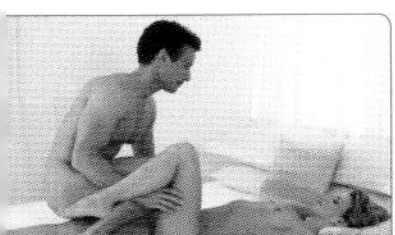
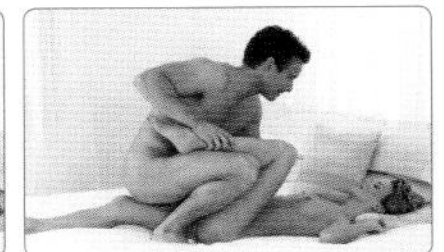
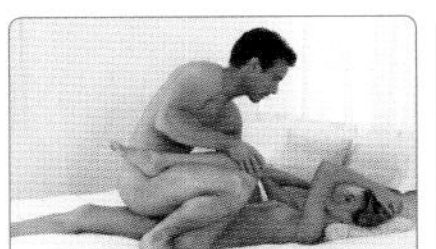
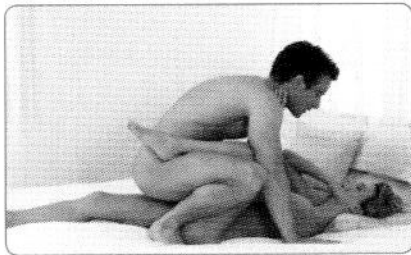
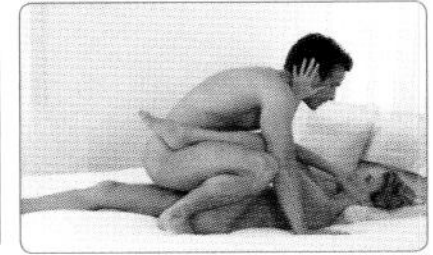
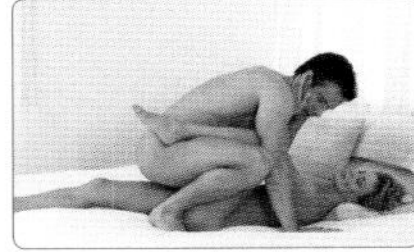

Pressing and Twining

☆☆☆☆ Kama sensation rating

Celebrate your love in these two emotionally charged positions. You're about to be locked in a passionate face-to-face clinch in which he does the pressing and she does the twining. So put the silk sheets on the bed, light the candles, and let the loving commence.

Why they work

– Although he's in the dominant position, sex stays interactive. She controls his passion by hugging his top half in her arms and enclosing his bottom half between her legs.

– Pressing and Twining flow seamlessly into each other. There are plenty of other leg positions she can experiment with too, such as moving her knee or straightening her leg.

– When he feels her heel on the back of his leg in Twining position, he knows that she wants him deeper inside her.

– You can be as physically and emotionally close as you like in these positions; they're perfect for the can't-keep-your-hands-off-each-other stage of a relationship.

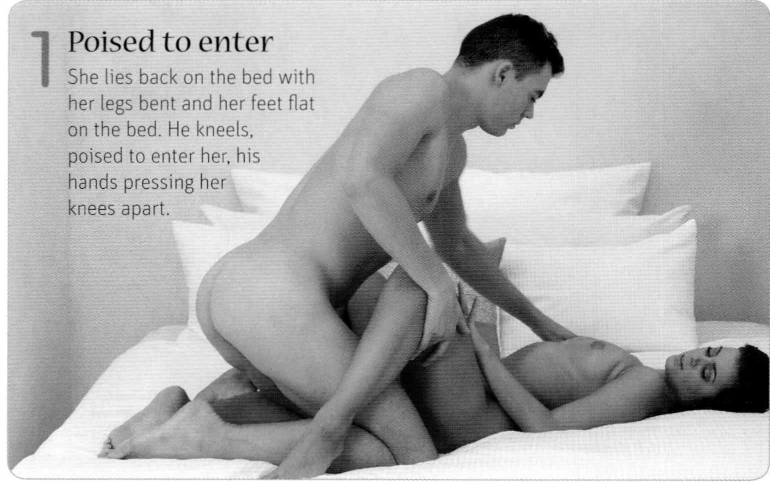

1 Poised to enter
She lies back on the bed with her legs bent and her feet flat on the bed. He kneels, poised to enter her, his hands pressing her knees apart.

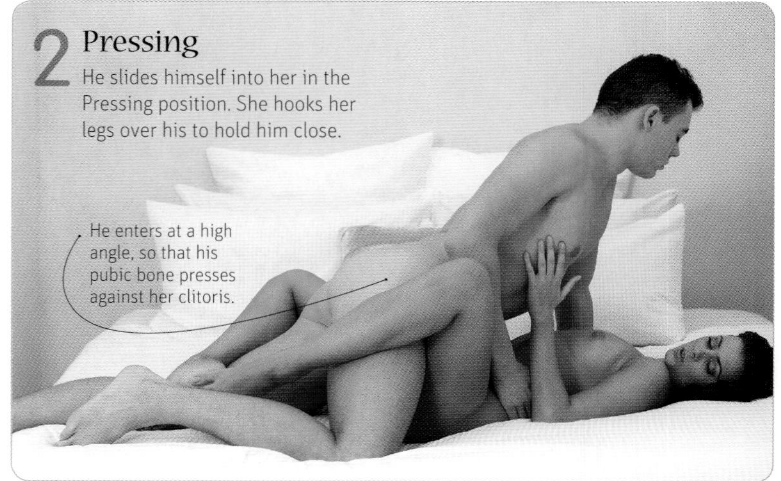

He enters at a high angle, so that his pubic bone presses against her clitoris.

2 Pressing
He slides himself into her in the Pressing position. She hooks her legs over his to hold him close.

Turn on...
... Mix up the rhythm of your thrusts: make some light and shallow, some plunging and deep.

Turn off...
... Don't forget that it's OK to have a break from thrusting during sex so that you can concentrate on enjoying the intimate, lovey-dovey stuff.

"Blind with passion, with no thought of pain or injury, they embrace as though they want to enter each other." KAMA SUTRA

3 Leg angle

She lifts one foot off the bed and angles her leg across the back of his thigh. She uses her heel to keep him pressed close.

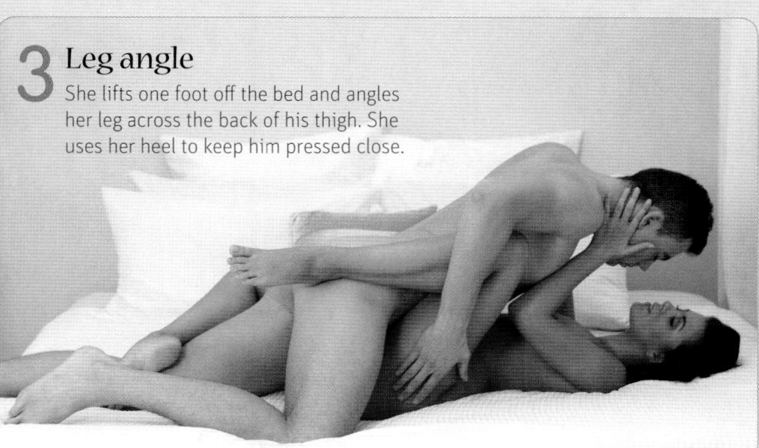

Taking it further

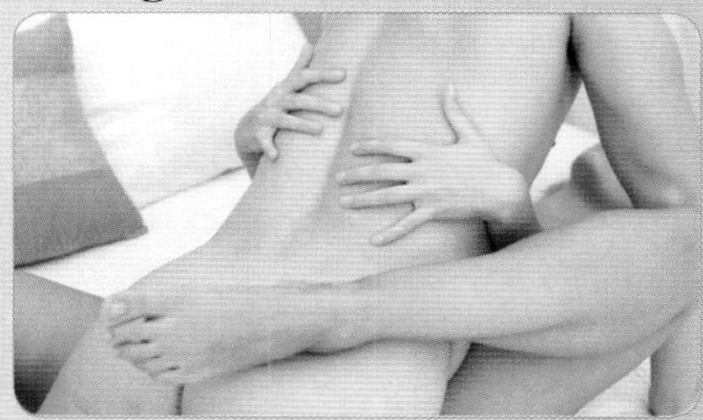

Deeper penetration

She slides her heel from the back of his thigh up over the curve of his buttocks and into the small of his back; this lets him in deeper.

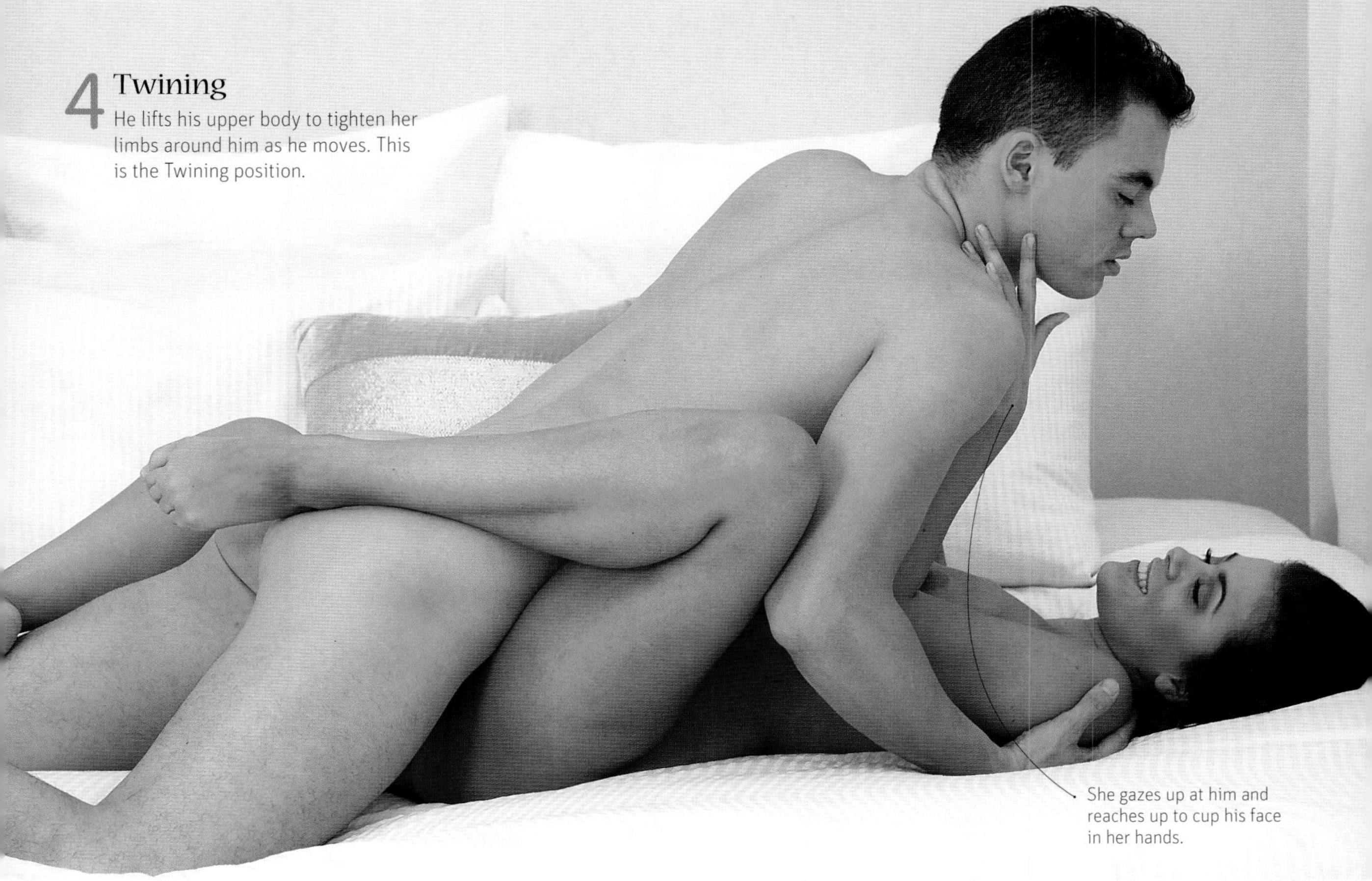

4 Twining

He lifts his upper body to tighten her limbs around him as he moves. This is the Twining position.

She gazes up at him and reaches up to cup his face in her hands.

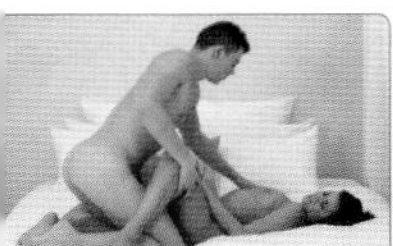
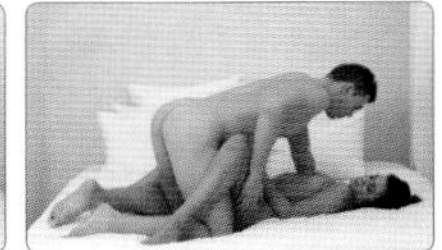
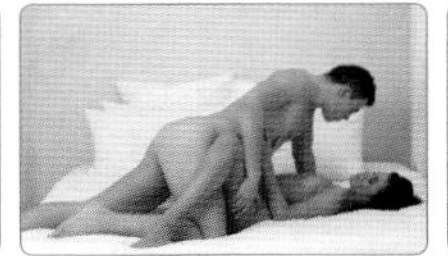
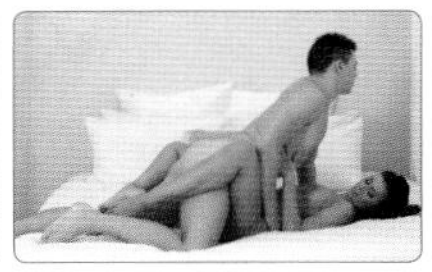
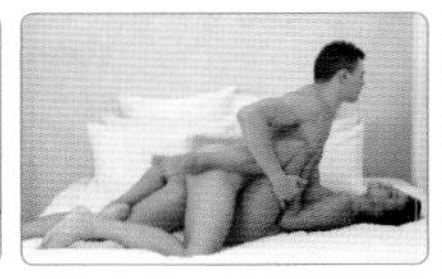
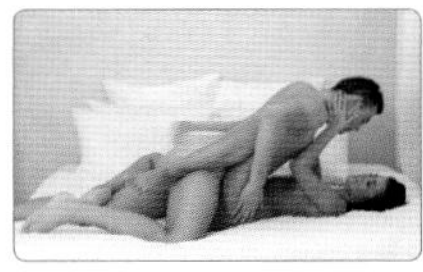

Butterflies in flight

☆☆☆ Kama sensation rating

Most popular woman-on-top positions feature her sitting or kneeling astride his waist and riding him cowgirl-style. Butterflies in Flight is more gentle and seductive. She remains in charge, while he gets the benefit of feeling all her erogenous zones moving gently down on his.

Why it works

– She can experiment and position herself so that his penis enters her at the most erotically satisfying angle.

– He experiences the excitement of taking a passive role during sex. He's pinned down by her body, and her hands and feet are on top of his, so it's difficult for him to move.

– It's a chance to have sex at a more sedate pace than usual; you can both relish the subtle movements and sensations.

– She can push herself up and down in small but sexy movements with her arms, legs, and core strength, using his feet as a platform.

Turn on...

... Use your dominant position to tease and seduce him. Brush him with your breasts. Kiss him, then pull away. Let your hair fall around his face. Tense your vaginal muscles to grip him tightly.

Turn off...

... Don't forget to satisfy yourself as well. Sustained up-and-down movements or circular grinding might produce enough friction for you to climax. You're in charge of the pace and tempo: enjoy it.

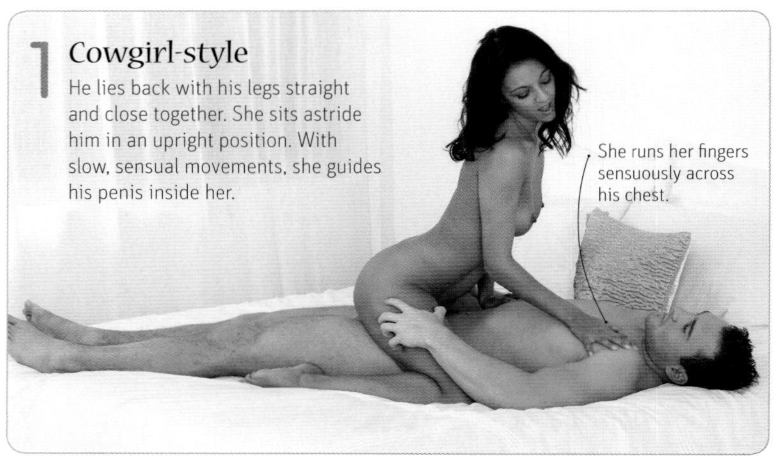
She runs her fingers sensuously across his chest.

1 Cowgirl-style
He lies back with his legs straight and close together. She sits astride him in an upright position. With slow, sensual movements, she guides his penis inside her.

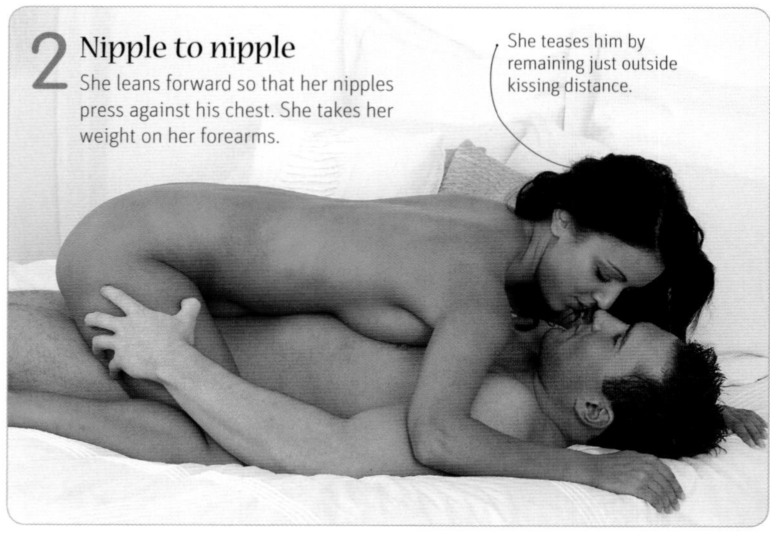
She teases him by remaining just outside kissing distance.

2 Nipple to nipple
She leans forward so that her nipples press against his chest. She takes her weight on her forearms.

"Once the member is gripped by the vagina, the man can no longer prevent the emission of semen, and the member is held tightly until it is drained." THE PERFUMED GARDEN

3 Top cover

She slides her legs down the bed so that her feet are level with his, then rests her legs on top of his and presses her toes against the tops of his feet.

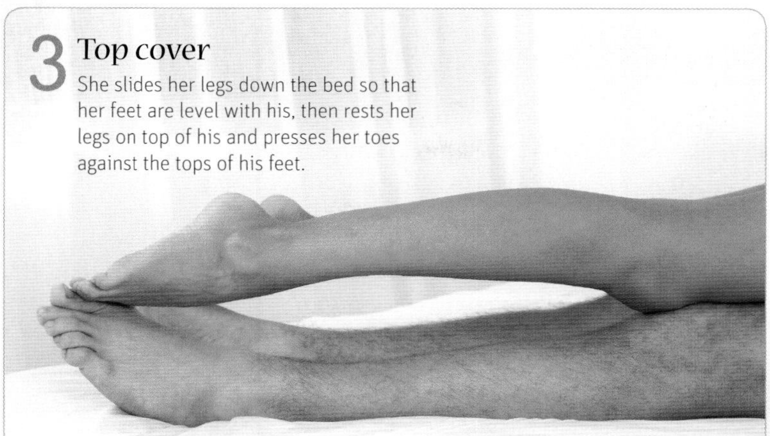

Taking it further

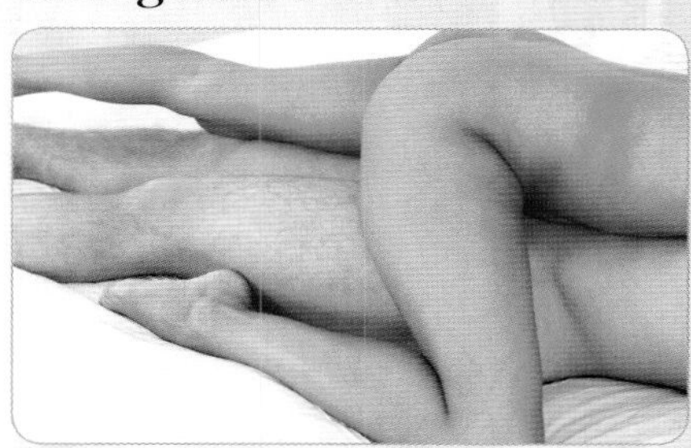

Allowing more movement

She moves into a position where she can grind her hips more freely by bending one leg so her knee is level with his waist.

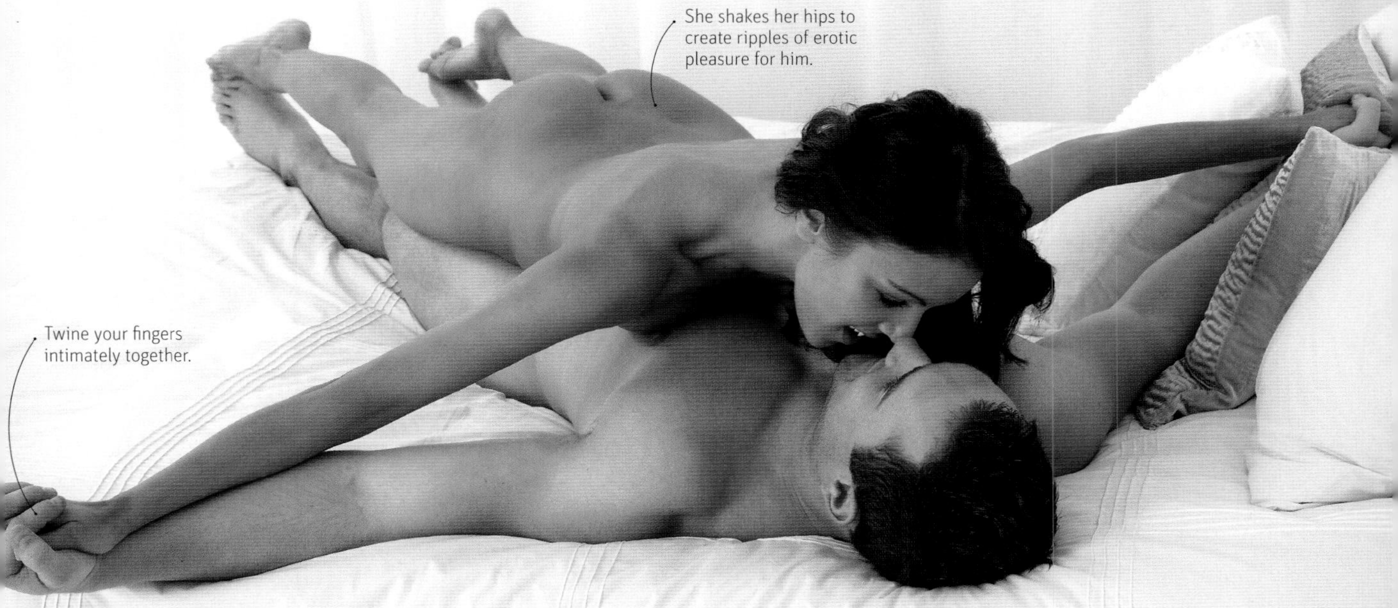

She shakes her hips to create ripples of erotic pleasure for him.

Twine your fingers intimately together.

4 Hands to the sides

He stretches his arms out to each side, and she puts her hands in his. She lifts her head and braces herself against his hands and feet as she moves.

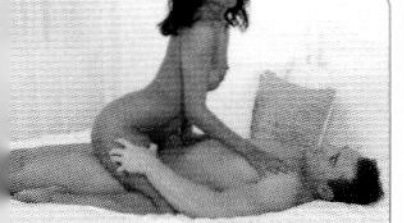
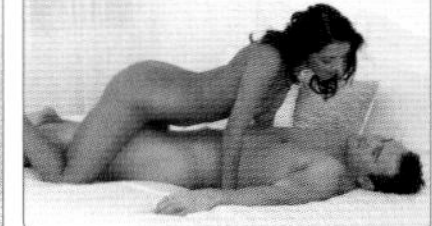
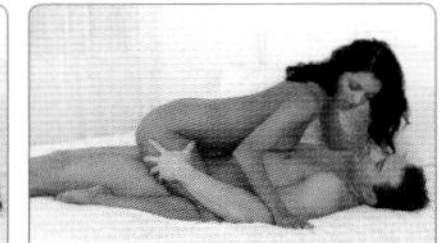
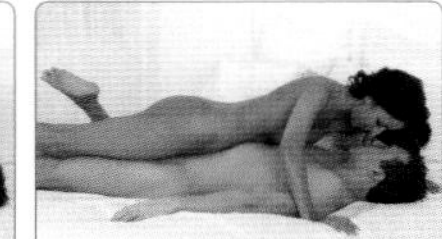
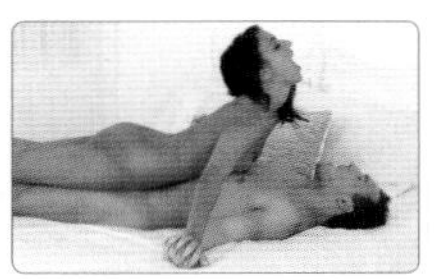

Gripping with toes

The closeness of Gripping with Toes comes from his strong predatory on-all-fours posture enclosing her vulnerability. Because she's half suspended with her legs around his torso, she's mostly dependent on him to make the moves. Sustaining this challenging position for an entire sex session depends on whether her thigh muscles can go the distance.

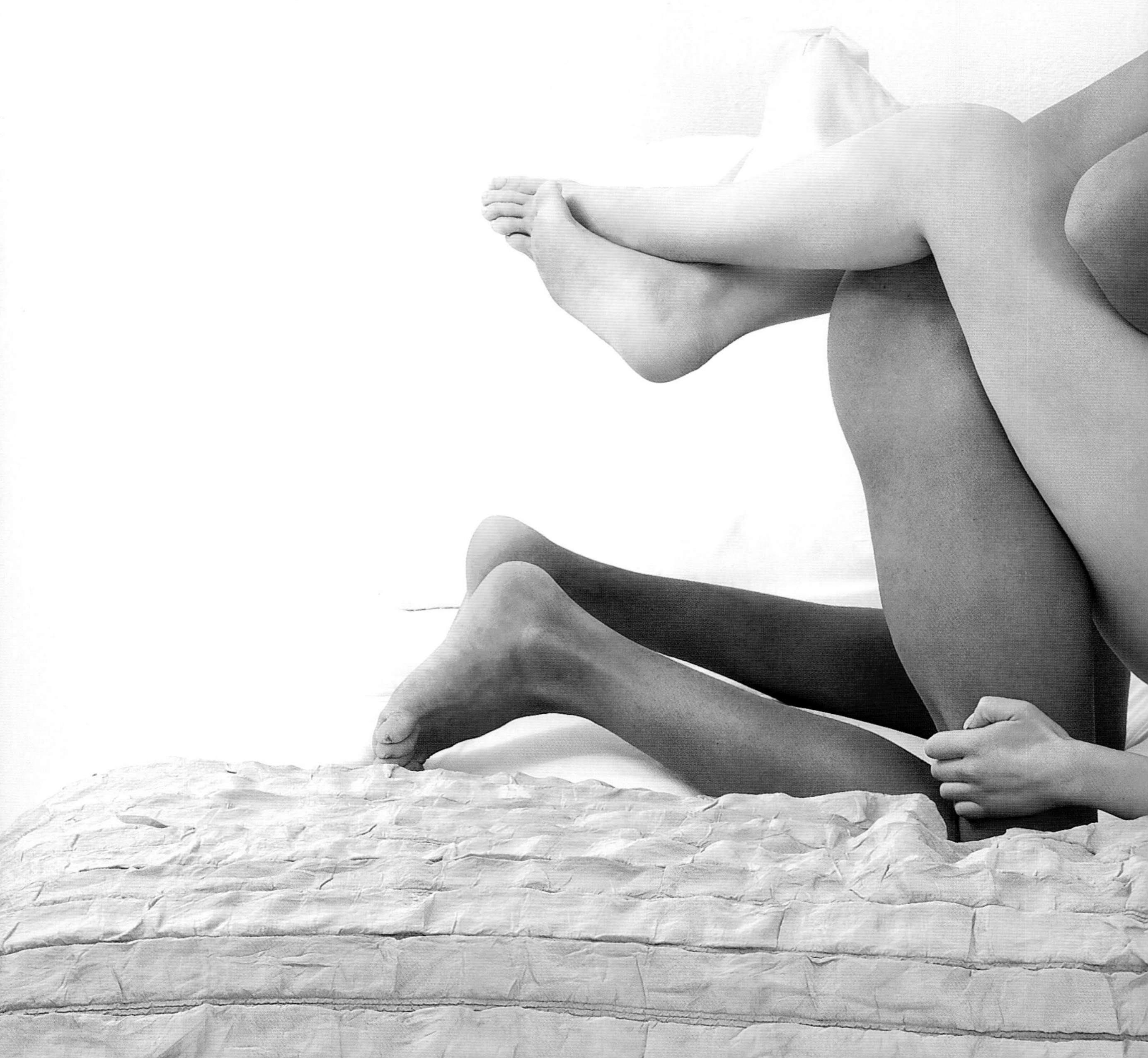

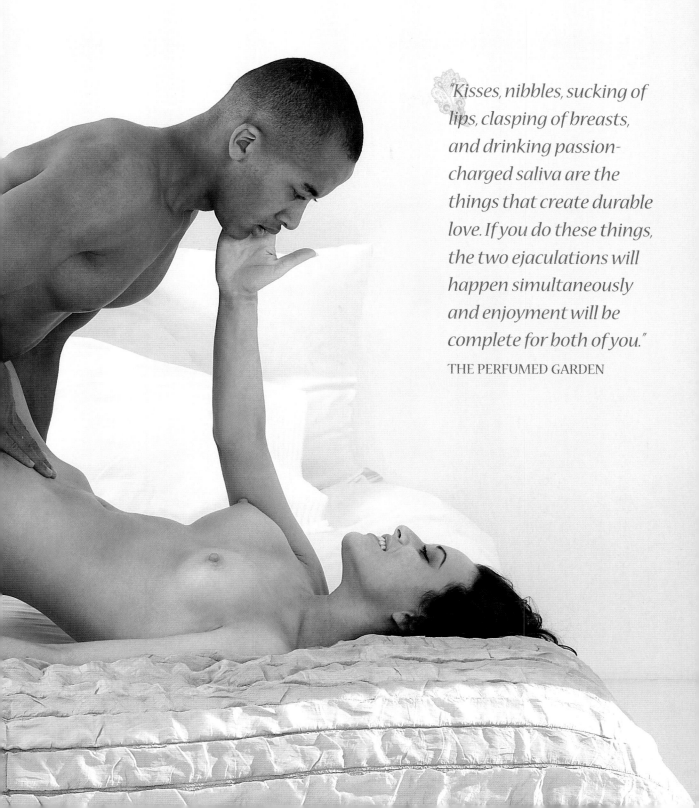

"Kisses, nibbles, sucking of lips, clasping of breasts, and drinking passion-charged saliva are the things that create durable love. If you do these things, the two ejaculations will happen simultaneously and enjoyment will be complete for both of you."

THE PERFUMED GARDEN

Gripping with toes

Kama sensation rating

Why it works

– If she has strong thigh muscles, she can give him delicious sensations by pulling herself up and down on his body (think of pull-ups on a gym bar).

– He loves the feeling of her legs locked passionately around his torso.

– You can both experience the heady thrill of novelty and the satisfaction of pulling off a tricky maneuver; it's not easy to have sex when she's partially suspended.

– Her head is lower than her feet, so she gets a rush from being slightly inverted.

– Athletic positions such as this require sexual cooperation. Once you've tried Gripping with Toes, you'll want to push your erotic boundaries even further.

Turn on...

... Relish the drama of the position. If you like to show off, this is your chance. She can throw her hands over her head, and, if she's really supple, she can pull herself up so high on his body that only her head and shoulders stay on the ground.

Turn off...

... Don't expect orgasms to come easily in this position. You're both more likely to be concentrating on holding the pose rather than surrendering to the throes of passion.

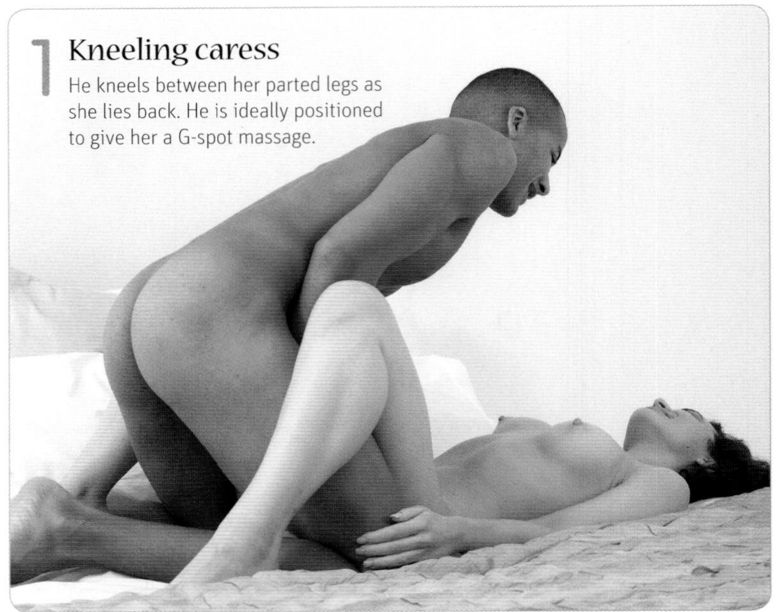

1 Kneeling caress

He kneels between her parted legs as she lies back. He is ideally positioned to give her a G-spot massage.

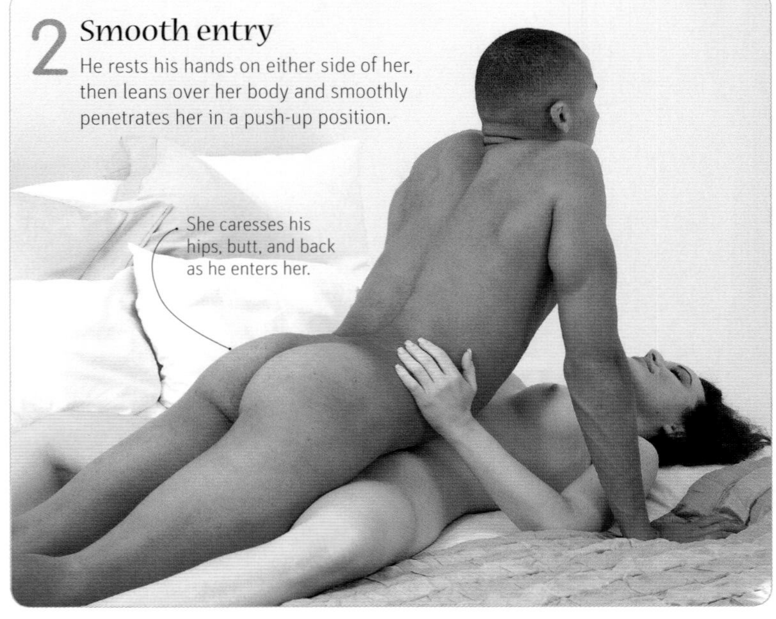
She caresses his hips, butt, and back as he enters her.

2 Smooth entry

He rests his hands on either side of her, then leans over her body and smoothly penetrates her in a push-up position.

"A man whose member gets strong and hard is relished and appreciated by women." THE PERFUMED GARDEN

3 Rising up

She wraps her legs around his waist and crosses her ankles behind his back. He raises himself onto all fours, lifting her with him as he goes.

Taking it further

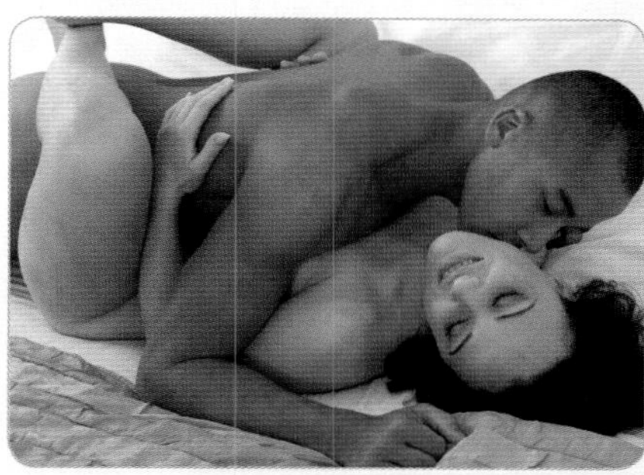

Moving in for a kiss

He lowers his body so that his chest is close to her breasts and his weight is on his elbows, allowing him to lean in for a passionate kiss.

She clings to his waist by tensing her thigh muscles and keeping her ankles in a tight lock.

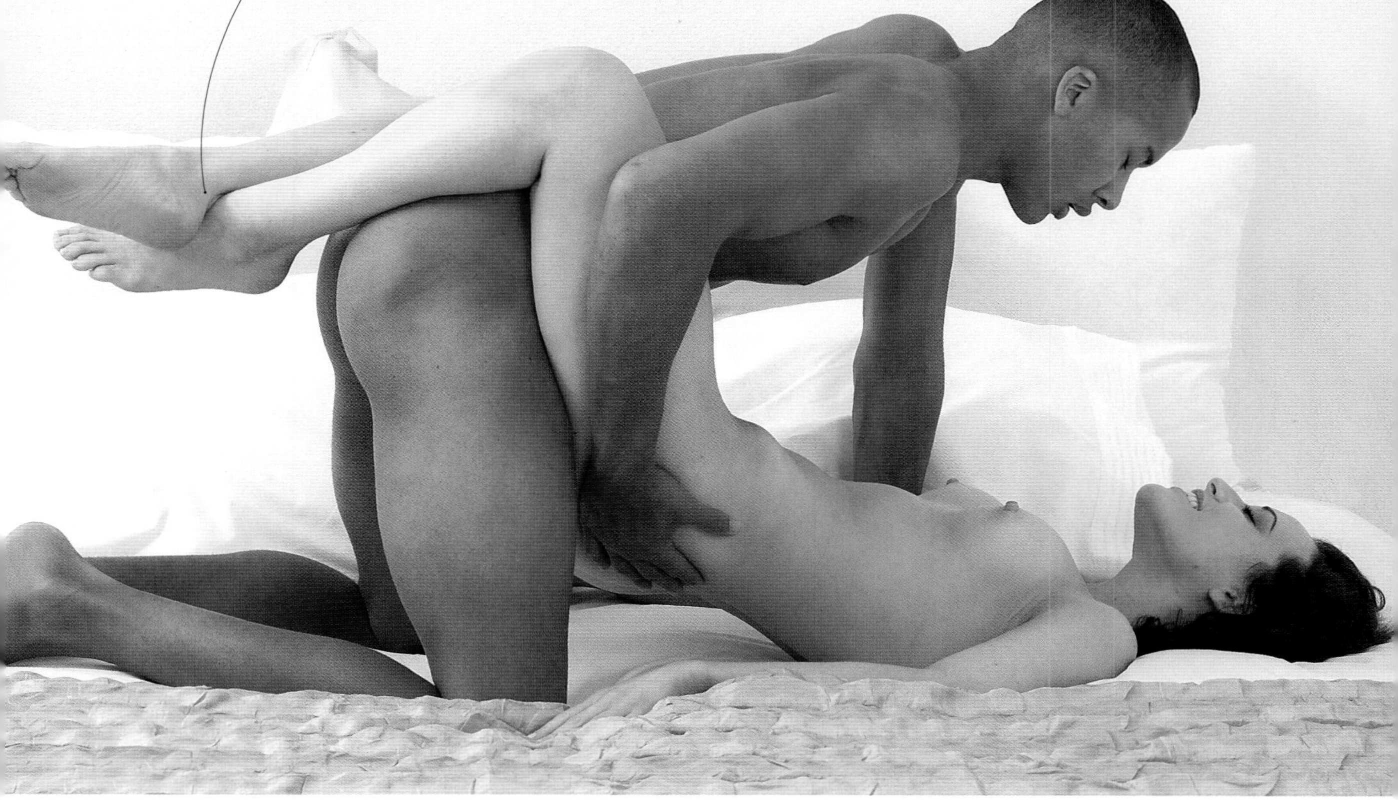

If you liked this, try...

- The Gaping Position, for similar penetration with a more solid grounding (see page 156).
- The Wife of Indra, for something more difficult (see page 204).

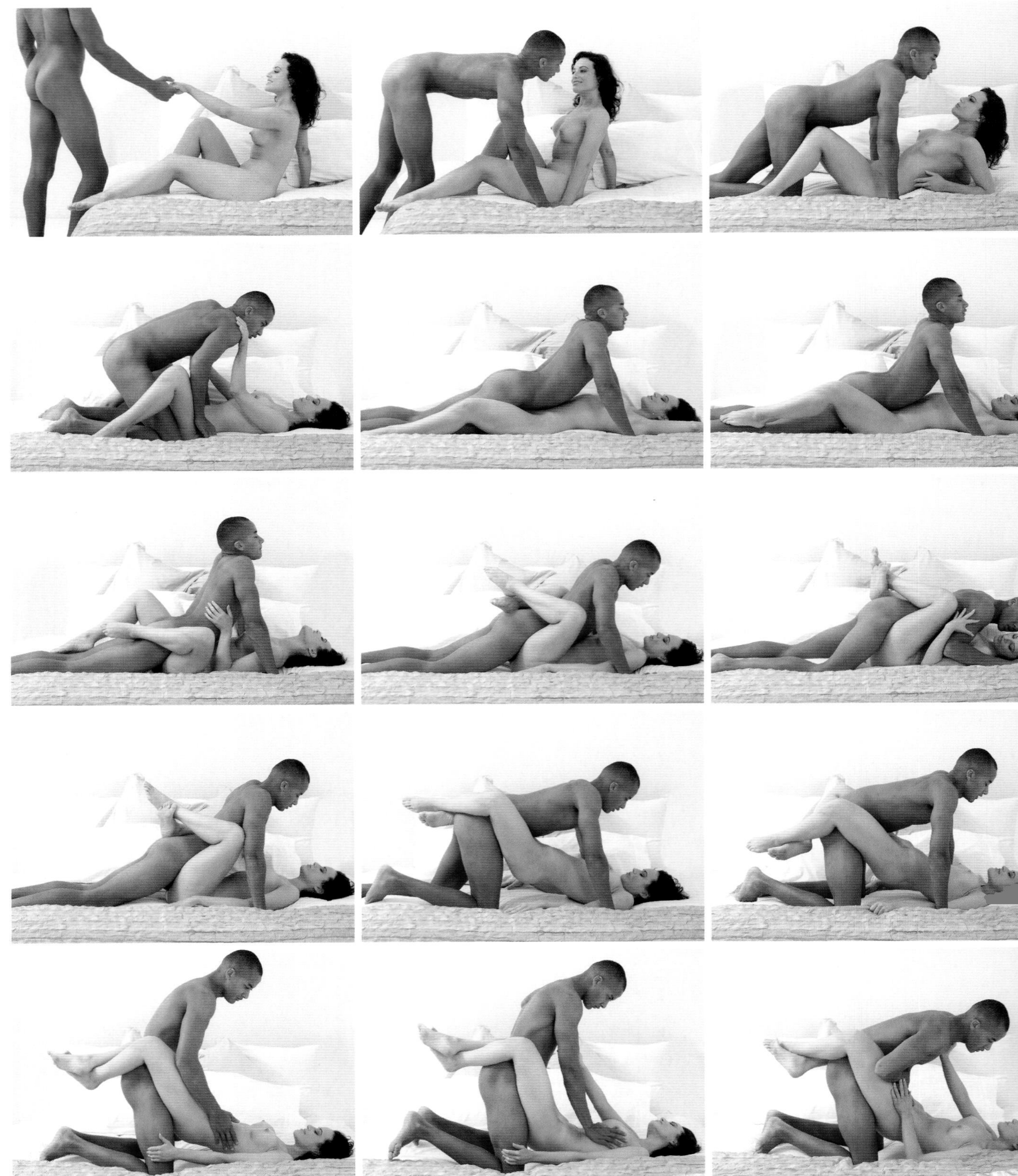

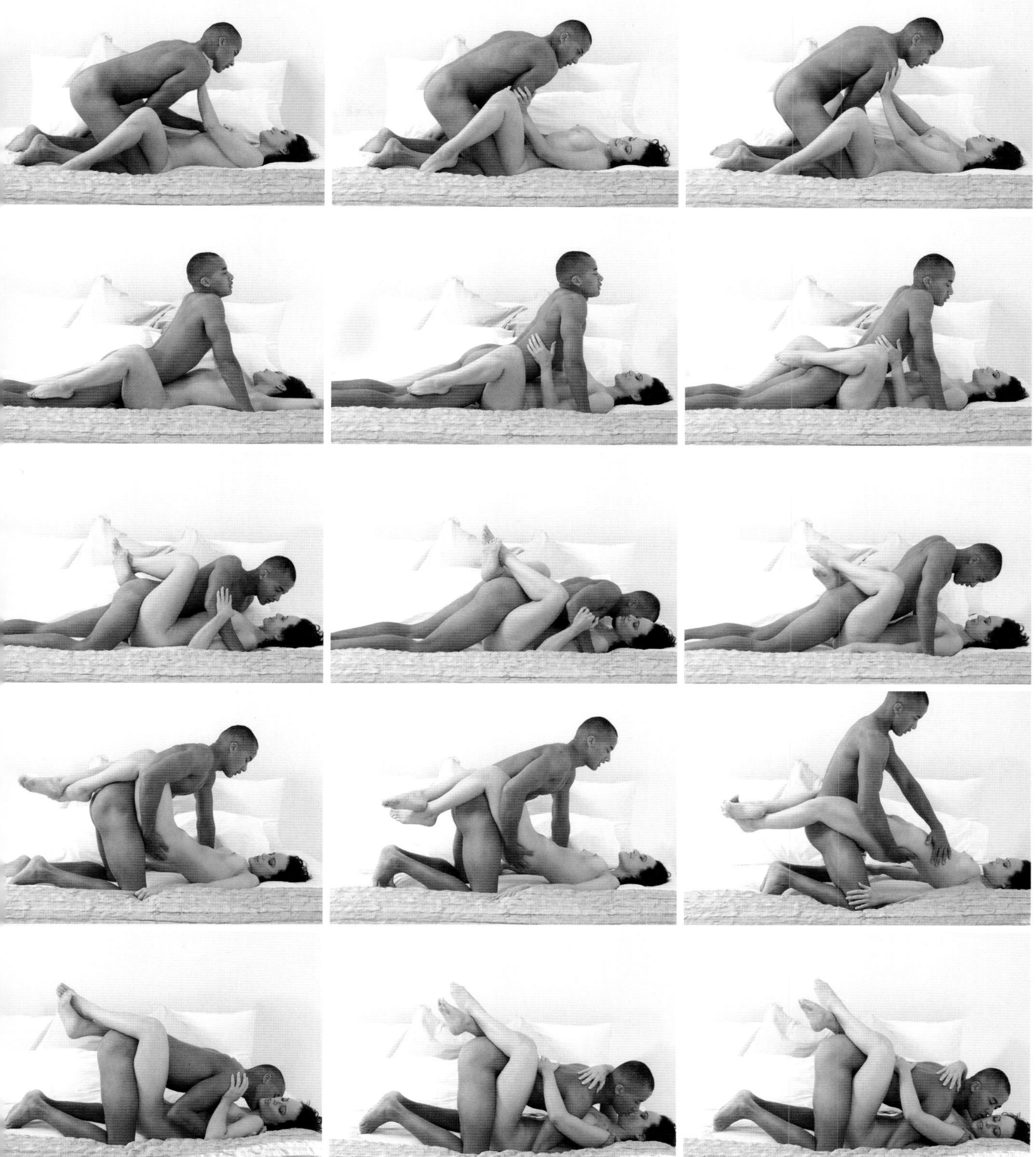

Transverse lute and Placid embrace

☆☆☆☆☆ Kama sensation rating

The mood is anything but placid in this mini-sequence. After an intense smooch lying on your sides, you both roll over by 90 degrees so that she's on her back. He then picks her up and guides her onto his ready and willing erection.

Why they work

– In the Placid Embrace he can penetrate deeply, and she can either watch the force of his desire or lean back and enjoy the ride.

– Side-by-side positions such as the Transverse Lute mean that either of you can take the lead in moving, kissing, and caressing.

– The Transverse Lute also gives you the chance to indulge in lots of spine-tingling foreplay and get under each other's skin before he actually penetrates.

– Moving from the Transverse Lute to the Placid Embrace creates a thrilling mood change: she is swept into his arms as he takes charge.

1 Side-on embrace

You both lie on your sides locked in a tight embrace. He rests his upper leg on top of her upper leg. He guides his erection between her thighs. This is the Transverse Lute.

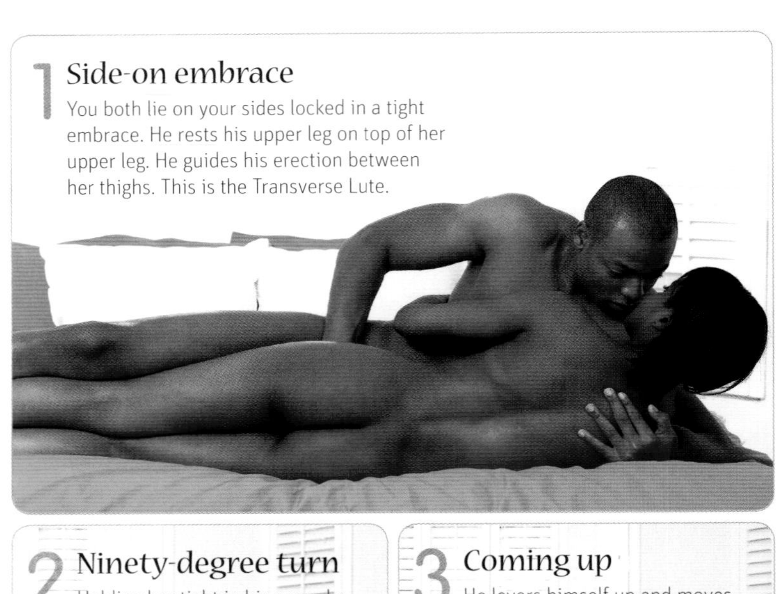

2 Ninety-degree turn

Holding her tight in his arms, he rolls her over by 90 degrees so that he's on top. He enters her, and you both lie still to savor the sensation.

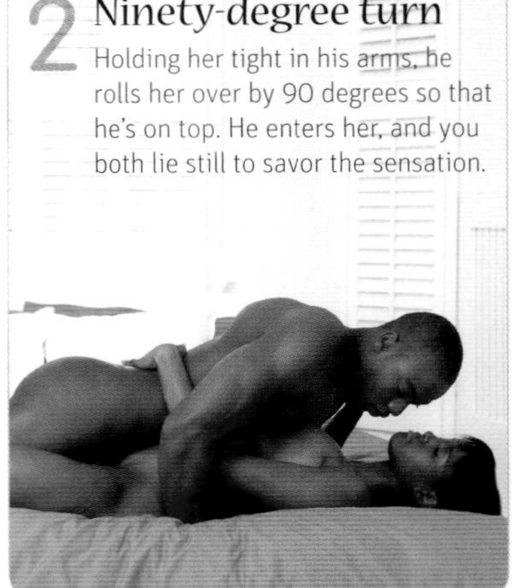

3 Coming up

He levers himself up and moves into an upright kneel between her legs. She wraps her legs around his hips and crosses her ankles.

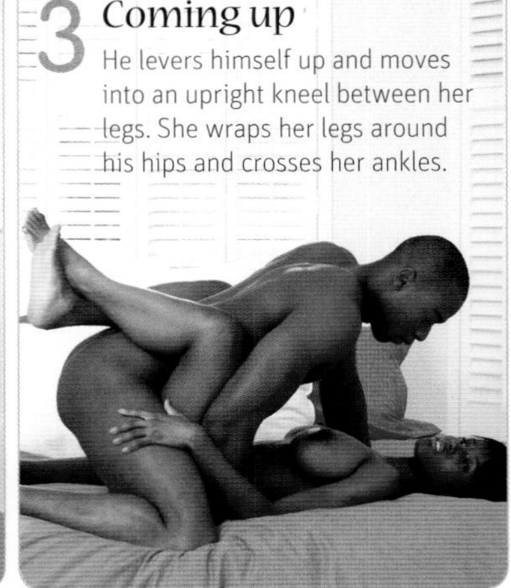

Turn on...

... Try these positions after a long and flirtatious evening out; several hours of smoldering glances, provocative remarks, and teasing touches will more than put you in the mood.

Turn off...

... Don't let the mood disperse after sex. Pay each other sexy compliments and touch each other affectionately until you fall asleep.

"If a man attempt any deed, he should do it with the spirit of a lion." ANANGA RANGA

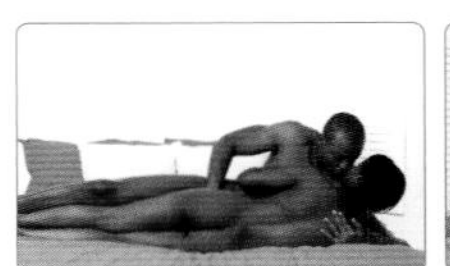

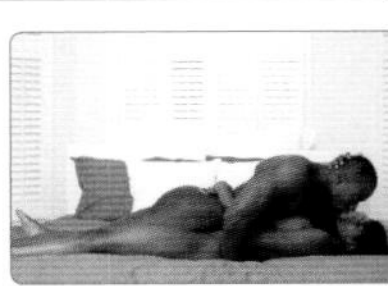

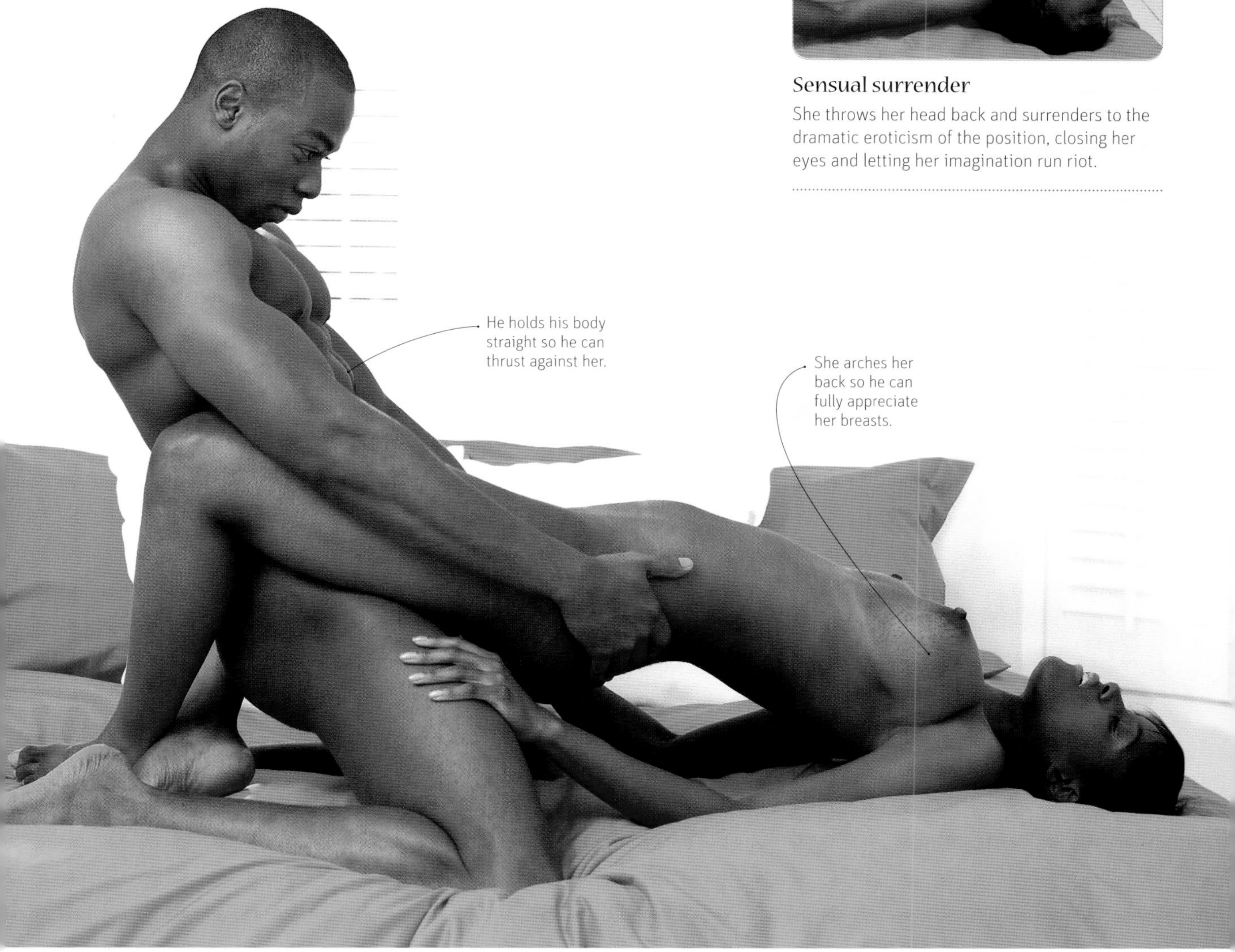

Taking it further

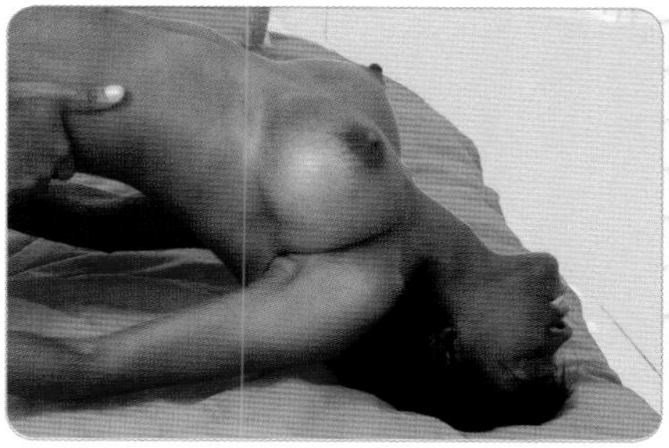

Sensual surrender

She throws her head back and surrenders to the dramatic eroticism of the position, closing her eyes and letting her imagination run riot.

4 Smooth lift

He puts his hands under her back and lifts her smoothly off the bed, making sure that he stays inside her. This is the Placid Embrace.

He holds his body straight so he can thrust against her.

She arches her back so he can fully appreciate her breasts.

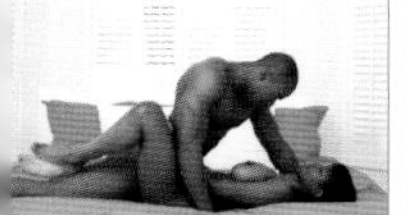
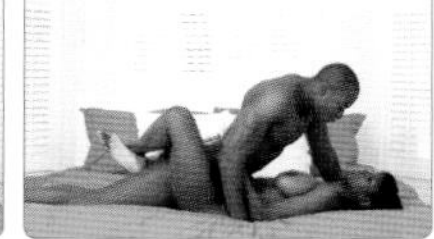
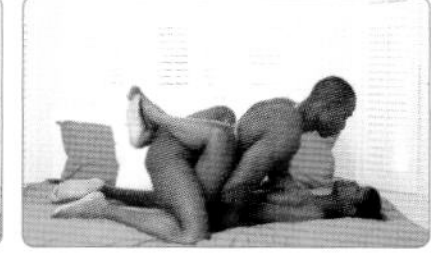
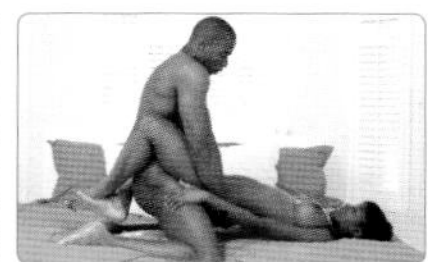
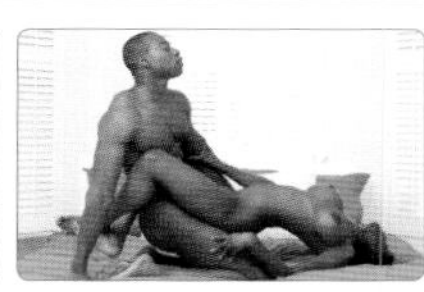

The pine tree

☆☆☆☆ Kama sensation rating

This sexy position is so-called because the woman's raised legs resemble the tall, elegant trunk of a pine tree; perfect for tree-huggers everywhere. Try The Pine Tree when you're in the mood for sex that's X-rated and hot, yet loving and intimate too.

Why it works

- He's in a stable position that lets him control how fast and deep his movements are. Any variations produce thrilling sensations for both of you.
- Lying on her back with her legs stretched straight in the air makes her feel not just supple and athletic, but sexy too.
- He gets an erotic frisson from being held at bay by her legs as he penetrates her.
- She can fix him with a provocative look as he gazes at her through her thighs.
- Her hands are free to pleasure both of you.

Turn on...

... Enjoy the intensity of the position. Tell her how gorgeous she is. Tell him how good he feels. Make as much noise as you want—moans and cries are the sexiest compliment you can pay a lover.

Turn off...

... Don't get carried away and push her legs too far over toward her body. Unless she's very supple, there's a line between feeling pleasantly stretched and uncomfortably pressured; ask her to warn you if you are about to cross it.

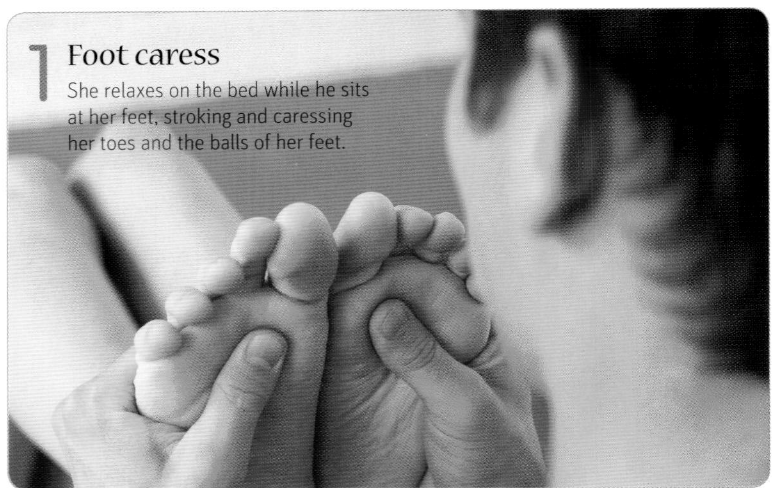

1 Foot caress
She relaxes on the bed while he sits at her feet, stroking and caressing her toes and the balls of her feet.

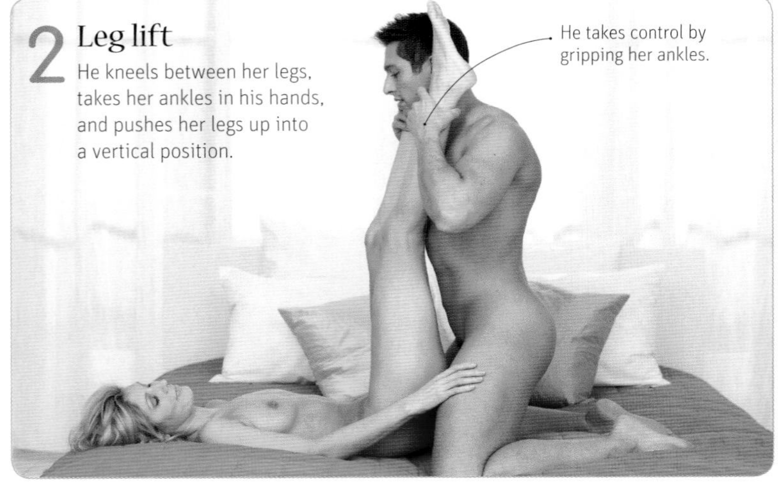

2 Leg lift
He kneels between her legs, takes her ankles in his hands, and pushes her legs up into a vertical position.

He takes control by gripping her ankles.

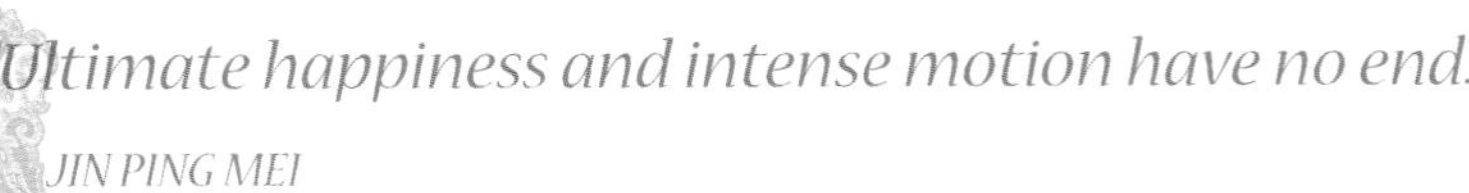

"Ultimate happiness and intense motion have no end."

JIN PING MEI

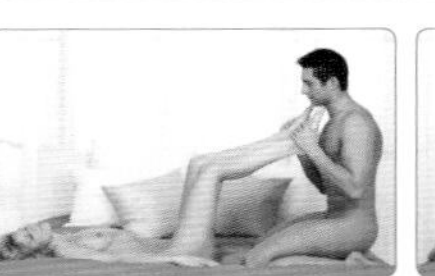

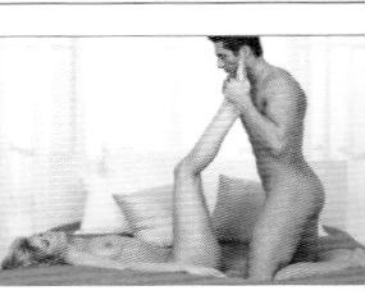

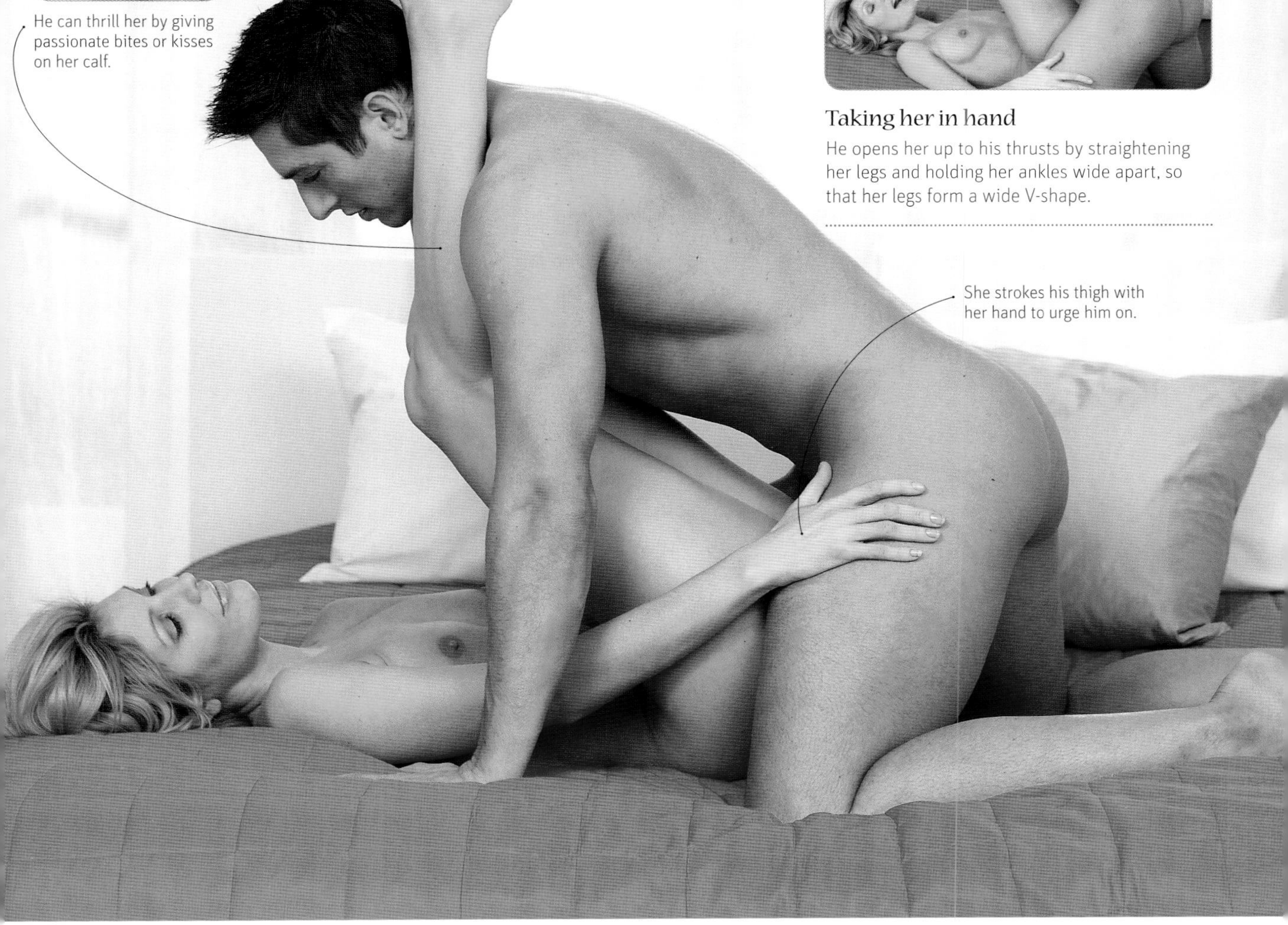

3 Kneeling entry

He moves into an upright kneel, supports her legs on his shoulders, and smoothly enters her.

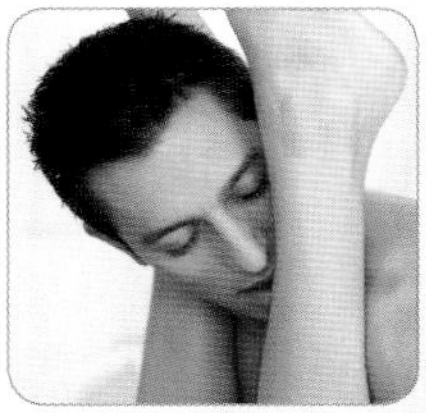

He can thrill her by giving passionate bites or kisses on her calf.

She strokes his thigh with her hand to urge him on.

Taking it further

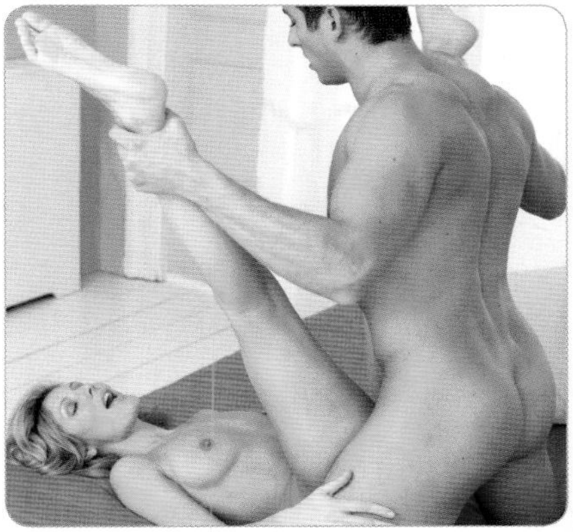

Taking her in hand

He opens her up to his thrusts by straightening her legs and holding her ankles wide apart, so that her legs form a wide V-shape.

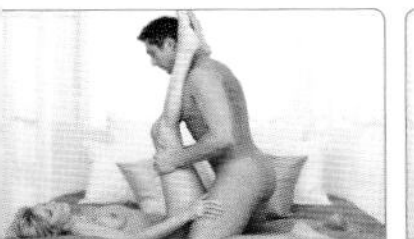
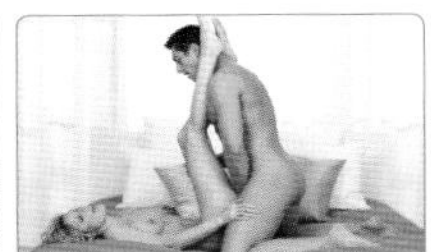
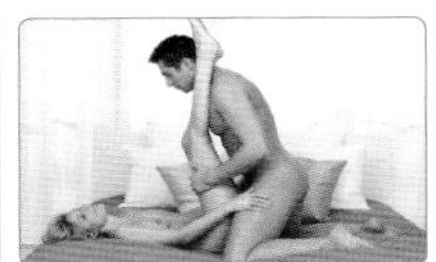
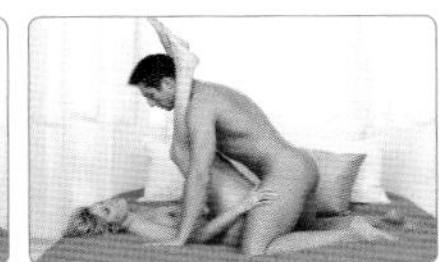
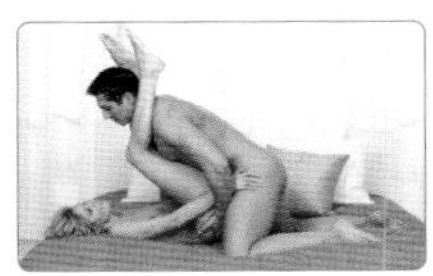

The fifth posture

☆☆ Kama sensation rating

This simple position is a wonderful sensual gift from him to her. His job is to lavish her naked body all over with breathtaking caresses while gently making love to her. Her job is simply to lie back and enjoy: what more could any girl ask for?

Why it works

- Because he doesn't penetrate her fully, the sensitive outer third of her vagina gets most of the attention.
- She can focus exclusively on her own pleasure with no pressure to reciprocate.
- He experiences the thrill of making her melt.
- It's perfect for early morning wake-up sex; you're both warm and sleepy, and you get a gentle yet erotic start to the day.
- If his erection comes and goes, it doesn't matter, because the emphasis is on sensual touch rather than hard and fast thrusting.

Turn on...

... Pull her leg up high on your hip (or make other adjustments) if you can't penetrate her easily. This position is most suitable for well-endowed men who have a long reach.

Turn off...

... Don't get too hung up on penetration. The emphasis in this position is on sensual touch and all the fantastic sensations you can give her with your hands. You can always roll over into a man-on-top position later, if you like.

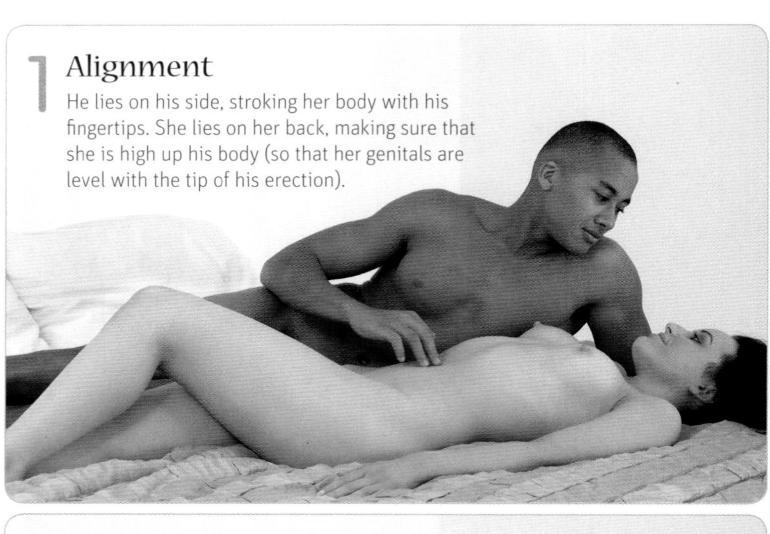

1 Alignment
He lies on his side, stroking her body with his fingertips. She lies on her back, making sure that she is high up his body (so that her genitals are level with the tip of his erection).

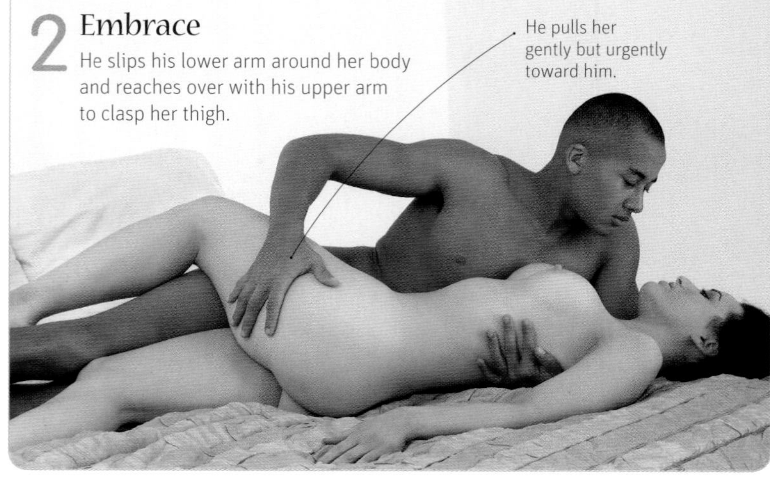

2 Embrace
He slips his lower arm around her body and reaches over with his upper arm to clasp her thigh.

He pulls her gently but urgently toward him.

"Give ear, and listen to the sighs, cries, and murmurs of the woman—these testify to the intensity of the pleasure you have given her." THE PERFUMED GARDEN

3 The connection

She rolls her hips toward him as he pulls her thigh over his legs and pushes himself between her legs.

He uses the palm of his hand to gently trace the curves of her body.

She does mini-pelvic thrusts to stimulate the tip of his penis.

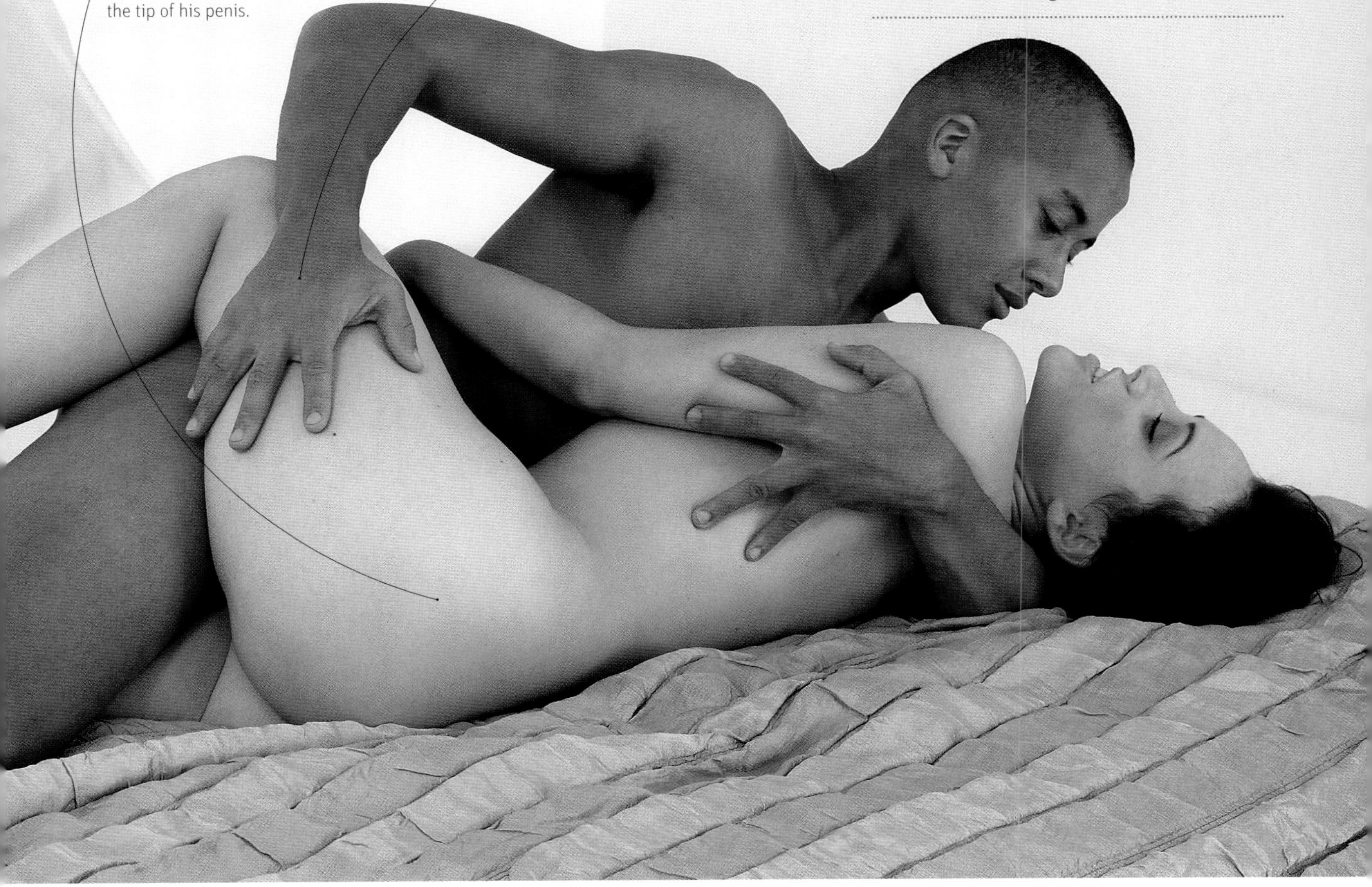

Taking it further

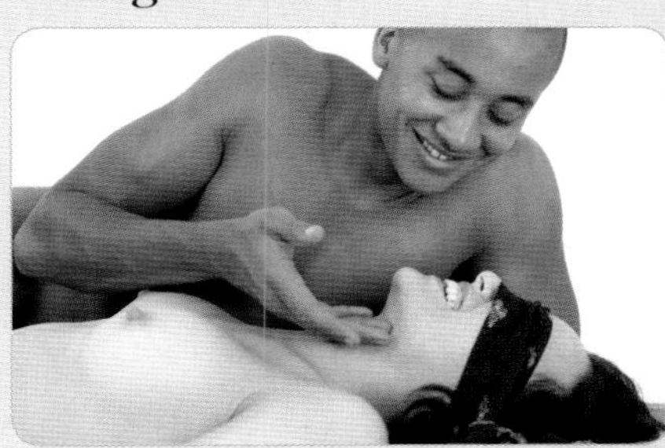

Heightening the senses

He puts a blindfold on her; this concentrates her attention on the delicious caresses and strokes she's receiving.

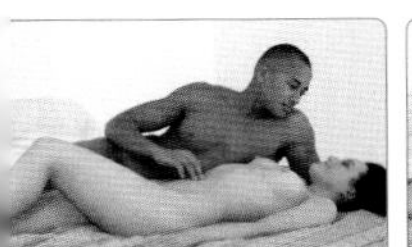
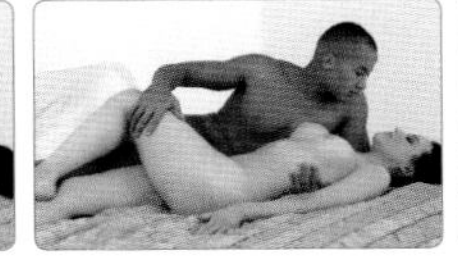
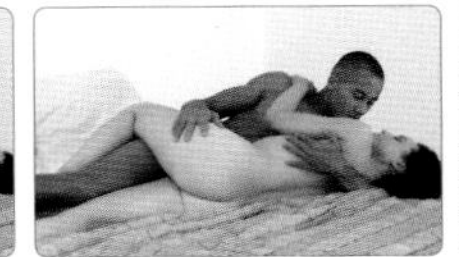
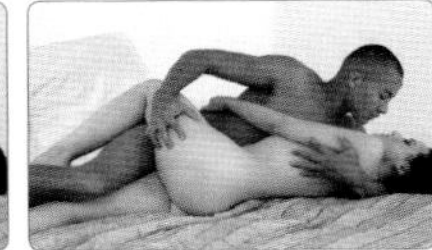
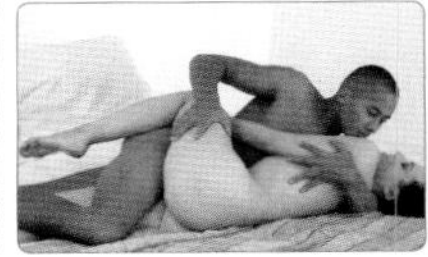
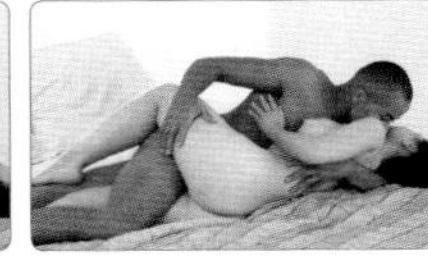

The movements of sex

The way you grind your pelvis, move up and down, or undulate your whole body can make the difference between predictable sex, and explosive sex that'll leave you limp and gasping. Here are some movement suggestions from the *Kama Sutra* and *The Perfumed Garden*.

If you usually pump your way to orgasm with no variation in style, pace, or rhythm, set yourself a challenge. Pretend you've never had sex before and have to figure out how to move from scratch. Try every type of movement from bouncing, rocking, rubbing, and circling to squirming, shaking, slithering, and rippling; and that means both of you. Even try staying still for the occasional moment during sex. If you feel silly, turn off the lights.

Churning This involves him taking the base of his shaft firmly in hand and swirling the tip of his penis along the length of her vulva. The main highlight of his tour should be her clitoris, using back-and-forth flicks or firm circles, with occasional detours to her vaginal entrance, where he presses and churns his glans.

This can lead on to another teasing stroke known as Love's Tailor, in which he slips the tip of his penis a little way inside her and rubs it up and down. It is great for her because, as the *Kama Sutra* says, a "woman's itch is most extensive in the outer part of her vagina." Then, just when she's getting used to shallow in-and-out movements, he can give her the thrill of the unexpected by suddenly plunging in all the way. He can vary his strokes from shallow to deep throughout sex.

Love's bond This is where he penetrates her so the full length of his penis is inside her, then pauses for a blissful maximum-penetration moment. This can lead on to the familiar in-and-out motion of intercourse; he can thrust repeatedly without withdrawing, which is known as Sporting of a Sparrow. The *Kama Sutra* says this takes place "at the end of intercourse." To make it as stimulating as possible, keep the movements light, fluid, and long.

Another mid-sex technique to try involves him withdrawing completely and then re-entering at top speed, known as Giving a Blow. It's not to everyone's taste, so, if you try it, choose a comfortable position in which you can be sure of a smooth re-entry.

A woman acting the part of a man All the strokes so far have been for men to do on women, but the roles can easily be reversed so she is the active party. The *Kama Sutra* also describes how she can twist around on his penis in The Top (see page 226), grip him tightly in The Mare (see page 126), and rock on his penis in The Swing (see page 126).

Rock with me Sex therapists often recommend a rocking technique to help women reach orgasm. She lies on her back with him on top. His exact position is important: he needs to "ride high" on her body so that the base of his penis is rubbing up against her clitoris. He can achieve this by penetrating her, then shimmying up her body until he can't get any higher without his penis slipping out. Now you start the all-important rocking. As she rocks her pelvis down toward the bed, he rocks his toward the ceiling. This pulls a large part of his shaft out of her. Next, she rocks her pelvis toward the ceiling as he rocks his toward the bed. This brings his entire penis back inside her, causing tight, sliding friction against her clitoris. Repeat until climax!

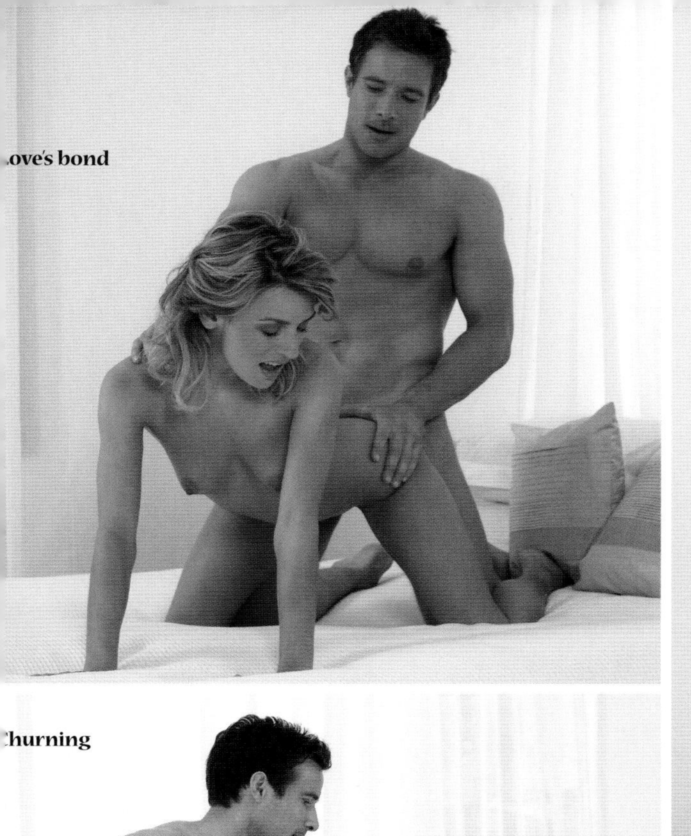

ove's bond

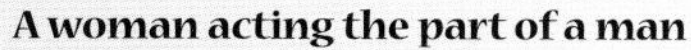

A woman acting the part of a man

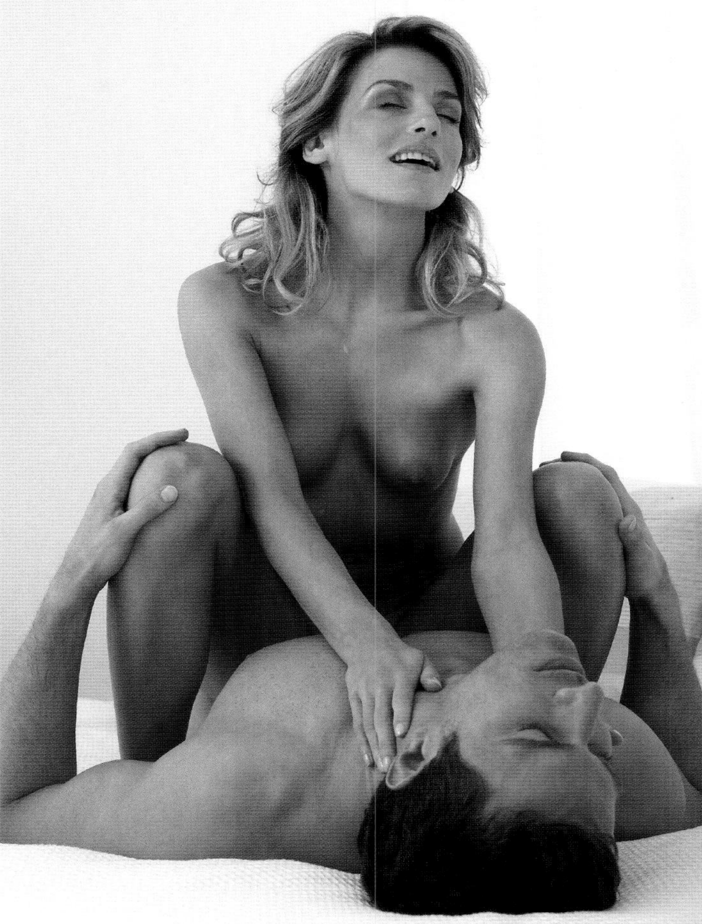

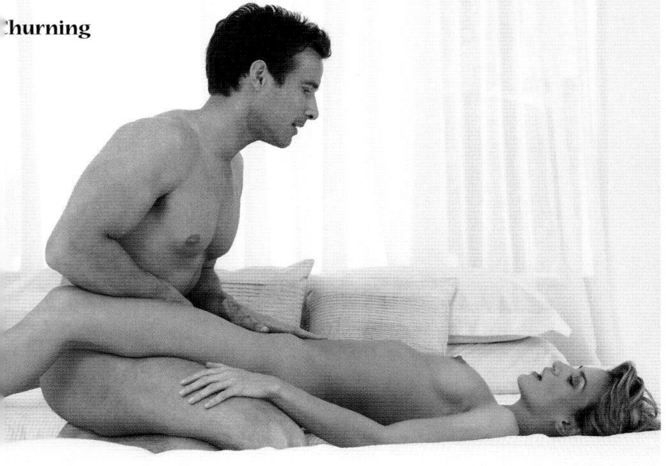

hurning

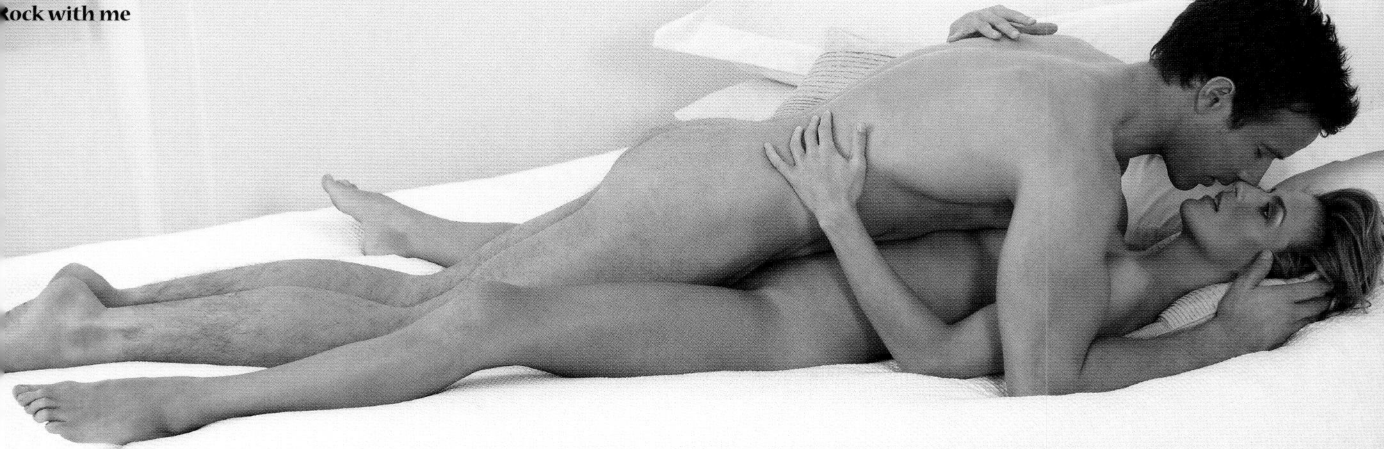

ock with me

Singing monkey

☆☆☆ Kama sensation rating

She takes control in this friendly yet provocative woman-on-top position. It's sex at its slowest and sauciest. It's also a great opportunity for her to treat him to an erotic performance in which she shows off her body. He, meanwhile, sits back and enjoys the ride.

Why it works

– Her legs are spread wide so that penetration is deep and easy, and she can easily stimulate her clitoris with her fingers.

– She can explore different sensations by leaning back on her hands to change the angle at which his penis enters her.

– It's a confident and sexy position in which you can take your time, lean back on your hands, and appreciate each other.

– You can kiss to your heart's content. Start with tentative lip and tongue touches, and progress to an intense mouth-melding that leaves you breathless.

Turn on...

... Try it in the bathroom. There aren't many sex positions that actually work in a standard bathtub; this is one of the few that does, so fill the tub, light some candles, and get steamy.

Turn off...

... Don't forget the lube. Sex in water can make penetration less smooth, so keep a tube of a silicone-based lubricant within reach. Don't use the water-based kind—it'll wash off.

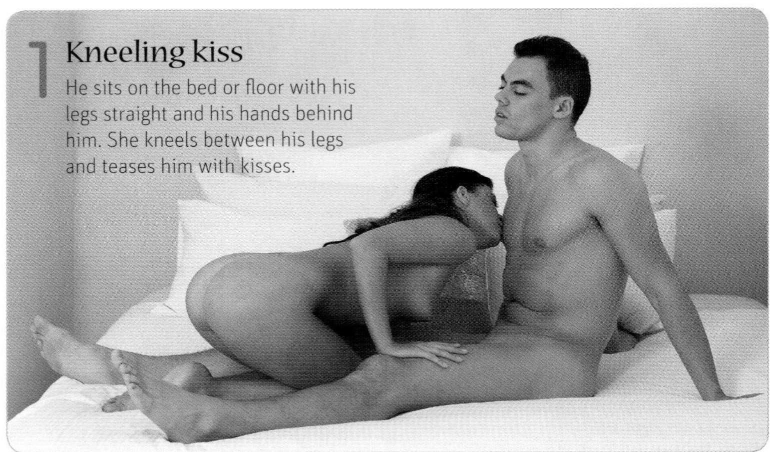

1 Kneeling kiss

He sits on the bed or floor with his legs straight and his hands behind him. She kneels between his legs and teases him with kisses.

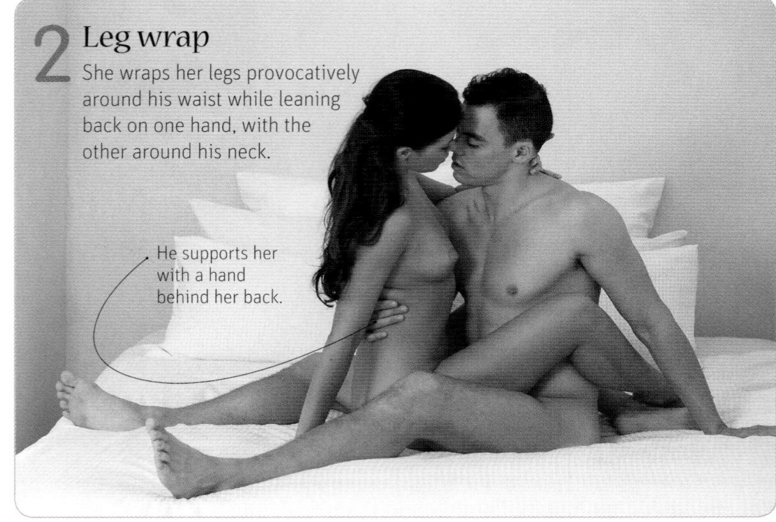

He supports her with a hand behind her back.

2 Leg wrap

She wraps her legs provocatively around his waist while leaning back on one hand, with the other around his neck.

"A kiss is one of the most potent stimulants that a man or woman can indulge in." THE PERFUMED GARDEN

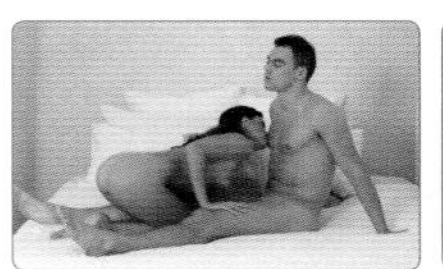

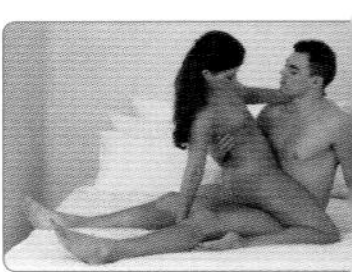

Taking it further

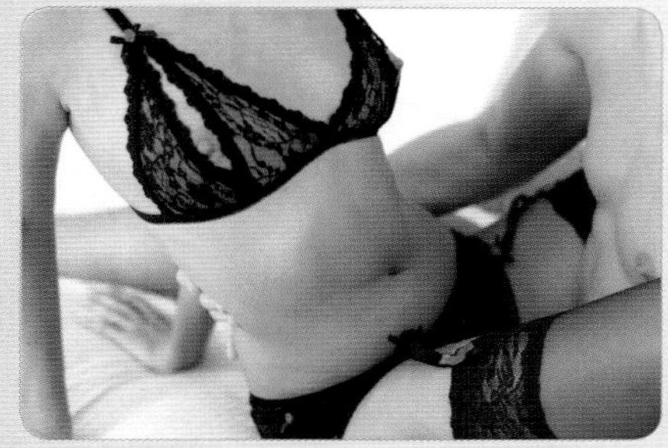

Putting on a show

She dresses for the occasion; wearing something erotic can elevate any sex from routine and mundane to truly memorable.

3 Monkey clasp

He pushes his legs together so that they are under her ass, then he puts one hand on the small of her back to guide her on to his penis. She wraps one arm around his shoulder and rests her other hand on his leg.

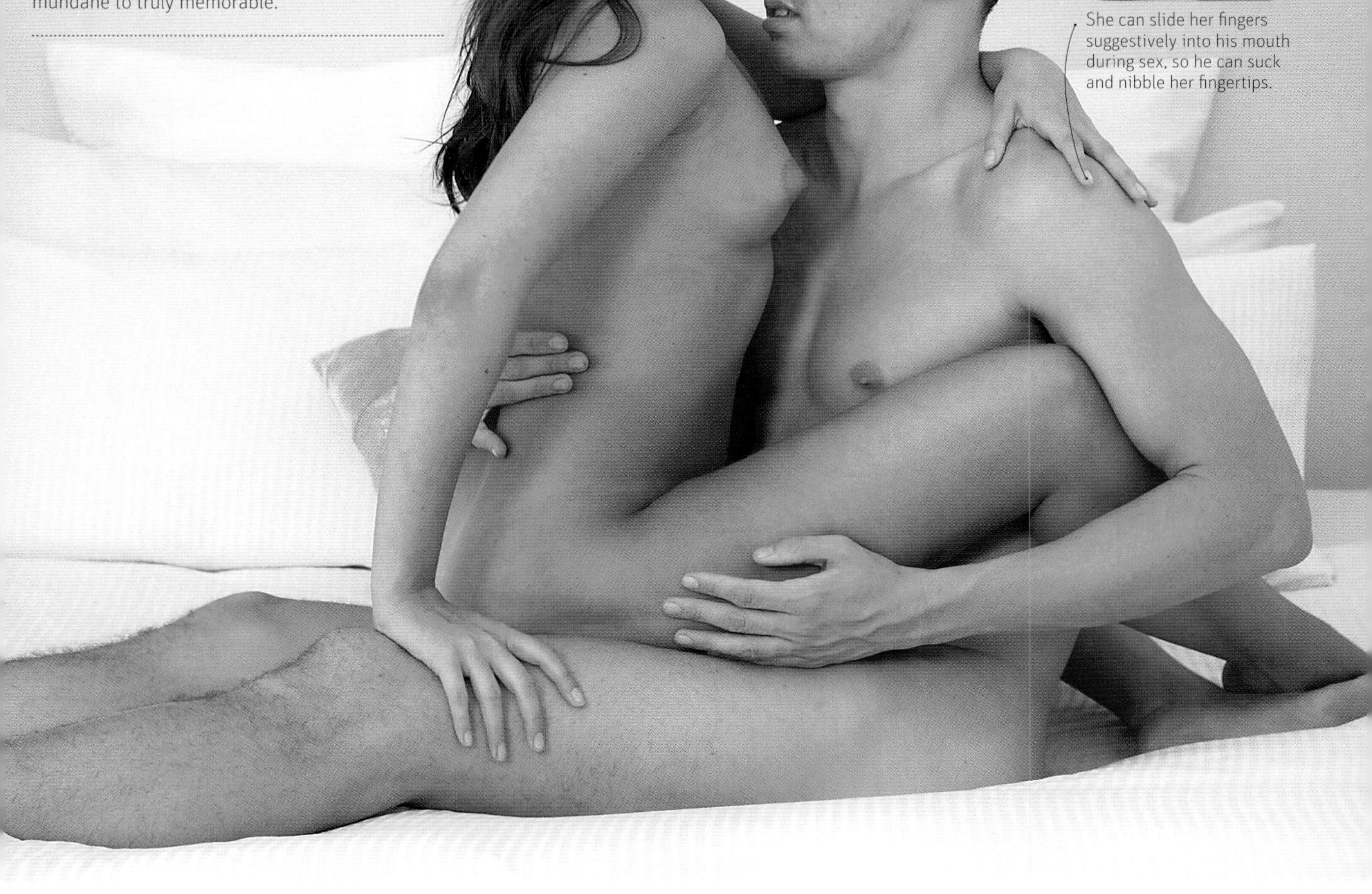

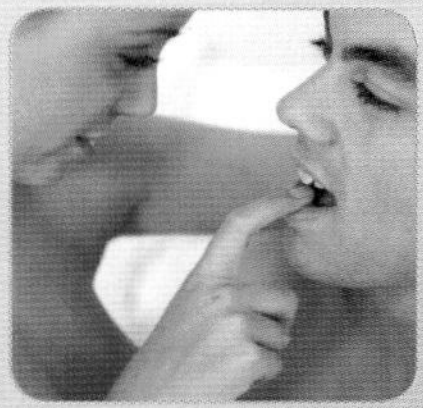

She can slide her fingers suggestively into his mouth during sex, so he can suck and nibble her fingertips.

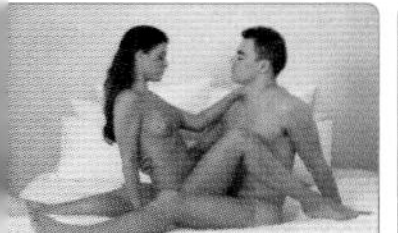
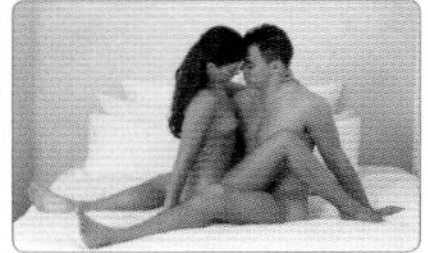
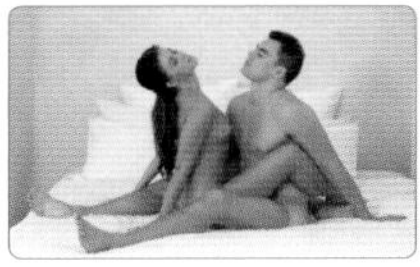
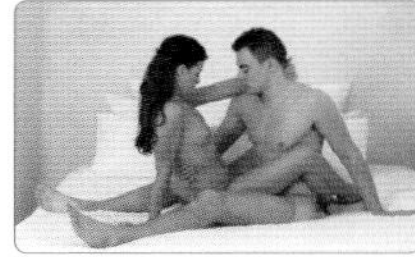
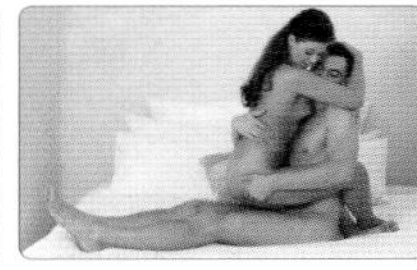
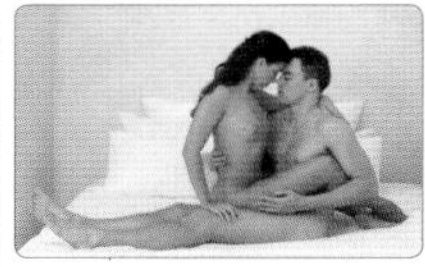

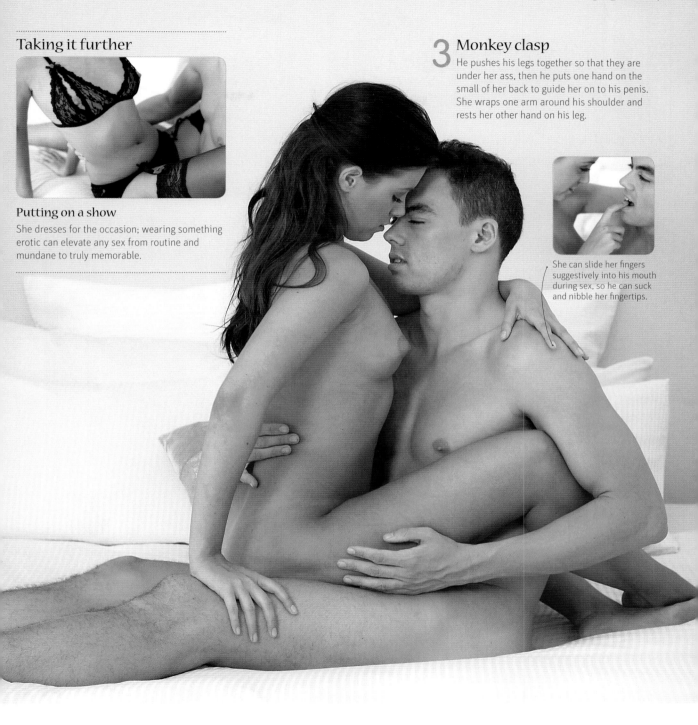

Cicada on a bough

☆☆☆☆ Kama sensation rating

He creeps up and takes her from behind in this slinky variant of sex from behind. You both get all the kinky sensations and benefits of rear-entry sex, but because you're not down on all fours it feels more dignified, gentle, and romantic.

Why it works

– She gets a potentially orgasmic G-spot massage from his penis as it slides against the front wall of her vagina on each thrust.

– It appeals to her "being taken" fantasies because she just has to lie still and receive him.

– He's got easy access and complete freedom of movement because he's lying in between her legs, plus he gets that feeling of control.

– The fact that you're not face-to-face makes it easy to indulge in a private fantasy.

– You can tailor the position to your mood: make it warm and romantic for tender loving; or playful and kinky for wild nights in.

Turn on...

... Put some cushions under her hips; this gives her some freedom to wiggle and thrust so she's not pinned into a stationary position by his body (unless you find being pinned is the point).

Turn off...

... Don't put too much weight on her body. Support some of your weight on your knees and elbows so that she's free to focus on the sensations of you inside her rather than on top of her.

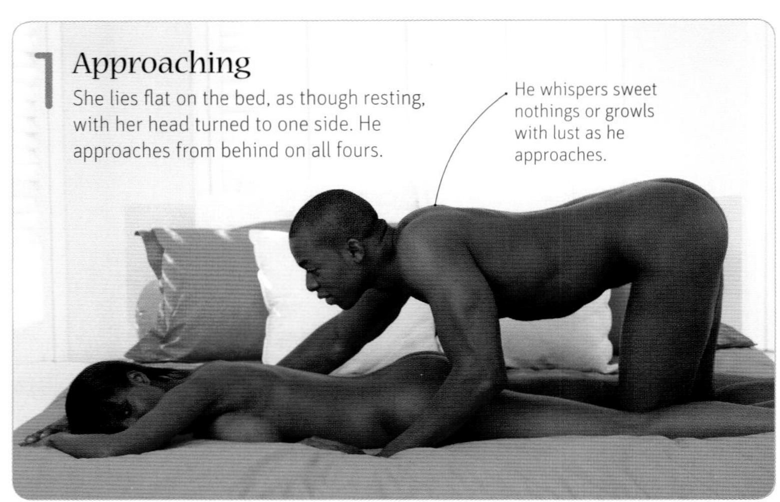

1 Approaching
She lies flat on the bed, as though resting, with her head turned to one side. He approaches from behind on all fours.

He whispers sweet nothings or growls with lust as he approaches.

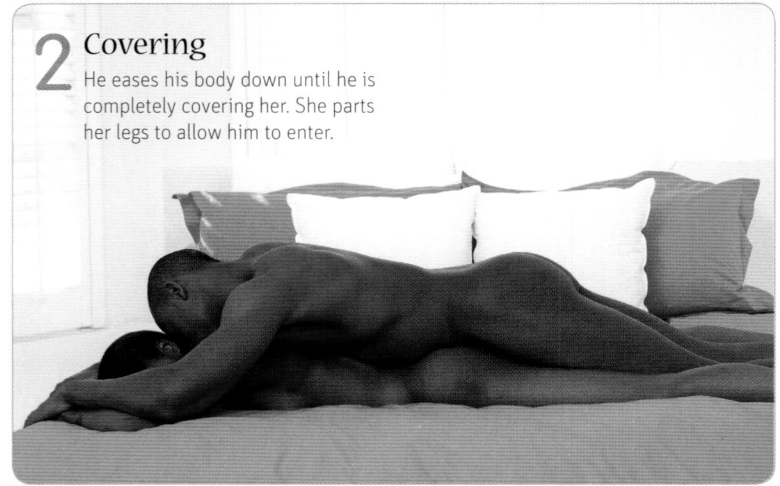

2 Covering
He eases his body down until he is completely covering her. She parts her legs to allow him to enter.

"A sign of enjoyment in a woman is a willingness to unite the two organs as closely together as possible." KAMA SUTRA

Taking it further

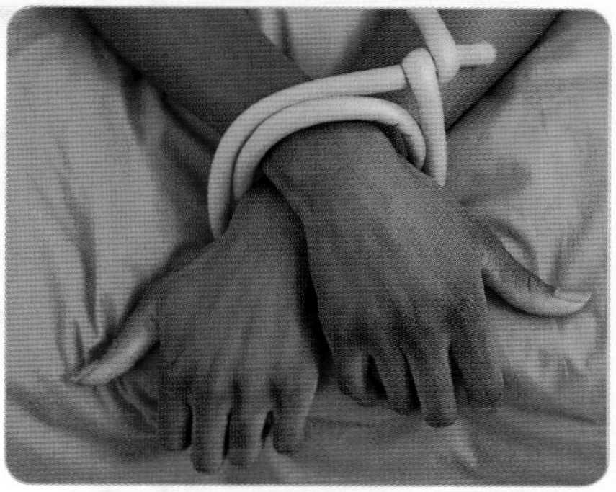

Bound to him

He ties or cuffs her wrists together to increase her feelings of vulnerability and switch from intimacy to kinkiness.

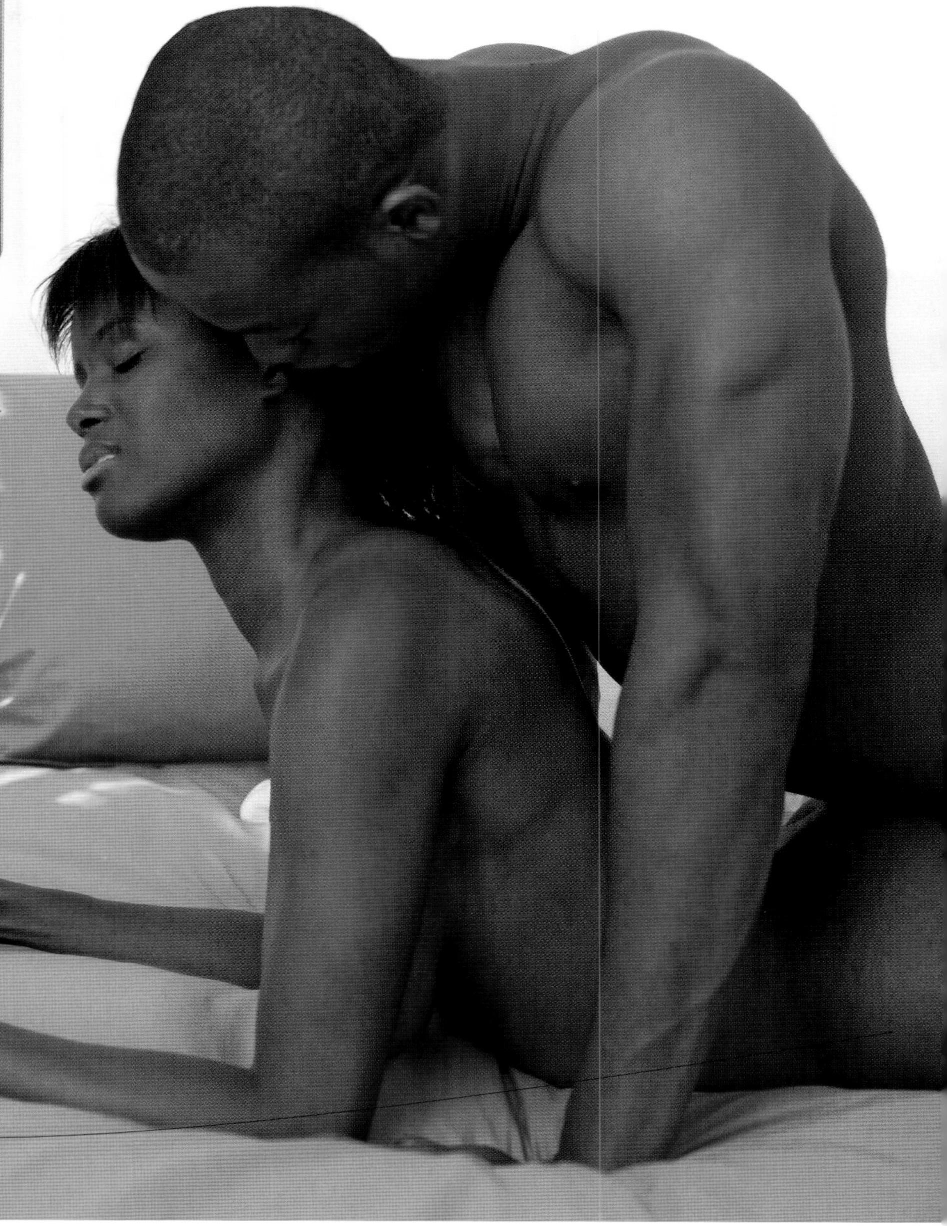

3 Chest raise

As he moves inside her she pushes herself up on her forearms; her head and chest are lifted off the bed, and her back brushes his chest.

She changes the tempo by wiggling her hips from side to side.

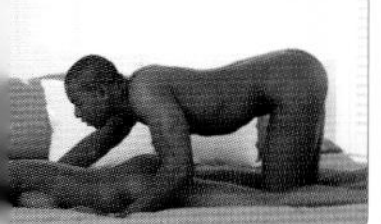
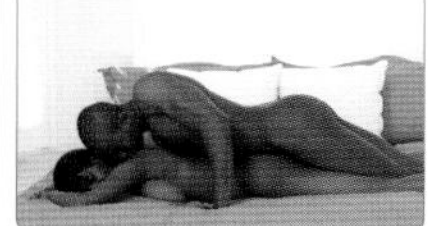
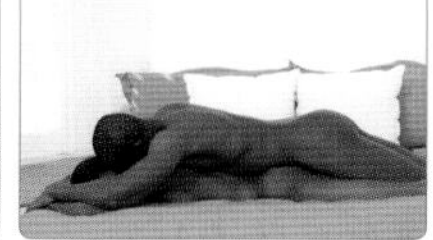
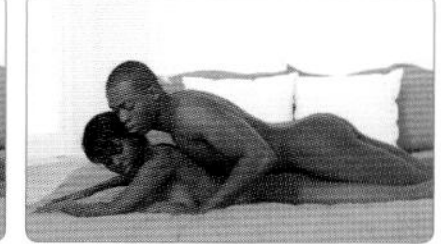
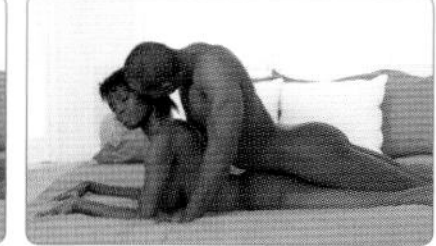
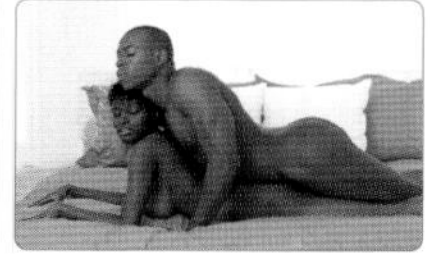

Kama's wheel

Kama's Wheel is a perfect part of a long sequence of sex positions; she can move seamlessly into almost any woman-on-top position from Kama's Wheel simply by lying back, pushing him back, or changing her leg position. It's not high on thrusting capacity, so this might be the position in which you sit up to take a break and kiss each other on the lips.

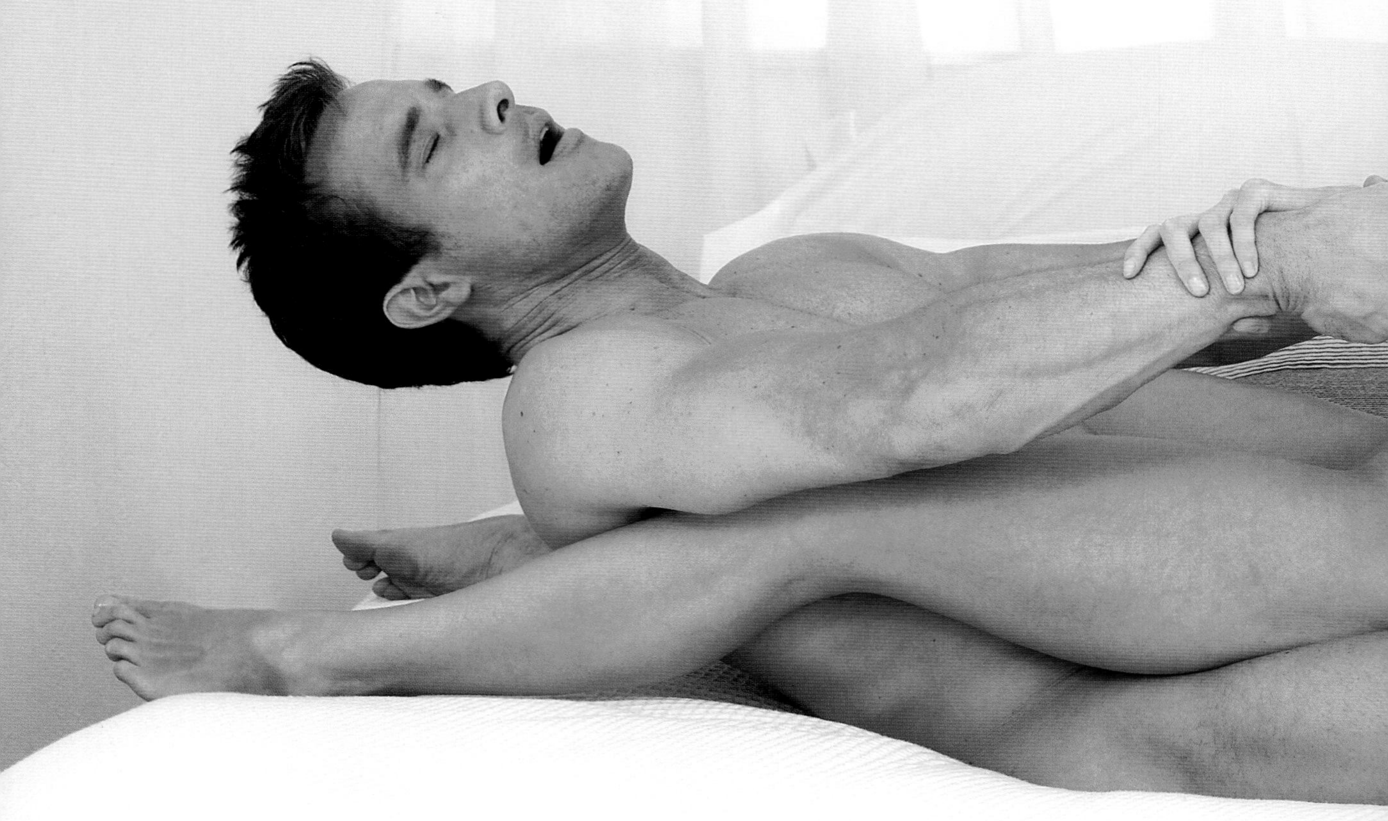

"If you see a woman heaving deep sighs, with her lips getting red and her eyes languishing, when her mouth half opens and her movements grow heedless… this is the moment for coition."
THE PERFUMED GARDEN

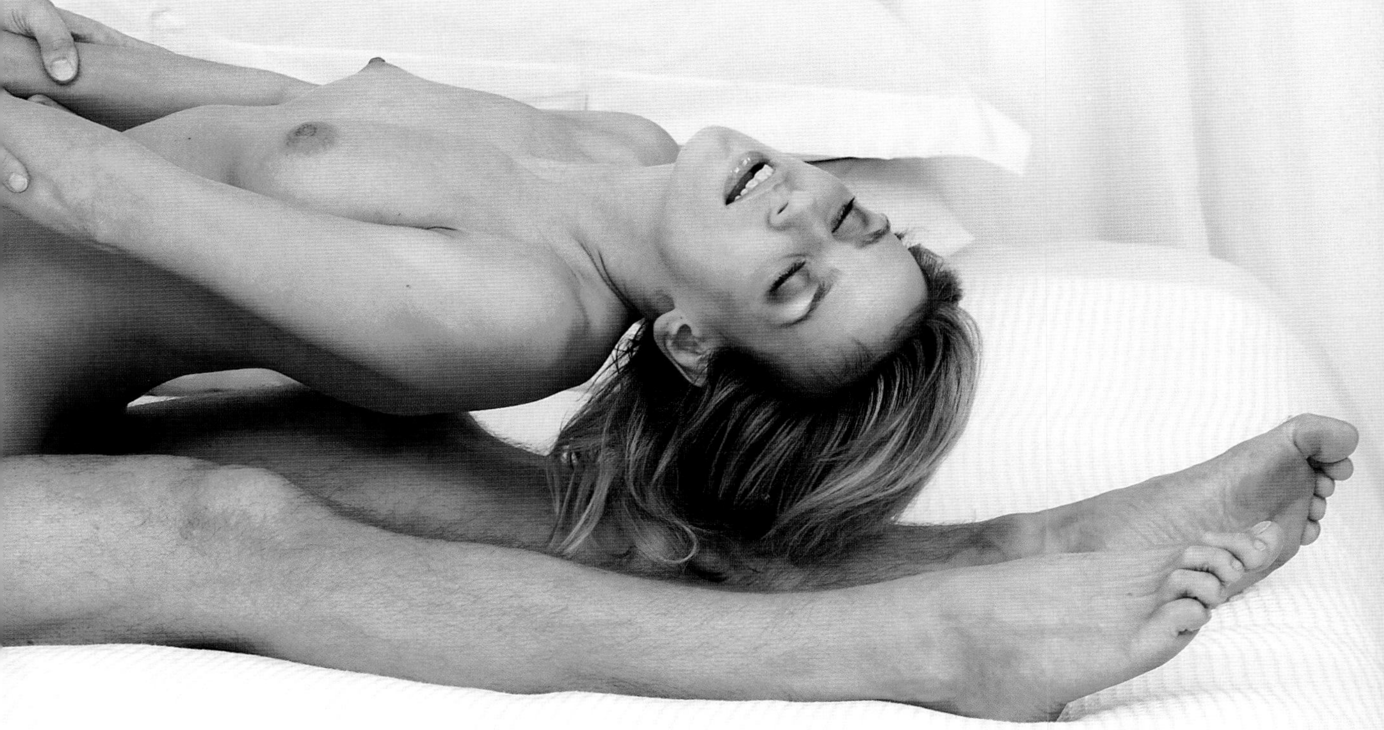

Kama's wheel

Kama sensation rating

Why it works

– She's centered directly on top of his penis, so she feels thoroughly penetrated.

– He can tense and relax the muscles of his penis to give her a sexy internal massage.

– She can reciprocate by squeezing him with her vaginal muscles.

– You both have your hands free to stroke and caress each other all over.

– She can lean back on her hands and thrust her hips up and down on top of him.

– You can customize this position in whatever way you like. Tantric sex enthusiasts can use it to delay orgasm and circulate sexual energy around the body. Exhibitionists can do it dressed in titillating fetish wear. Lovers enjoying a reunion can use it to merge in romantic bliss.

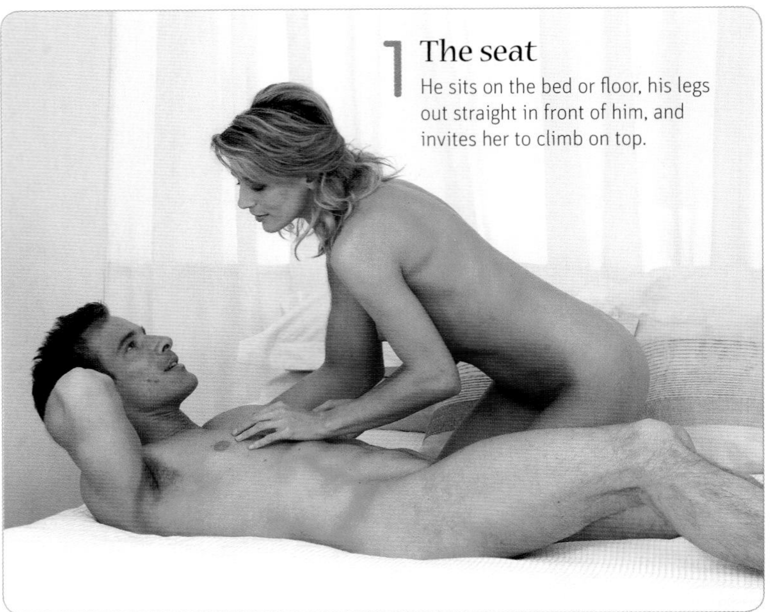

1 The seat
He sits on the bed or floor, his legs out straight in front of him, and invites her to climb on top.

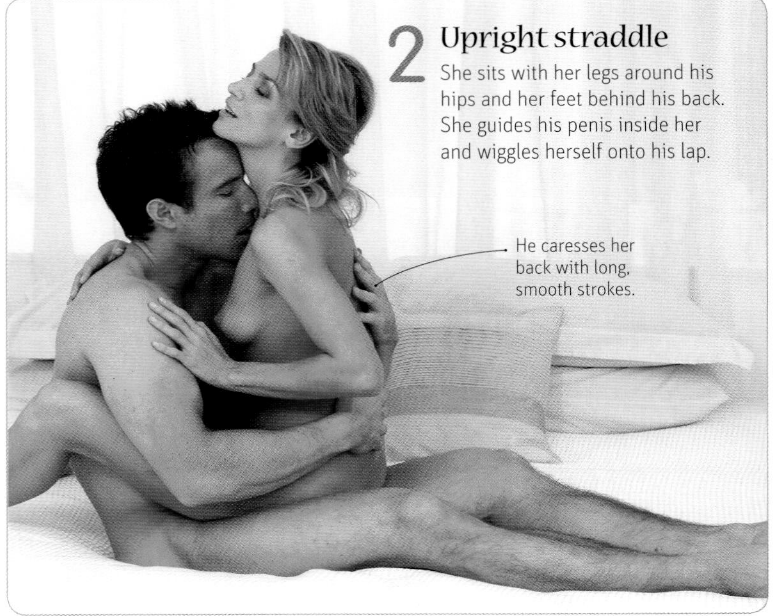
He caresses her back with long, smooth strokes.

2 Upright straddle
She sits with her legs around his hips and her feet behind his back. She guides his penis inside her and wiggles herself onto his lap.

Turn on...

... Use your mouth. He can lean forward to kiss and lick the space between her breasts. She can press her lips to his face as the passion mounts.

Turn off...

... Don't expect raw genital stimulation to keep you going in this position. The movements are subtle, so your arousal levels may go down a notch.

"Do not unite with a woman until you have excited her with playful caresses." THE PERFUMED GARDEN

3 The wheel in motion

He puts his hands firmly on her back, and she rests her hands on his thighs. Now you both push and pull against each other.

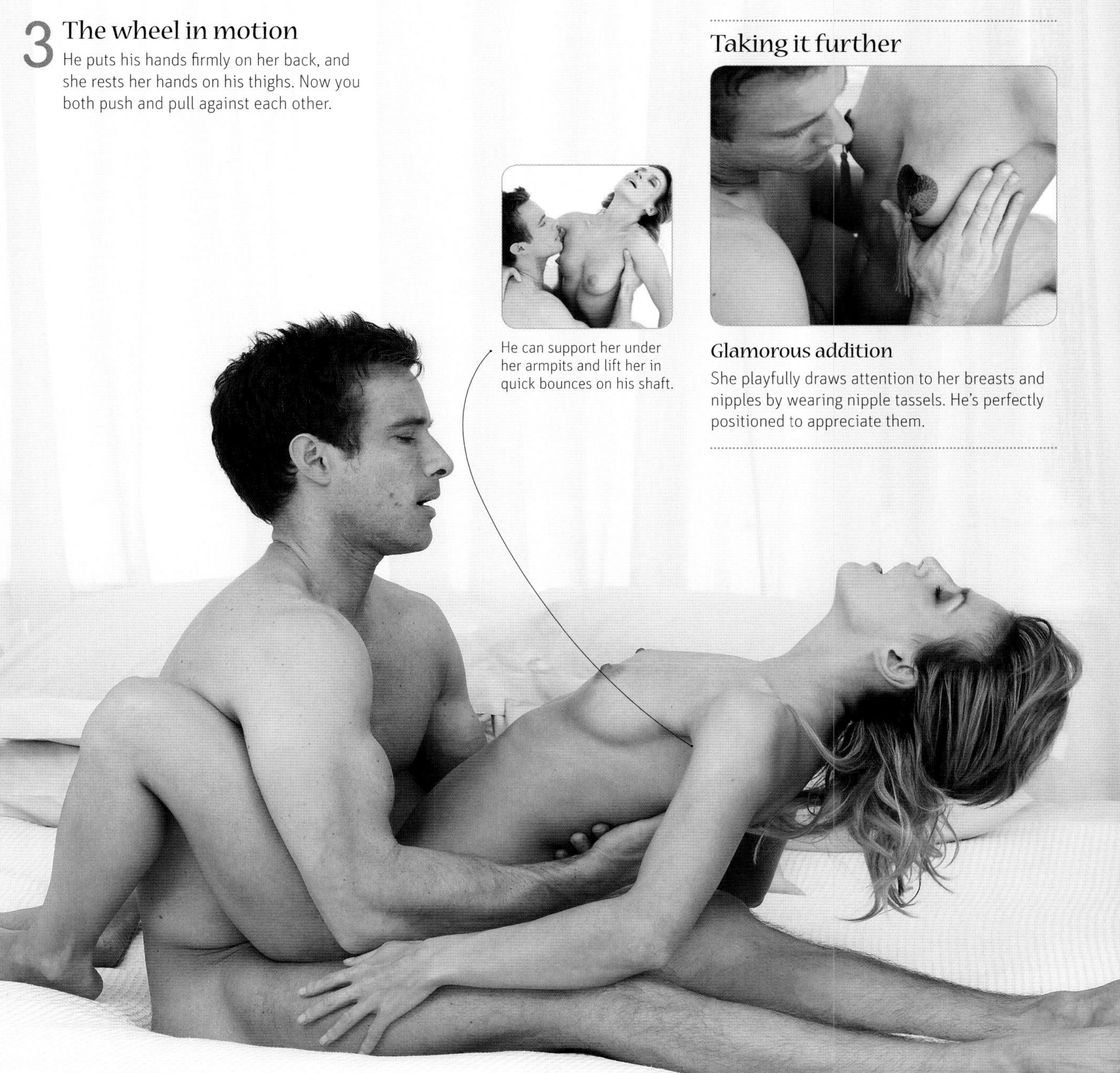

He can support her under her armpits and lift her in quick bounces on his shaft.

Taking it further

Glamorous addition

She playfully draws attention to her breasts and nipples by wearing nipple tassels. He's perfectly positioned to appreciate them.

If you liked this, try…

– The cosier Pounding on the Spot (see page 76).
– The super-hard Frog (see page 100).

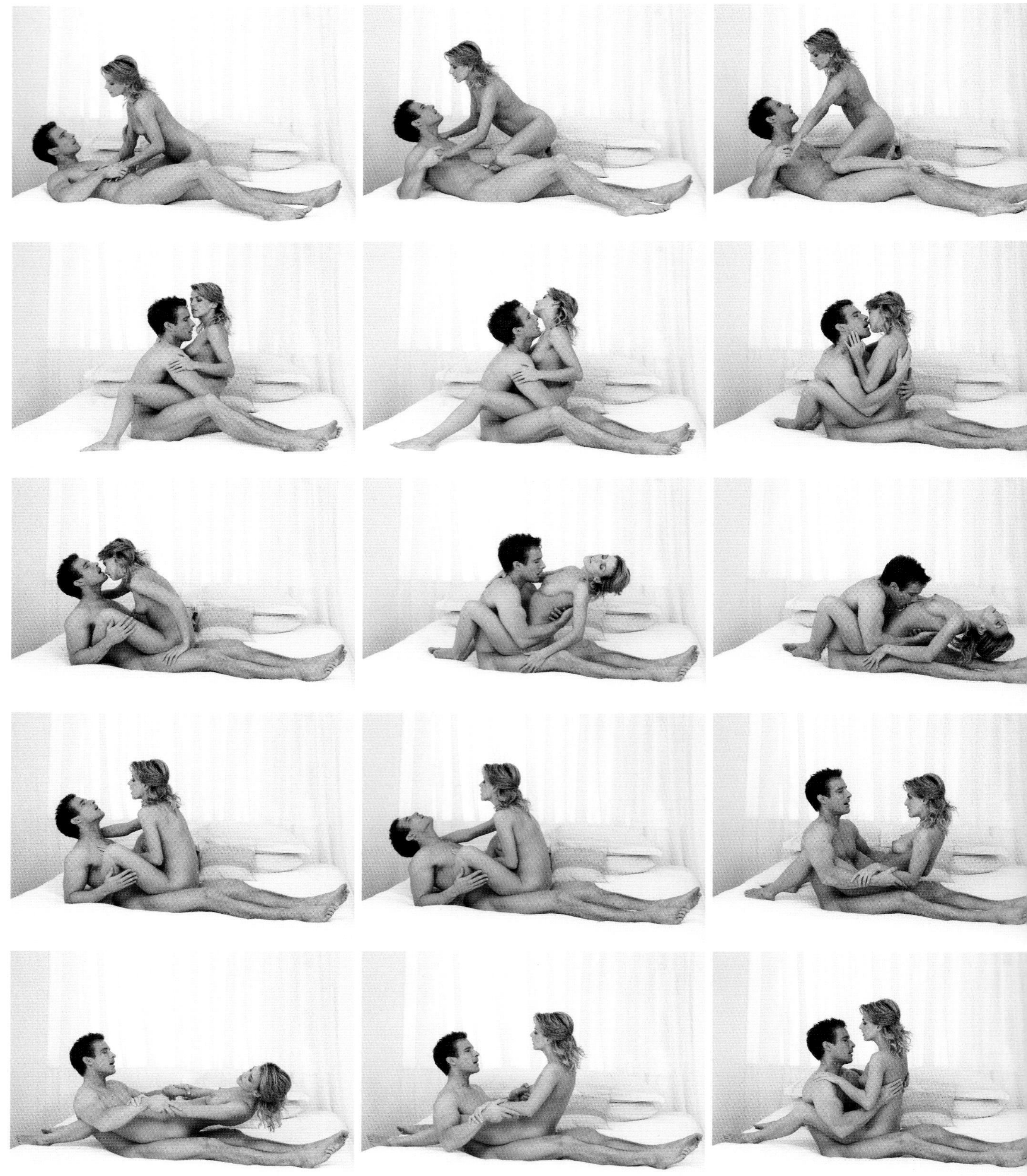

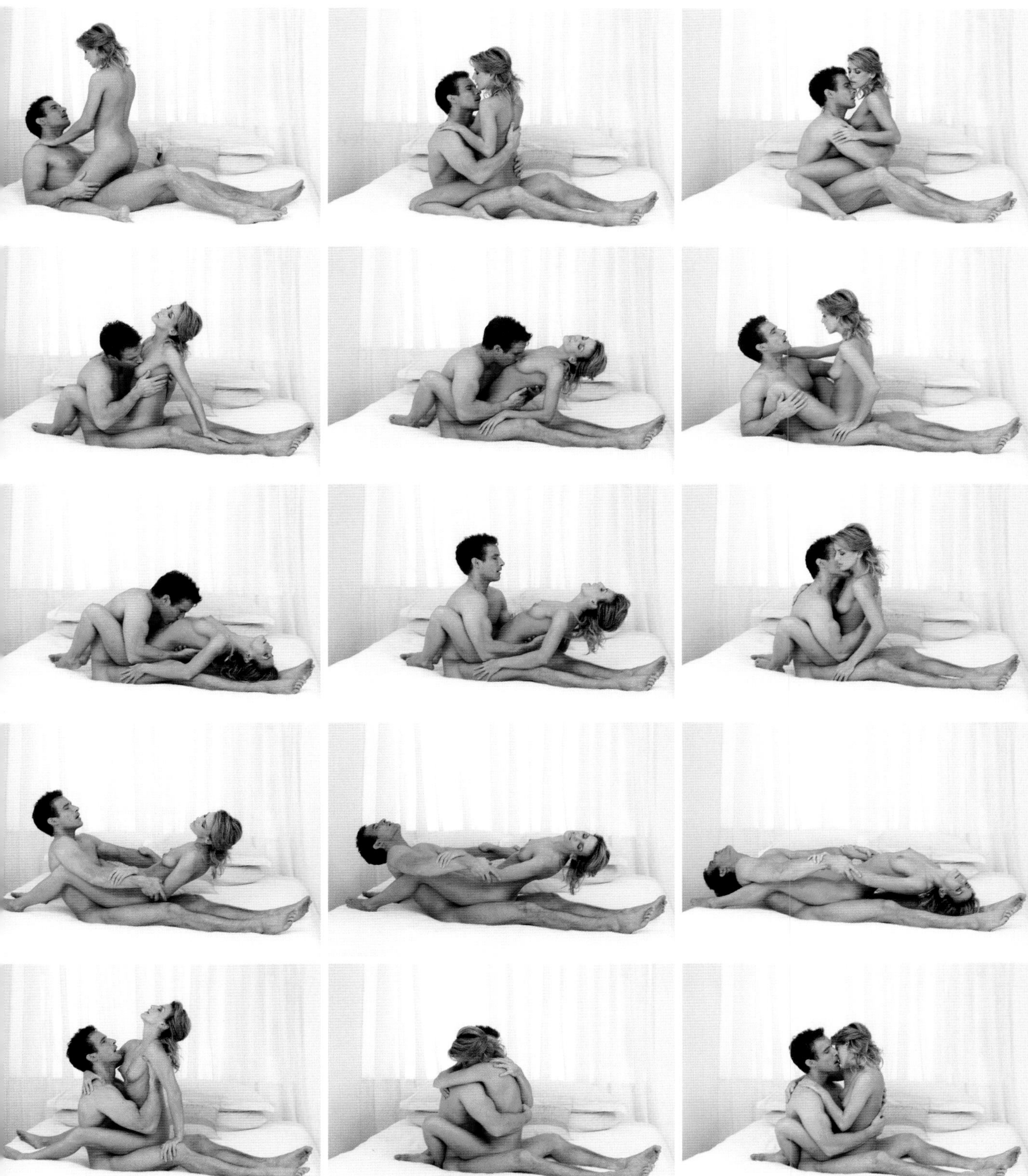

Silkworm spinning a cocoon

☆☆☆☆ Kama sensation rating

If the standard missionary position feels too sedate for you, try its raunchier relation. The woman is more active because she's got her legs in the air and wrapped tightly around him. He finds it exciting because he can directly feel the strength of her desire.

Why it works

– It's a staple sex position that hits all the right spots for him and her. The shaft of his penis caresses her clitoris on each thrust.

– He can try long, slow, deep strokes or teasing shallow ones.

– She can use the power of her thigh muscles to slam him in fast on each thrust.

– It's easy to change the sensations and the depth of penetration; she just raises or lowers her legs. Experiment to see what works for you.

– If you both hang on tight, you can roll over 180 degrees into a woman-on-top position.

Turn on...

... Try to pace yourselves. If he gives in to temptation and thrusts hard and fast, it's easy for him to come very quickly. If you want a more relaxed sex session, take the slow and scenic route, and pause for breaks if you need to.

Turn off...

... Don't tense up in the quest to avoid ejaculation. If your buttock muscles are locked tight, try to relax a bit. Try delaying ejaculation by gently tugging your balls instead.

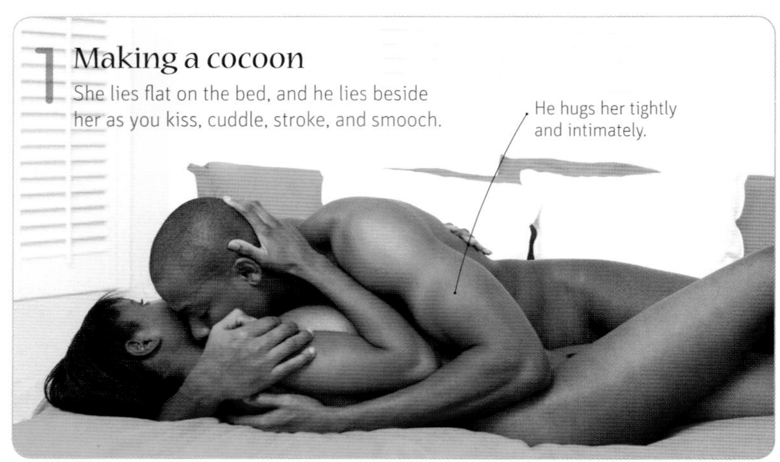

1 Making a cocoon
She lies flat on the bed, and he lies beside her as you kiss, cuddle, stroke, and smooch.

He hugs her tightly and intimately.

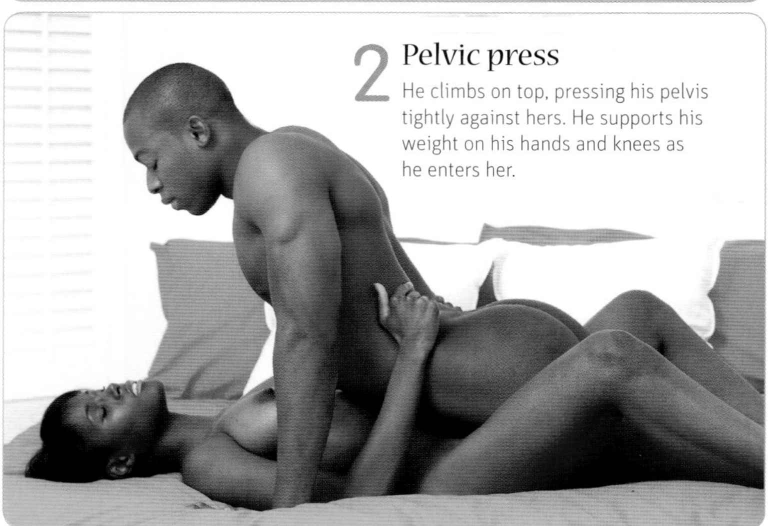

2 Pelvic press
He climbs on top, pressing his pelvis tightly against hers. He supports his weight on his hands and knees as he enters her.

"If anyone should think that the number of positions given is too small, all he needs to do is invent some more." THE PERFUMED GARDEN

3 Tight wrap

She bends her knees and wraps both legs around his body, crossing her ankles behind his bum. She puts her arms around his shoulders.

After he enters, he stays still for several seconds to savor the feeling of deep connection.

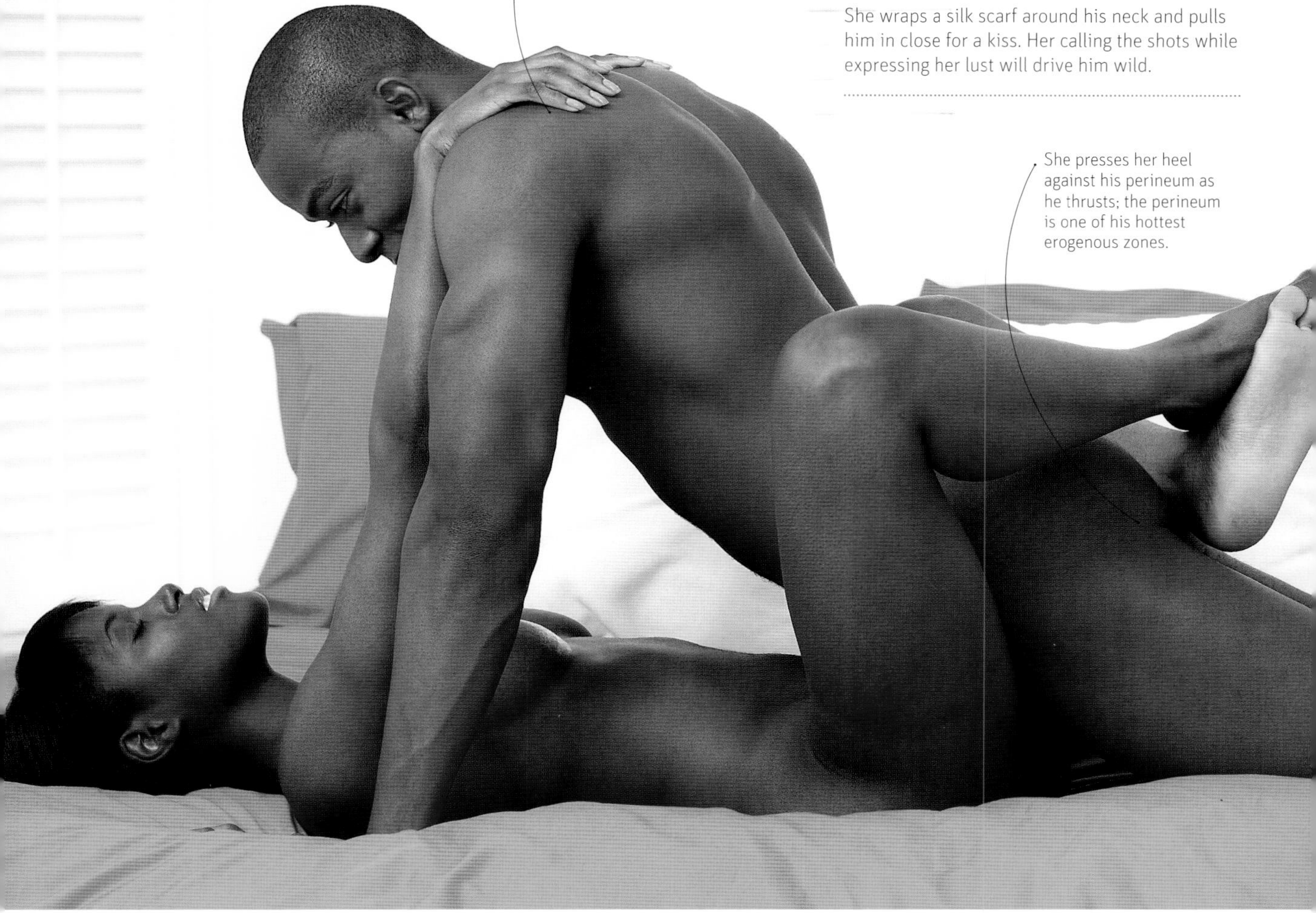

She presses her heel against his perineum as he thrusts; the perineum is one of his hottest erogenous zones.

Taking it further

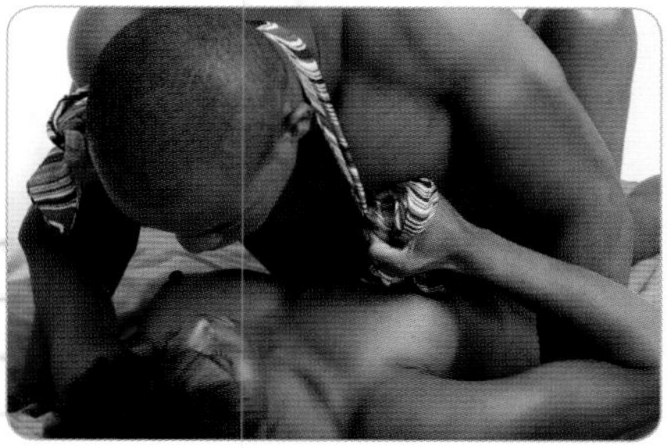

Silken caress

She wraps a silk scarf around his neck and pulls him in close for a kiss. Her calling the shots while expressing her lust will drive him wild.

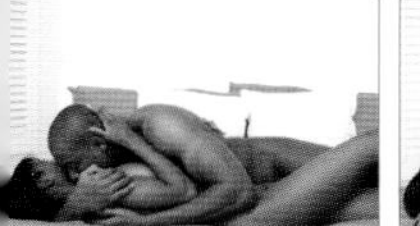
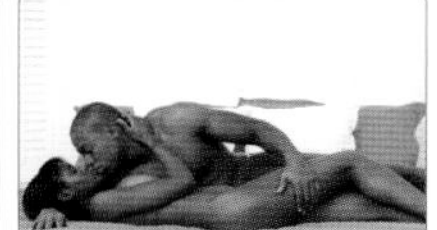
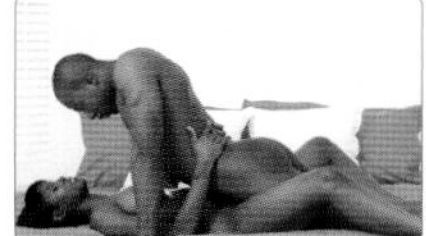
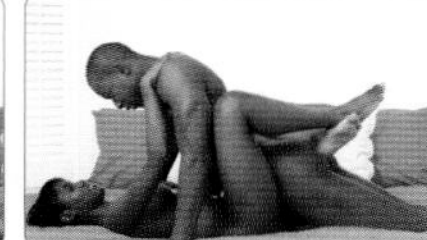
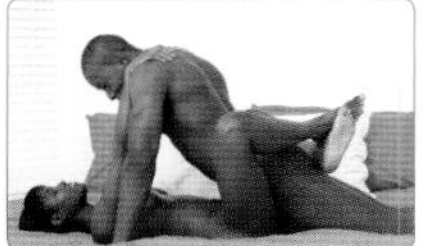
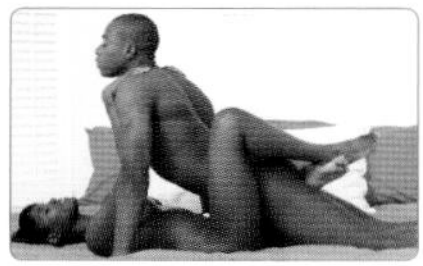

The inverted embrace

☆☆ Kama sensation rating

A woman should "place her man supine on the bed or carpet, mount his person, and satisfy her desires," according to the ancient texts. The Inverted Embrace is not only great for satisfying desires, but it's also good for getting up-close and intimate.

Why it works

- With her knees braced on the bed, she can bump, hump, and grind her way to orgasm.
- He's free to lie back and watch her in performance mode, and at her sexiest.
- You can bask in the intimacy of full-body contact and give yourselves up to kissing and cuddling; before, during, and after.
- It's great when he's tired and she's full of energy. But don't be surprised if he miraculously makes a recovery.
- If he's come and she hasn't, she can make the most of the final moments of his erection.

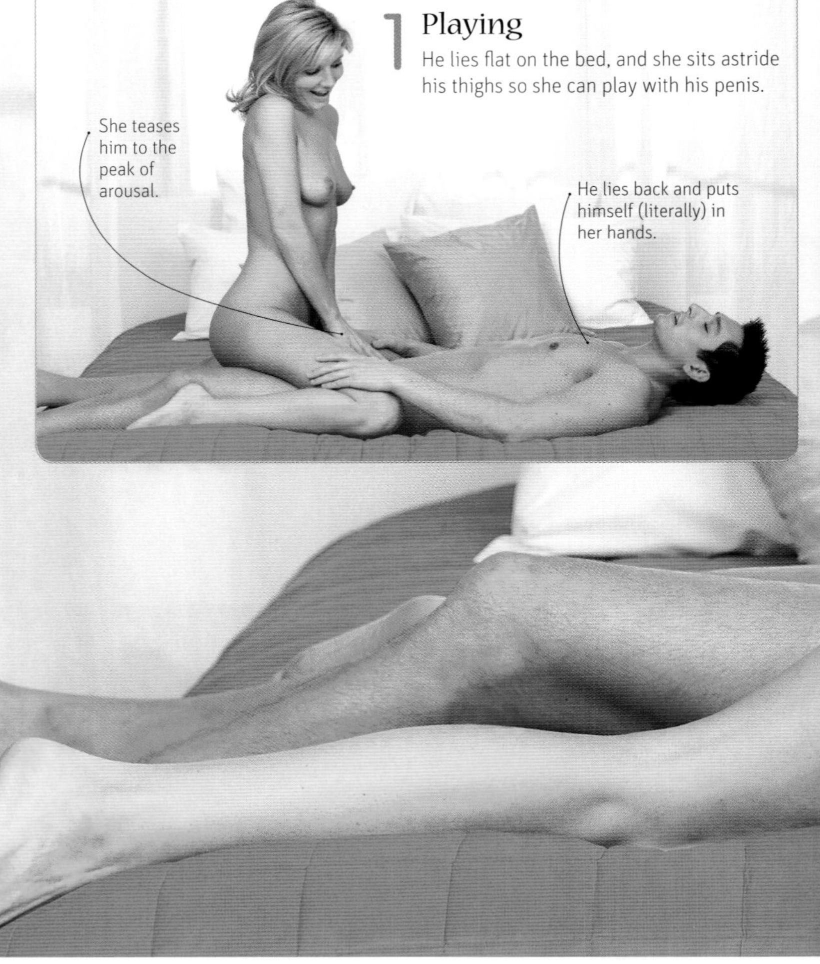

1 Playing

He lies flat on the bed, and she sits astride his thighs so she can play with his penis.

She teases him to the peak of arousal.

He lies back and puts himself (literally) in her hands.

Turn on...

... Find a pace and rhythm that will take you to the peak. In particular, try to find the angle that creates maximum pressure and friction between your clitoris and the shaft of his penis. Or try rubbing against his pubic bone.

Turn off...

... Don't worry if intercourse alone doesn't take you there. Simply add your hand (or his) or a vibrator to turbocharge your arousal.

"She lies straight upon the outstretched person of her lover and enjoys him by moving her hips sharply in various directions." ANANGA RANGA

2 All fours

She kneels upright, sinks slowly on to his penis, then puts her hands on either side of his shoulders so that she's on all fours.

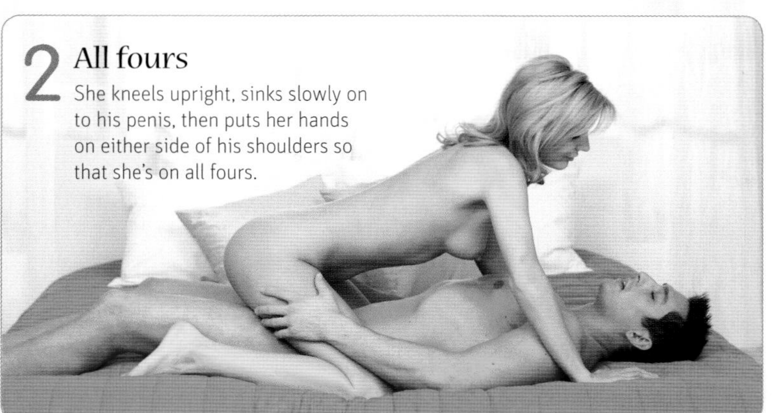

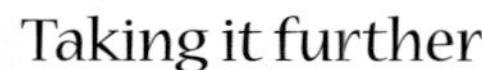

Taking it further

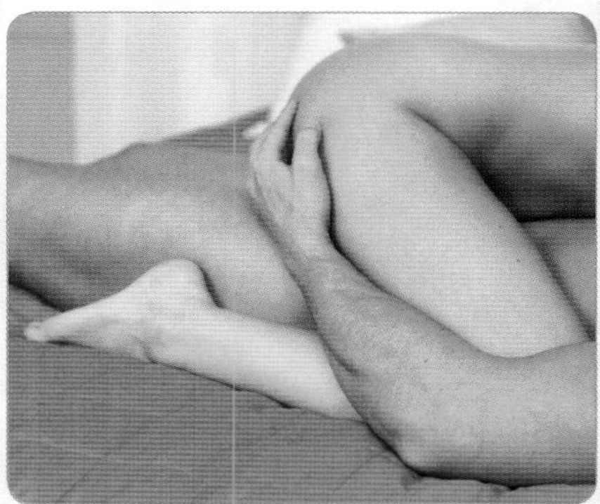

Moving toward the climax

She expands her range of movement by bending one knee so that her calf runs parallel to the side of his body and her foot is level with his buttock.

3 Slow slide

She slides her body slowly down to meet his. She puts her knees outside his and rests her elbows on the bed or floor.

When she's at the peak of arousal, he runs his fingers down her back to make her shiver with pleasure.

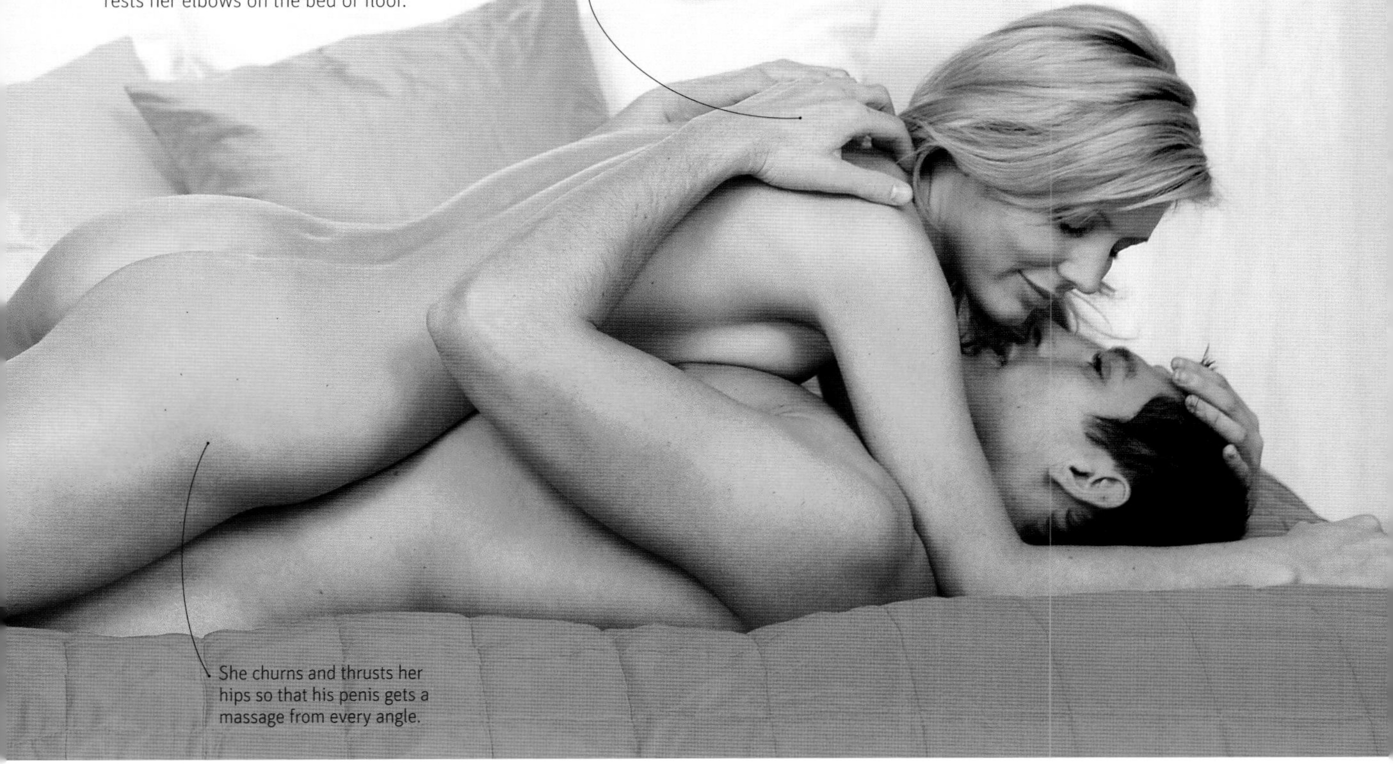

She churns and thrusts her hips so that his penis gets a massage from every angle.

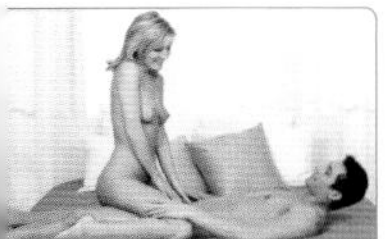
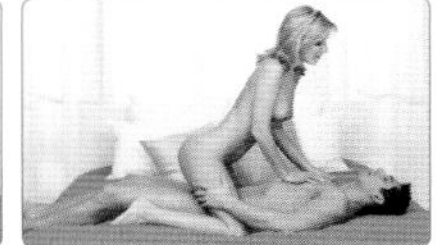
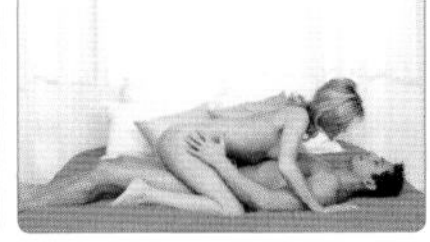
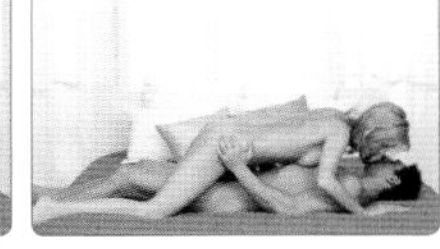
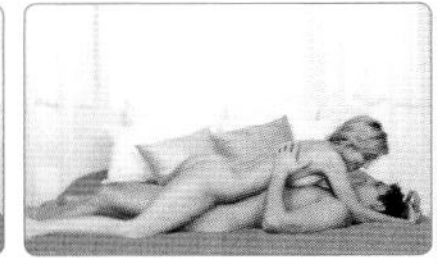

Pounding on the spot

☆☆☆ Kama sensation rating

Pounding on the Spot was considered by some of the ancient sex gurus to be the position that delivered the most satisfaction. It is certainly tender, if a bit restricting. If you find you can't move as freely as you want, just enjoy the mounting sense of sexual tension.

Why it works

– She's positioned directly on top of his penis, so she feels thoroughly filled and he feels powerfully enclosed.

– Your upright, cuddling position makes you feel intensely bonded.

– He enjoys the sensation and sight of her breasts caressing his face.

– You experience sublime internal tinglings as she flutters her vaginal muscles against his shaft, and he flexes his penis in response.

– He can put his hands under her butt to move her up and down or back and forth.

Turn on...

... Concentrate on your breathing. Try breathing in time while gazing deeply into each other's eyes. Feel the boundaries between you dissolve. This is a tantric sex practice that works well in positions where she sits upright in his lap.

Turn off...

... Don't worry if you don't merge with each other or connect blissfully with the universe. Tantric skills can take time to learn; they rarely come instantly (and neither do the practitioners!).

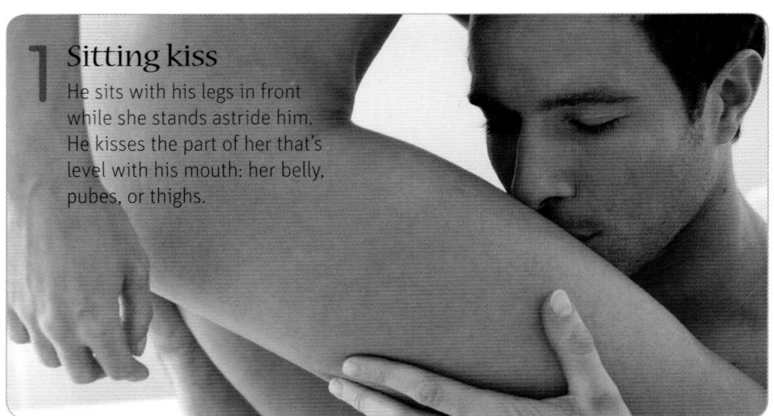

1 Sitting kiss
He sits with his legs in front while she stands astride him. He kisses the part of her that's level with his mouth: her belly, pubes, or thighs.

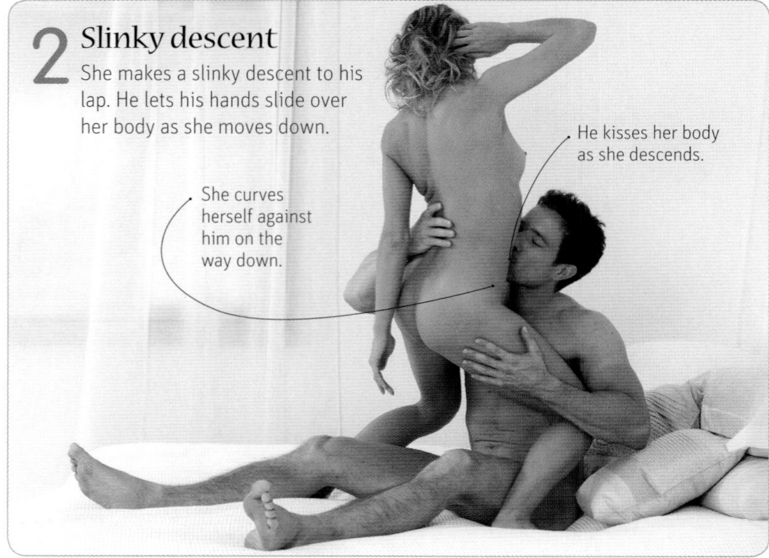
He kisses her body as she descends.
She curves herself against him on the way down.

2 Slinky descent
She makes a slinky descent to his lap. He lets his hands slide over her body as she moves down.

"The man tried different postures, but when he came to Pounding on the Spot he noticed that the woman's pleasure was intense, and he felt his member powerfully gripped."
THE PERFUMED GARDEN

Taking it further

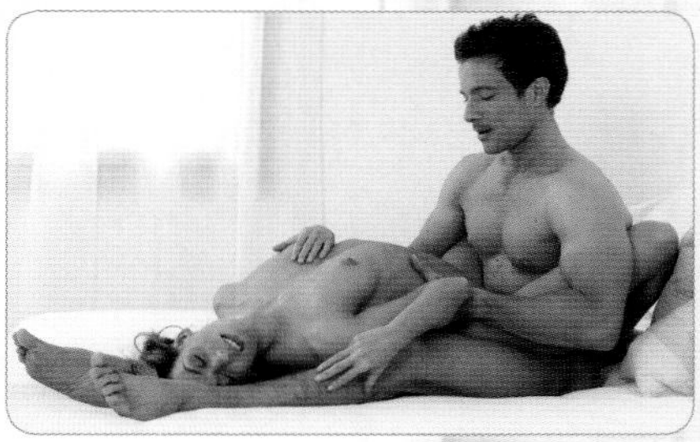

Taking in the view

She lies back across his lap so she can thrust her hips and give him the thrill of seeing his penis moving in and out.

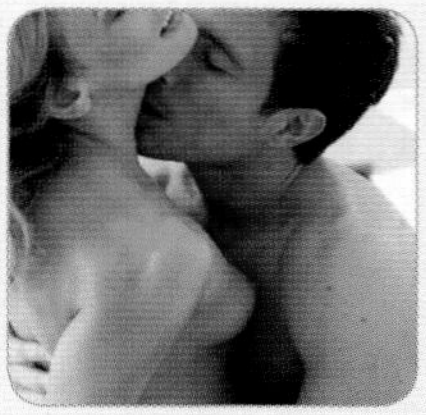

She can throw her head back for him to devour her neck with hungry bites and kisses.

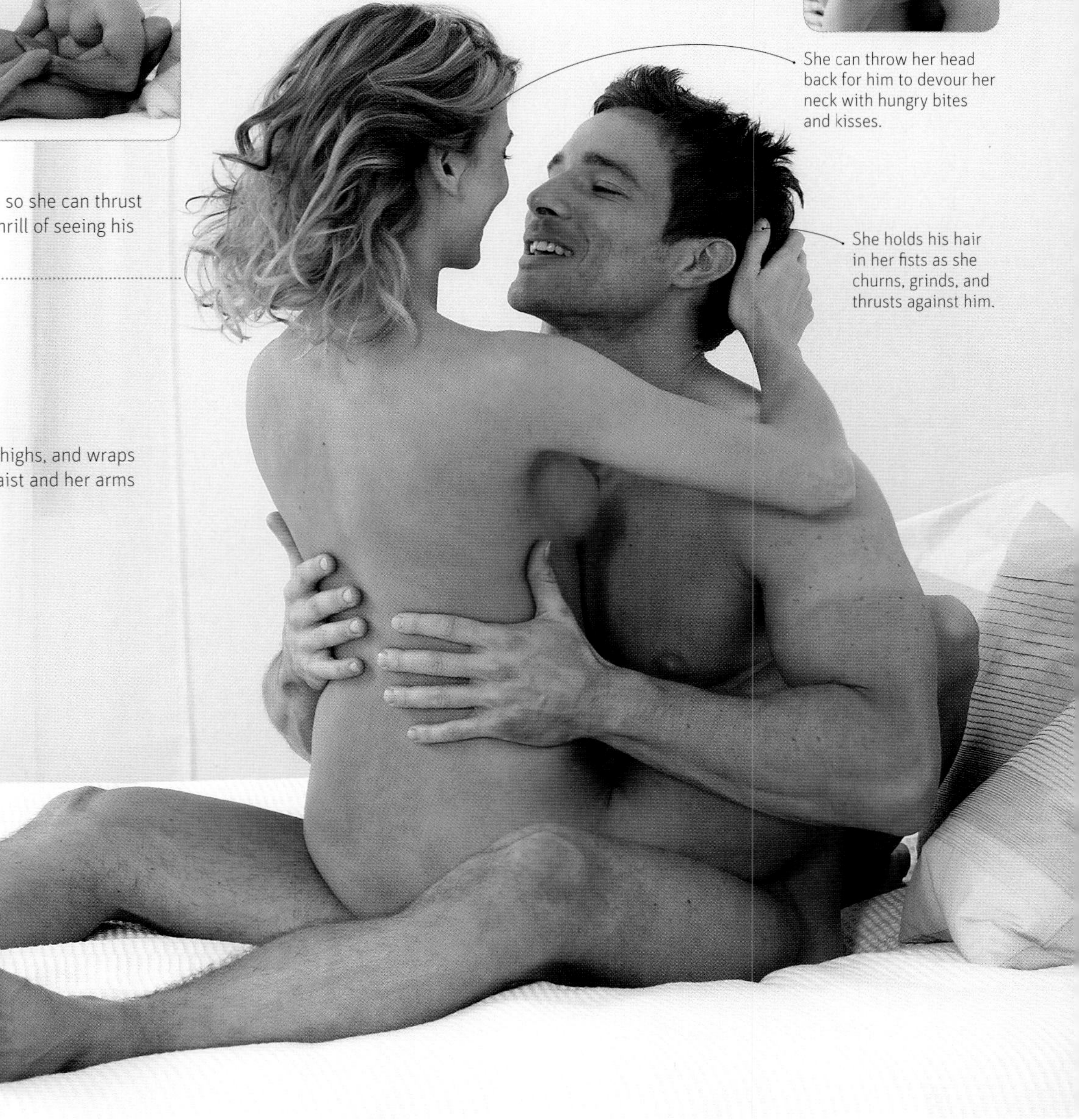

She holds his hair in her fists as she churns, grinds, and thrusts against him.

3 Close hug

She sits between his thighs, and wraps her legs around his waist and her arms around his shoulders.

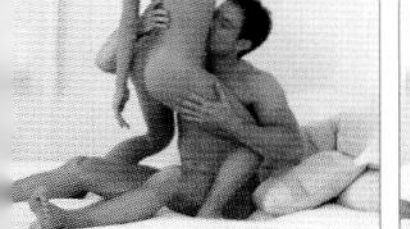
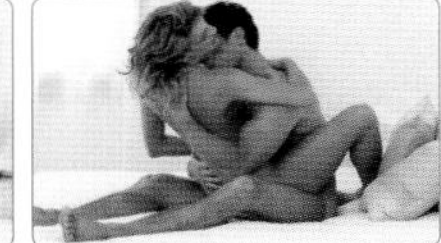
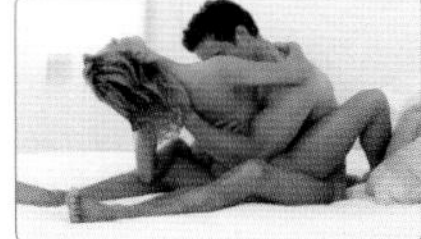
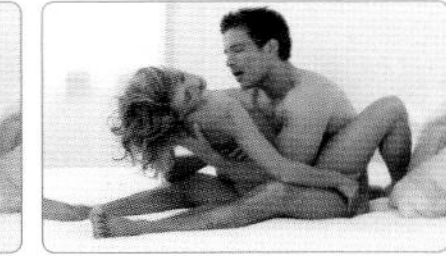
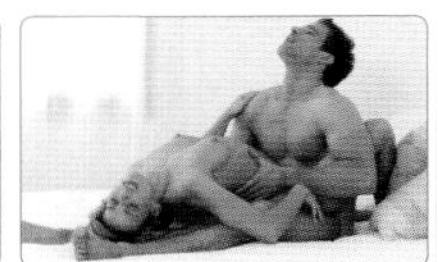
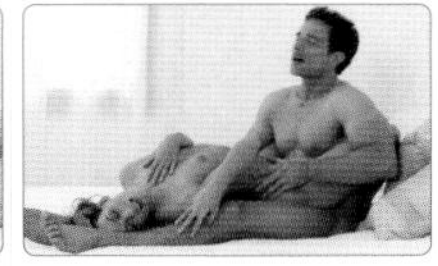

The pair of tongs

☆☆☆☆ Kama sensation rating

The Pair of Tongs is a staple position in most lovers' sex lives for the simple reason that it feels fantastic for both you. In honor of its name, she should use her vaginal muscles to grip his member as hard as a pair of tongs.

Why it works

– The Pair of Tongs is one of the most popular positions for women to reach orgasm as there is plenty of clitoral friction.

– He has his hands free, so he can spice things up with some creative handiwork on her breasts, clitoris, butt, or thighs.

– As she squeezes her vaginal muscles, the contractions give him an intensely erotic sensation.

– She's in complete control of the movement.

– He will love the view from below.

– She can turn sex into a sensual treat by leaning forward and massaging him.

Turn on...

... Encourage her to let go of her inhibitions. If you know she's shy about being on top, show your appreciation vocally. If you abandon yourself to lust, she will too.

Turn off...

... Don't stare at her. A fixed, unwavering gaze, however appreciative, may give her performance anxiety and put her off her stroke.

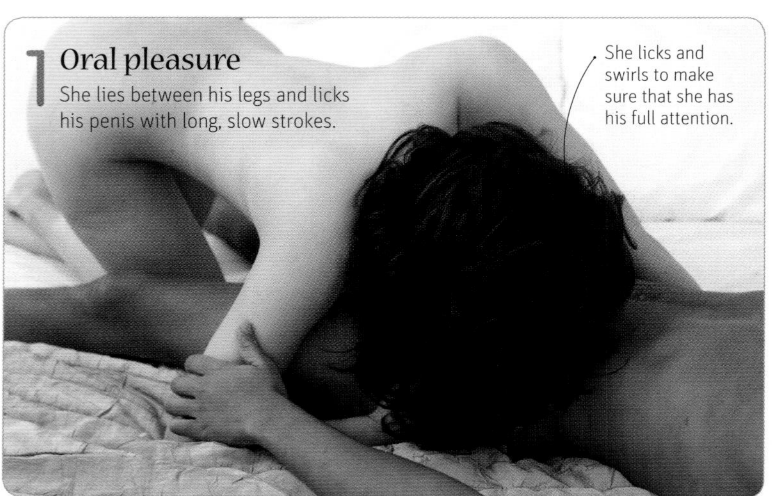

1 Oral pleasure
She lies between his legs and licks his penis with long, slow strokes.

She licks and swirls to make sure that she has his full attention.

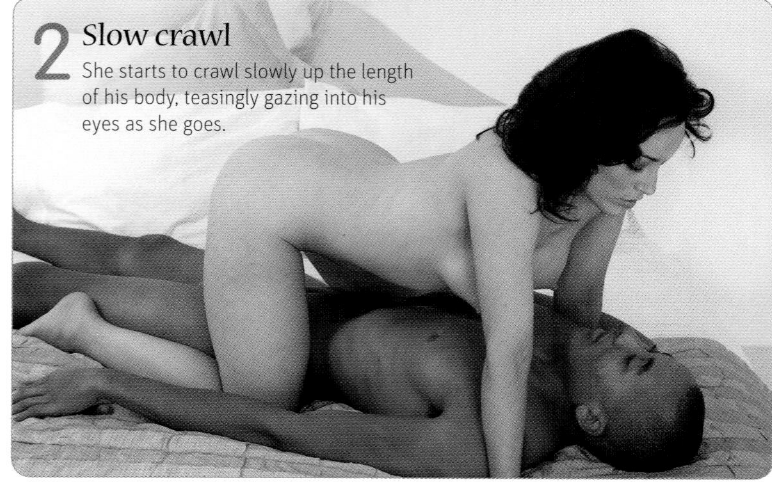

2 Slow crawl
She starts to crawl slowly up the length of his body, teasingly gazing into his eyes as she goes.

"The connoisseur of copulation should try all the postures..." THE PERFUMED GARDEN

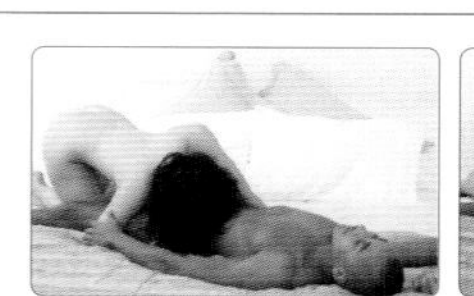

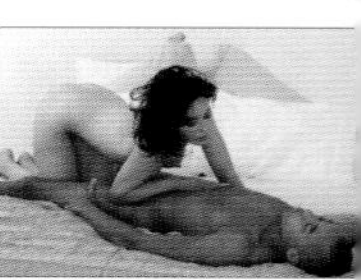

Taking it further

Provocative massage

She drizzles massage oil provocatively across his chest before giving him a sensual massage, which will send him wild with desire.

3 Straddling

When her face is level with his, she moves into an upright straddling position and lowers herself on to his penis.

She awakens sensation in his nipples and chest by moving her hands in light swirly movements.

He surprises her with a playful spank on the side of her buttock.

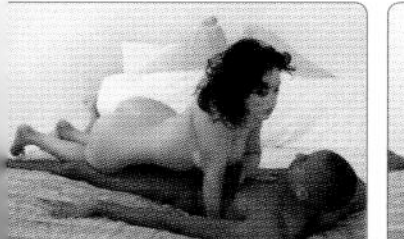
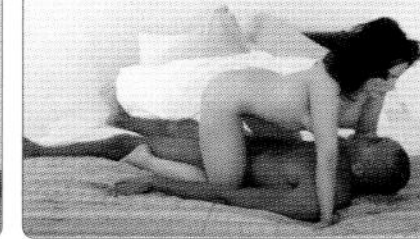
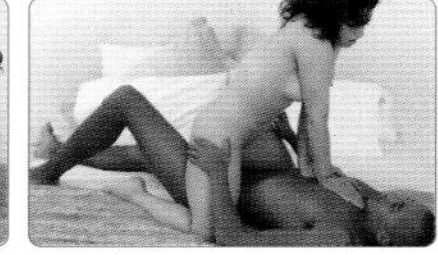
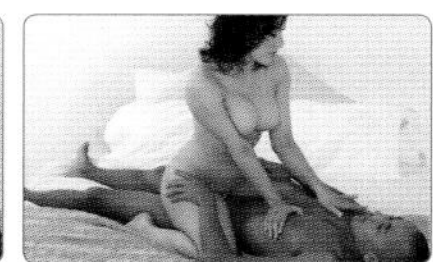
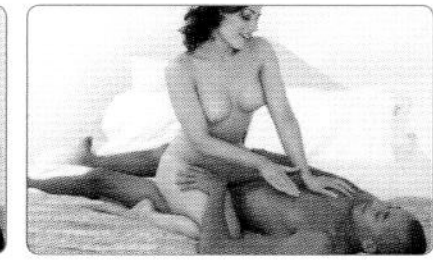
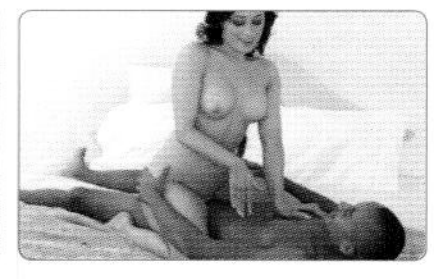

The one who stops at home

☆☆☆☆ Kama sensation rating

This position gives you a compelling reason to stop at home. The erotic atmosphere crackles as she moves with fluid undulations or fast hip flicks. Close the curtains, tear off each other's clothes, throw yourselves on the bed, and enjoy a noisy night in.

Why it works

- She can tease him by taking him to the brink with rapid hip jerks, then slowing things down with slow pelvic circles.
- She can brush her hands lightly along the sides of his body to make him tingle.
- He feels strong and dominant, but she gets a kick from being the prime mover.
- She adds to the erotic intensity by gazing into his eyes as she moves up and down.
- If she gets tired, you can take a quick break in the missionary position.

Turn on...

... Make this position just one part of a long, sexy evening at home. Indulge each other with food, wine, massage, and at least an hour of foreplay. Make love in a sequence of positions that flow on naturally from each other.

Turn off...

... Don't get into a competitive mind-set about how many positions you have to perform. If things are starting to feel soulless after your 10th twist/spin/leg extension/body inversion, you'll know that you've taken it too far, and it's time to relax.

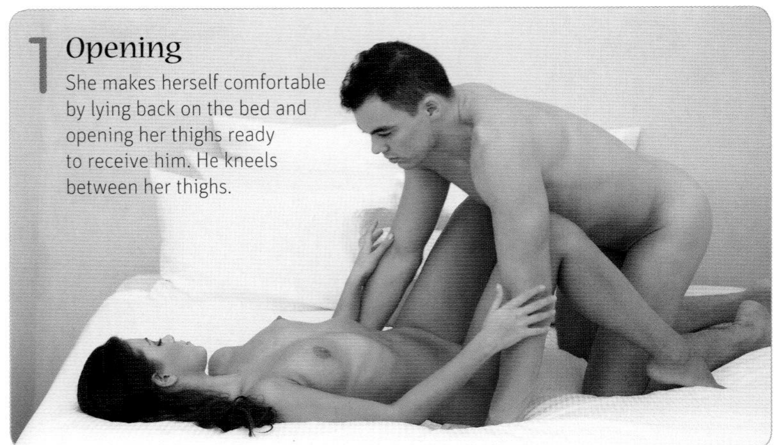

1 Opening
She makes herself comfortable by lying back on the bed and opening her thighs ready to receive him. He kneels between her thighs.

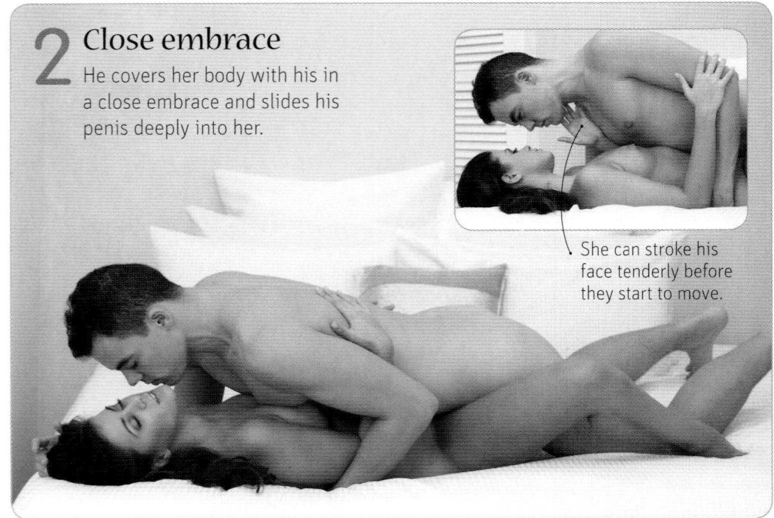

2 Close embrace
He covers her body with his in a close embrace and slides his penis deeply into her.

She can stroke his face tenderly before they start to move.

"When the introduction has taken place, the woman raises her buttocks as far as possible from the bed, and the man accompanies her in the movement..." THE PERFUMED GARDEN

3 Coming home

Staying joined to her, he raises himself on to all fours. She pushes up her hips so that her body rises in unison with his.

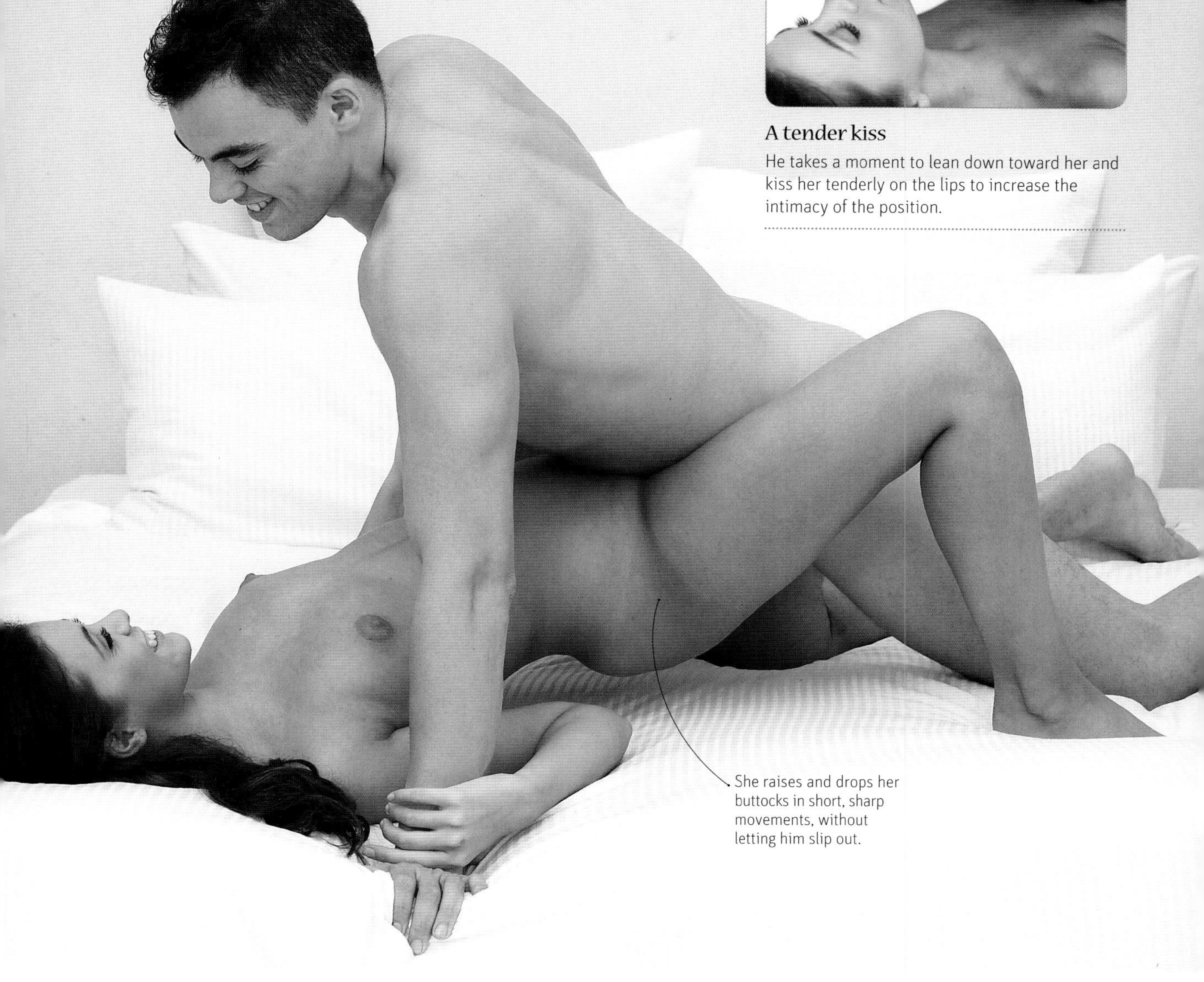

She raises and drops her buttocks in short, sharp movements, without letting him slip out.

Taking it further

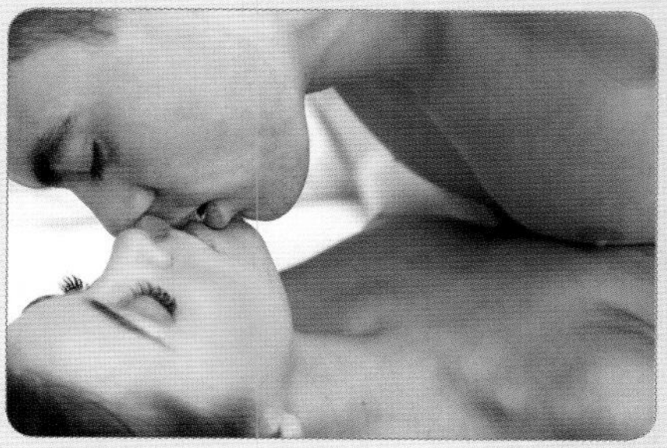

A tender kiss

He takes a moment to lean down toward her and kiss her tenderly on the lips to increase the intimacy of the position.

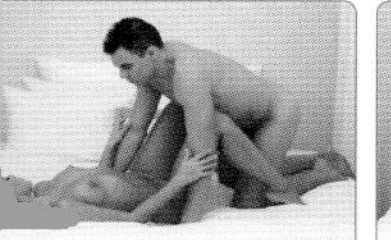
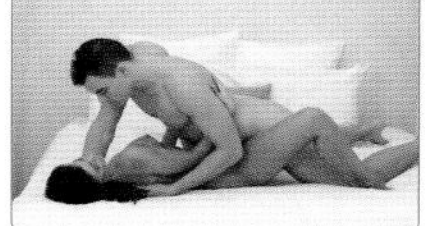
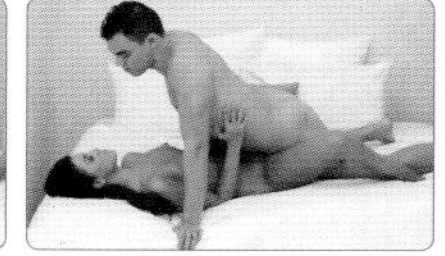
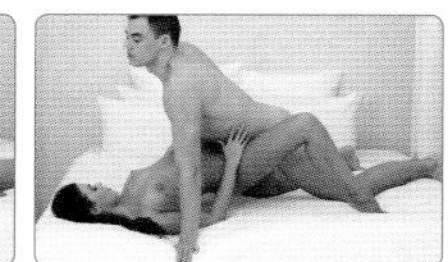
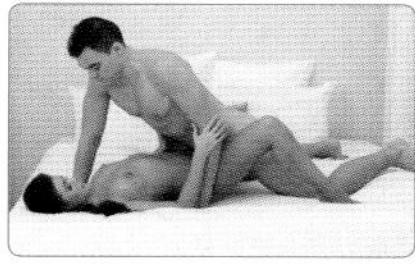

The eleventh posture

☆☆☆☆☆ Kama sensation rating

This slight twist on the missionary position is the perfect all-rounder for different moods of loving. It's great for satisfying sudden sex urges and moments of extreme lust, and it also works for long, slow, lazy love when time is no object.

Why it works

– Her feet on the backs of his legs give him a kinky trapped sensation.

– She can slide her feet up and down his legs to vary the depth of penetration.

– It's romantic, intimate, and warm; you can kiss, press your bodies close, and feel connected.

– You fit together perfectly, and it's easy to find a rhythm that fires up both of you.

– Both of your bodies are comfortable and supported, so you can stay in the position for a long time, and abandon yourselves to pleasure along the way.

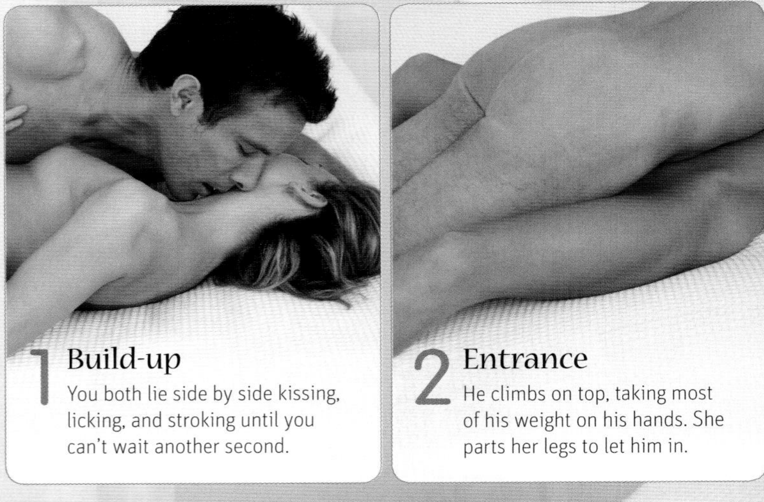

1 Build-up
You both lie side by side kissing, licking, and stroking until you can't wait another second.

2 Entrance
He climbs on top, taking most of his weight on his hands. She parts her legs to let him in.

Turn on…

… Enjoy this position for its glorious simplicity. Get into a groove and concentrate on the sensations inside your body; not just your genitals, but other parts, such as your belly and your chest. Let the pleasure spread through you.

Turn off…

… Don't let sex become so rhythmically repetitive that your mind wanders off the job. If you start thinking about work or how late it is, it's probably time for a change of pace or position.

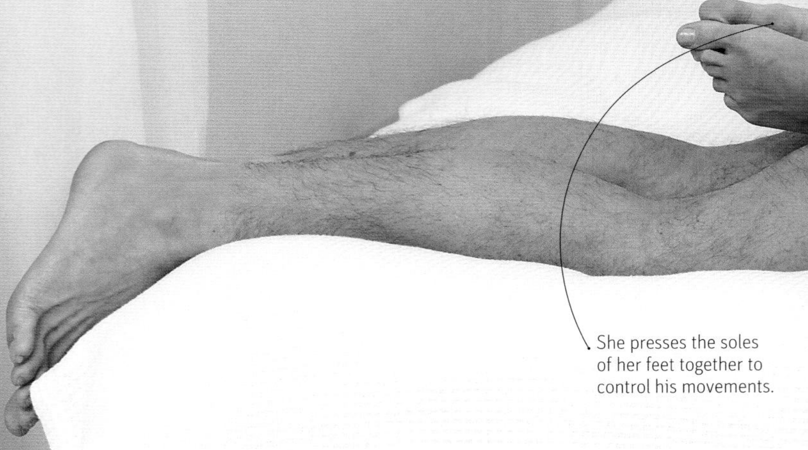

She presses the soles of her feet together to control his movements.

"According to your taste you may choose the position that delights you most." THE PERFUMED GARDEN

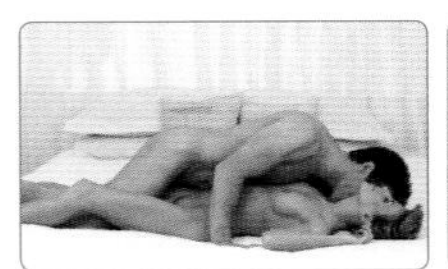

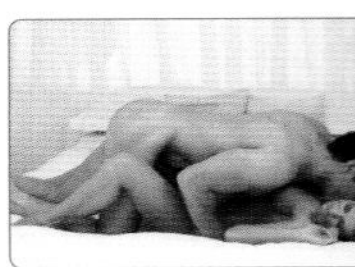

3 Sole to sole

She raises her legs and puts the soles of her feet together behind his calves. She drops her knees to the sides as he thrusts.

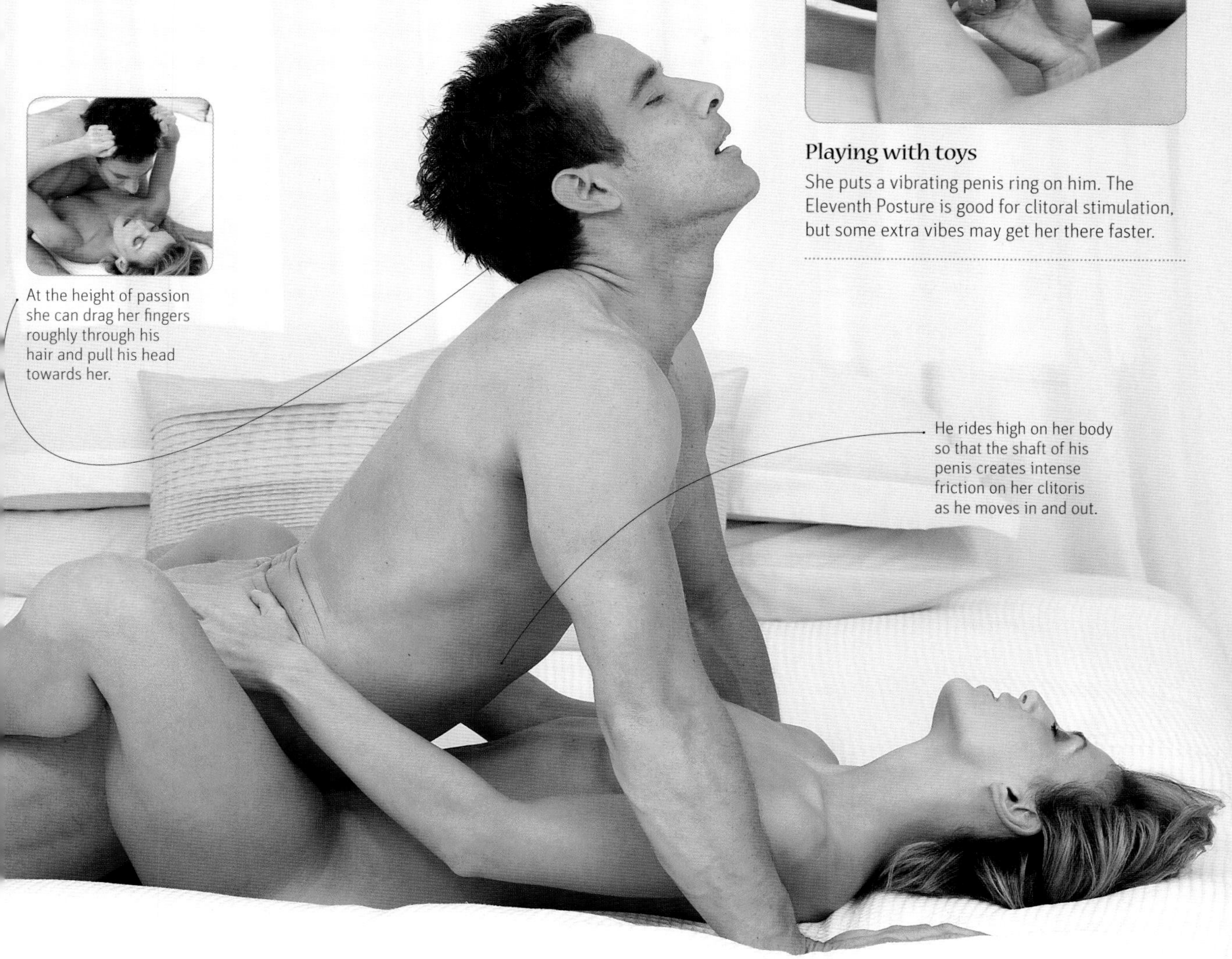

At the height of passion she can drag her fingers roughly through his hair and pull his head towards her.

He rides high on her body so that the shaft of his penis creates intense friction on her clitoris as he moves in and out.

Taking it further

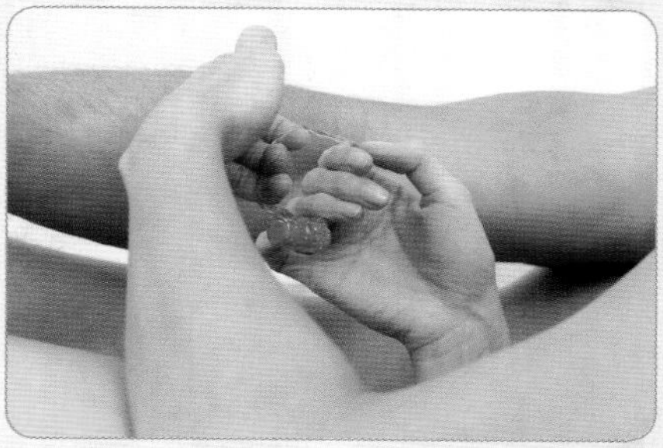

Playing with toys

She puts a vibrating penis ring on him. The Eleventh Posture is good for clitoral stimulation, but some extra vibes may get her there faster.

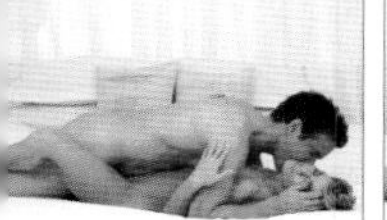
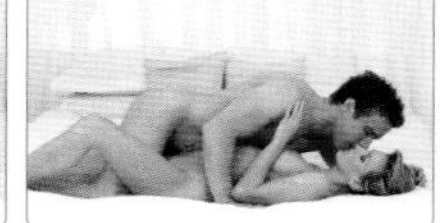
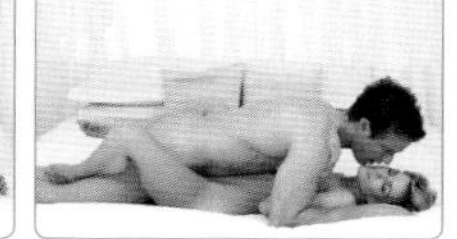
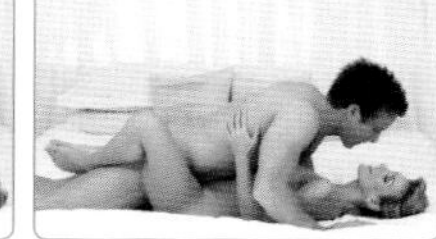
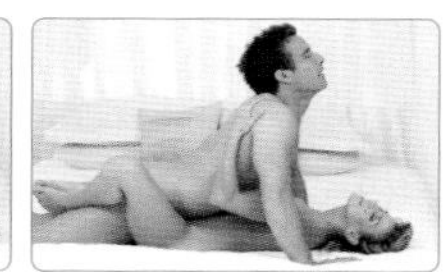

Splitting the bamboo

Splitting the Bamboo is erotic performance art meets yoga workout. She lies on her back and lifts each leg in turn throughout sex. This gives him a subtle but erotic massage as her vagina moves around his penis. It's also a turn-on for him if he loves the sight and sensation of her legs against him. If so, she should perform her moves with professionally slow raunchiness.

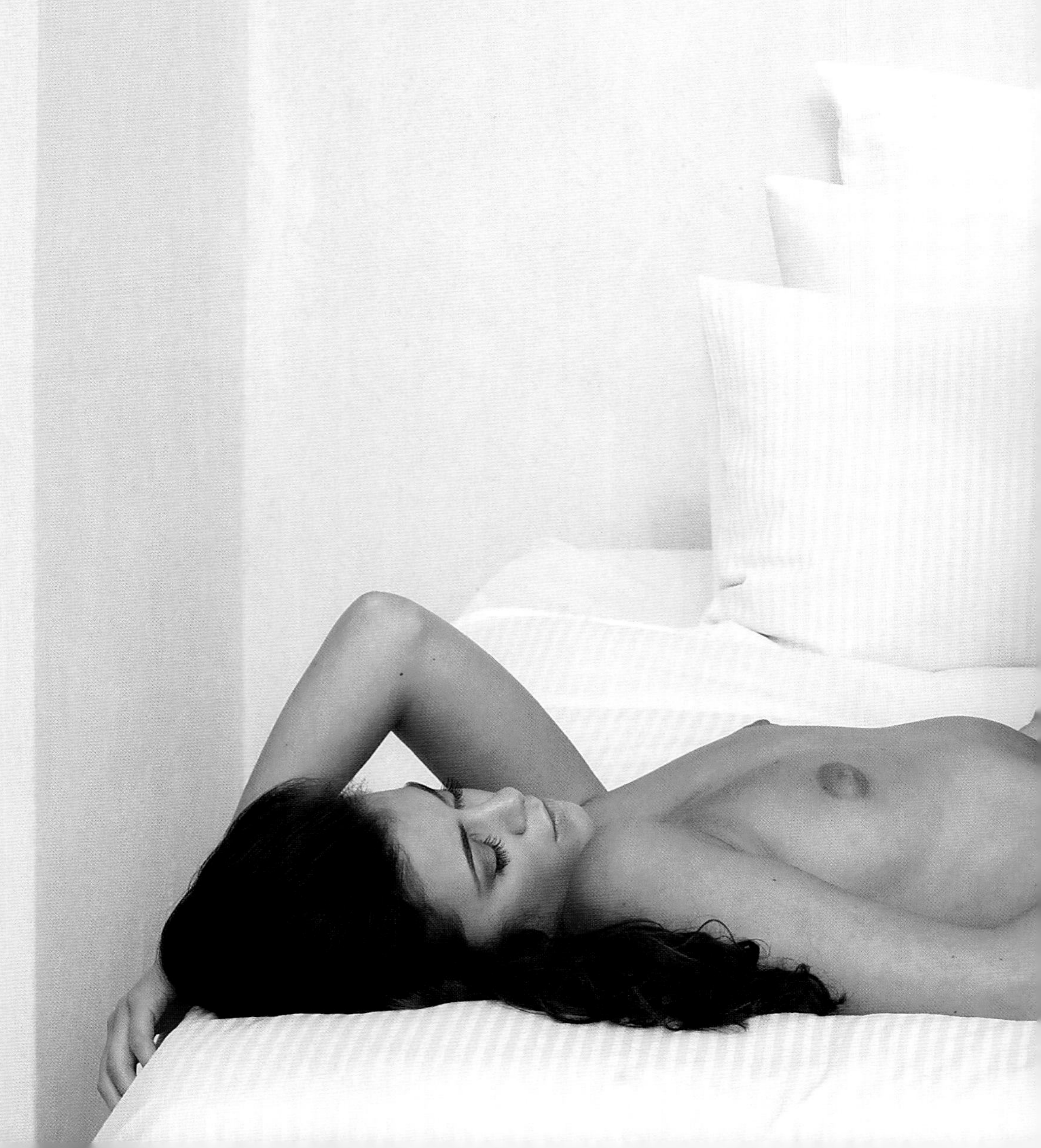

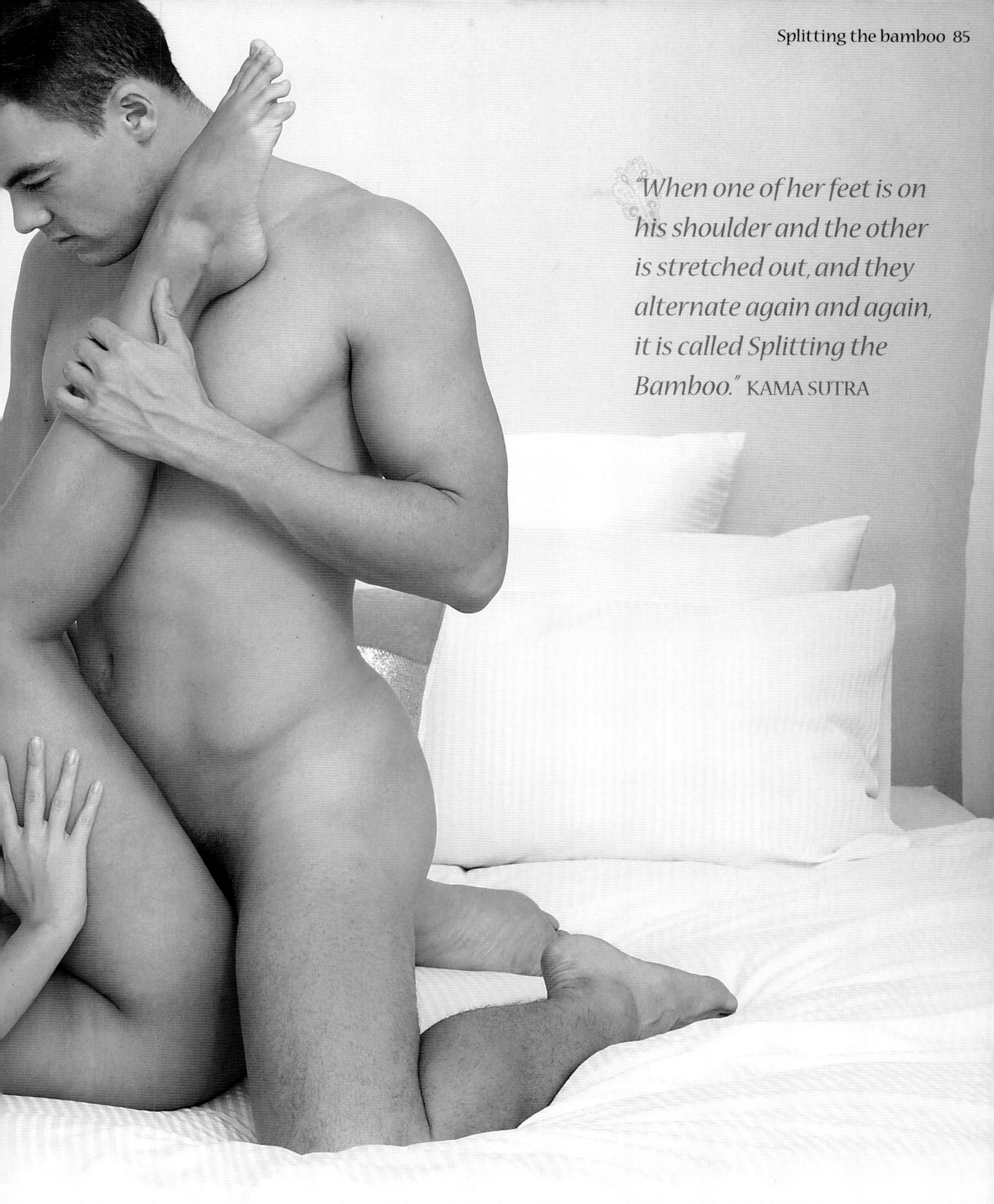

"When one of her feet is on his shoulder and the other is stretched out, and they alternate again and again, it is called Splitting the Bamboo." KAMA SUTRA

Splitting the bamboo

Kama sensation rating

Why it works

– Each time she raises and lowers her legs, her vagina moves around his penis, which changes the internal sensations for both of you. She feels pressure on both sides of her vagina. He feels as though his penis is being gently rolled inside her.

– It gives her a chance to perform some sexual acrobatics to an extremely receptive audience, and to get some very intimate and direct appreciation.

– Her leg positions give him the erotic sensation of being allowed in, yet held back.

– Although he's on top, she's the one making the moves. She enjoys kindling his desire, while he enjoys the titillation of watching her.

– It's great if he's close to orgasm because the subtle penis massage he's getting can pull him back from the very peak of arousal.

Turn on...

... This is a chance for her to show off and enjoy her sexual power. If she gets off on exhibitionism, set up a camera so that you can watch it all again later.

Turn off...

... Don't pursue the leg-lifting ritual if it feels more like exercise than sex, or if you're bored and craving some good old-fashioned thrusting.

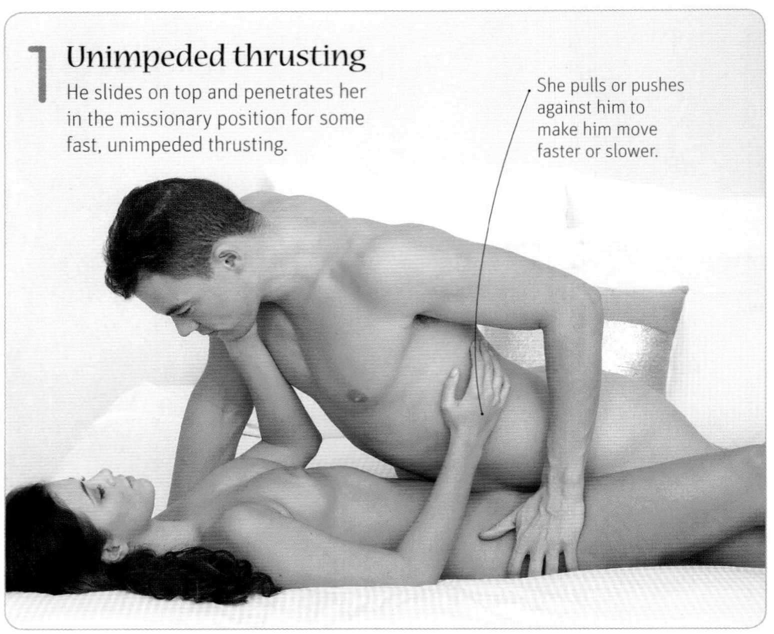

She pulls or pushes against him to make him move faster or slower.

1 Unimpeded thrusting

He slides on top and penetrates her in the missionary position for some fast, unimpeded thrusting.

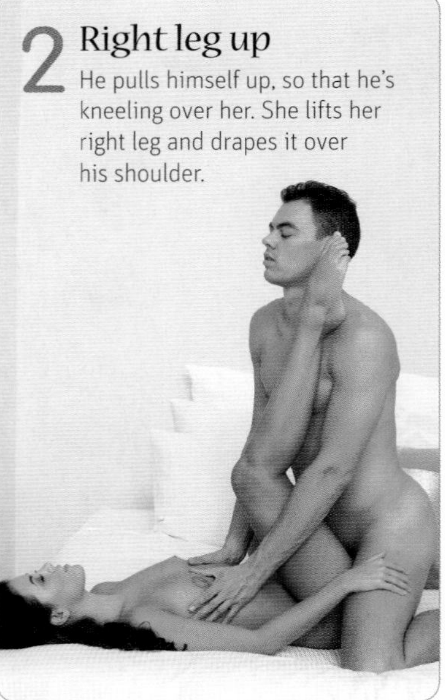

2 Right leg up

He pulls himself up, so that he's kneeling over her. She lifts her right leg and drapes it over his shoulder.

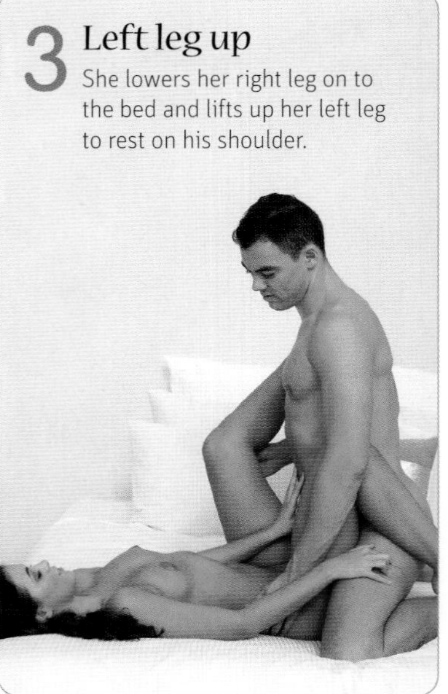

3 Left leg up

She lowers her right leg on to the bed and lifts up her left leg to rest on his shoulder.

"If she desires the coming of the tide of yin, her body will be shaking and holding him tight." THE TAO

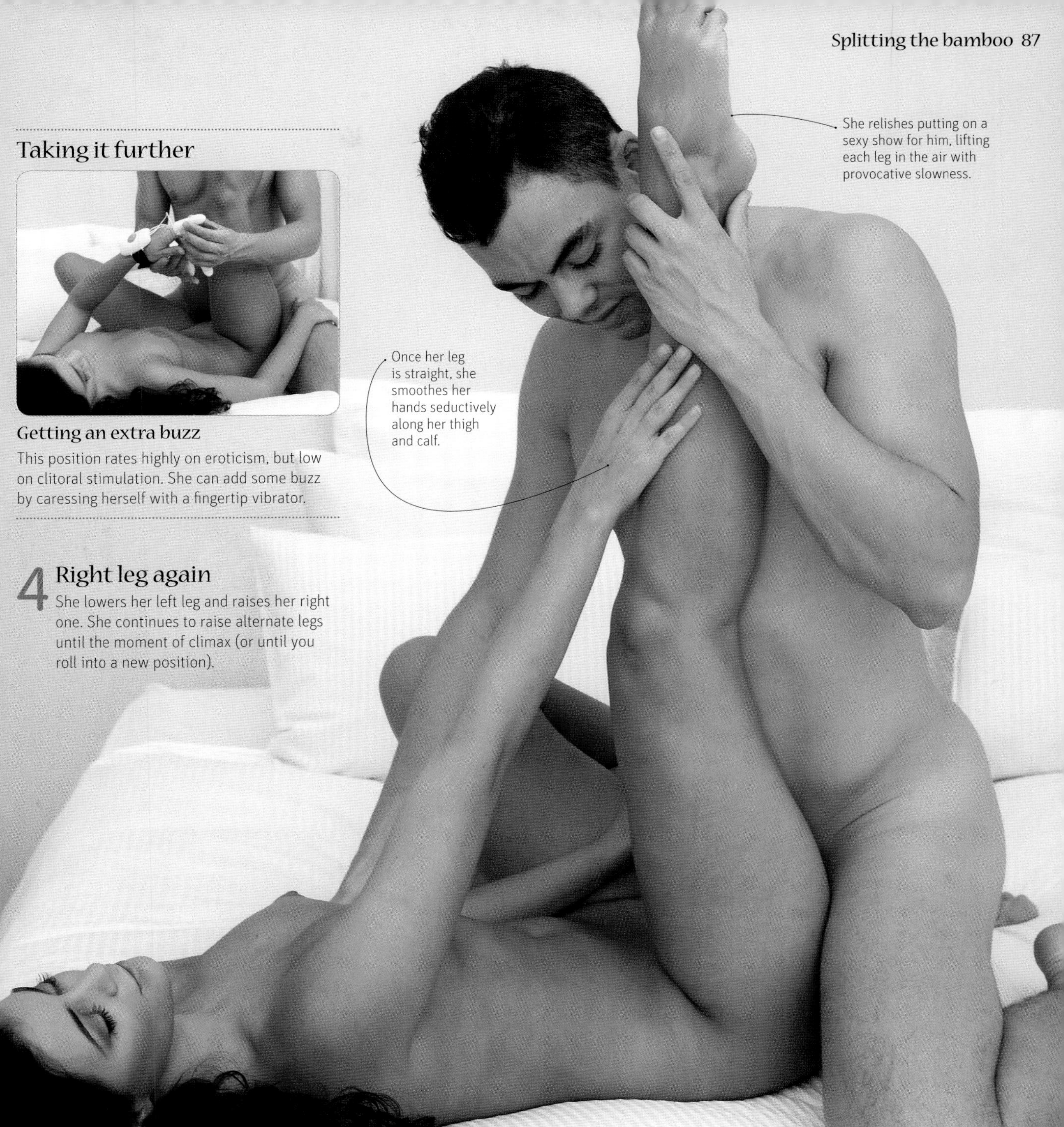
She relishes putting on a sexy show for him, lifting each leg in the air with provocative slowness.
Once her leg is straight, she smoothes her hands seductively along her thigh and calf.

Taking it further

Getting an extra buzz

This position rates highly on eroticism, but low on clitoral stimulation. She can add some buzz by caressing herself with a fingertip vibrator.

4 Right leg again

She lowers her left leg and raises her right one. She continues to raise alternate legs until the moment of climax (or until you roll into a new position).

If you liked this, try...

- Rising to the challenge of a half shoulder stand in Tail of the Ostrich (see page 190).
- The more intimate Third Posture (see page 202).

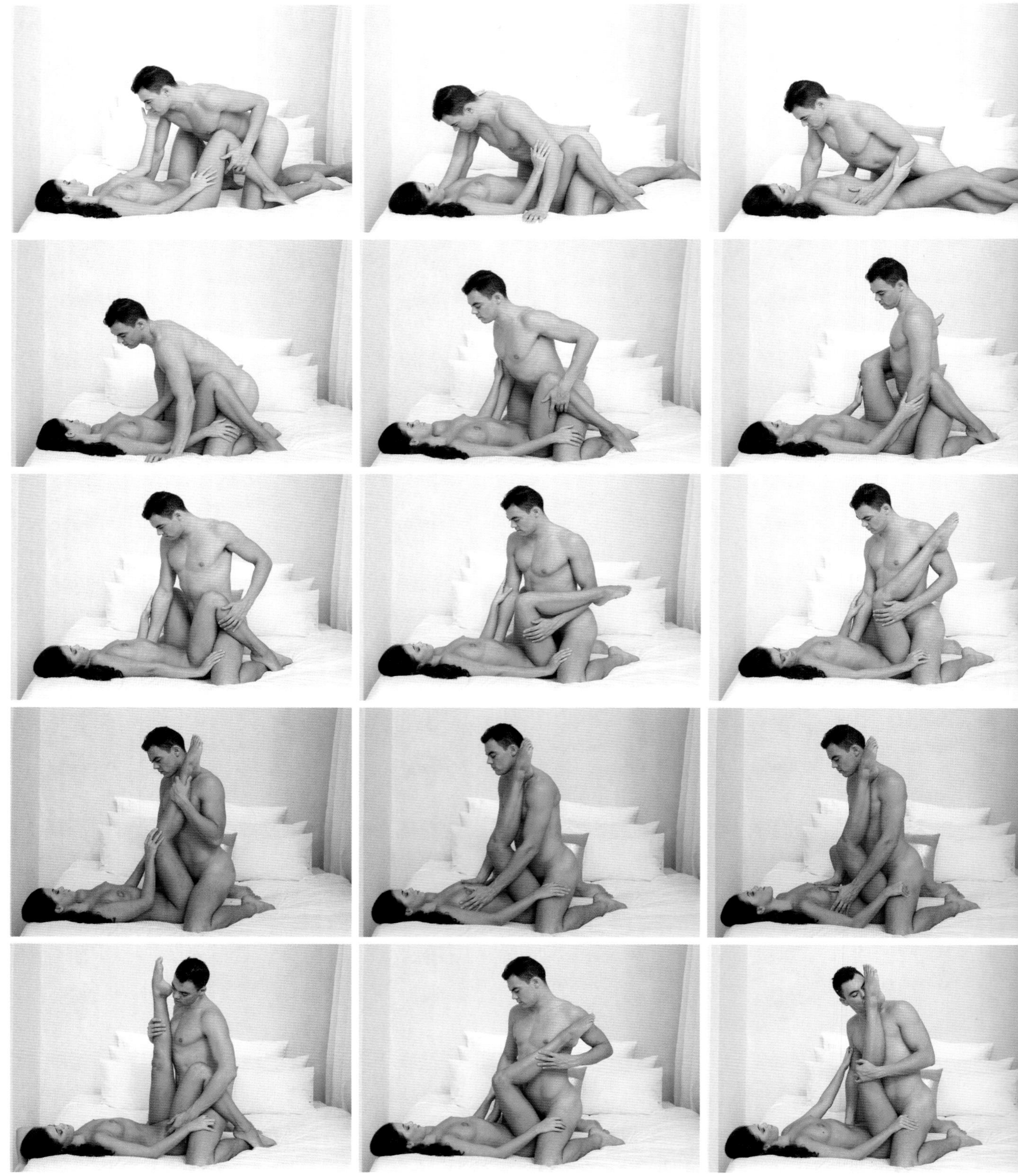

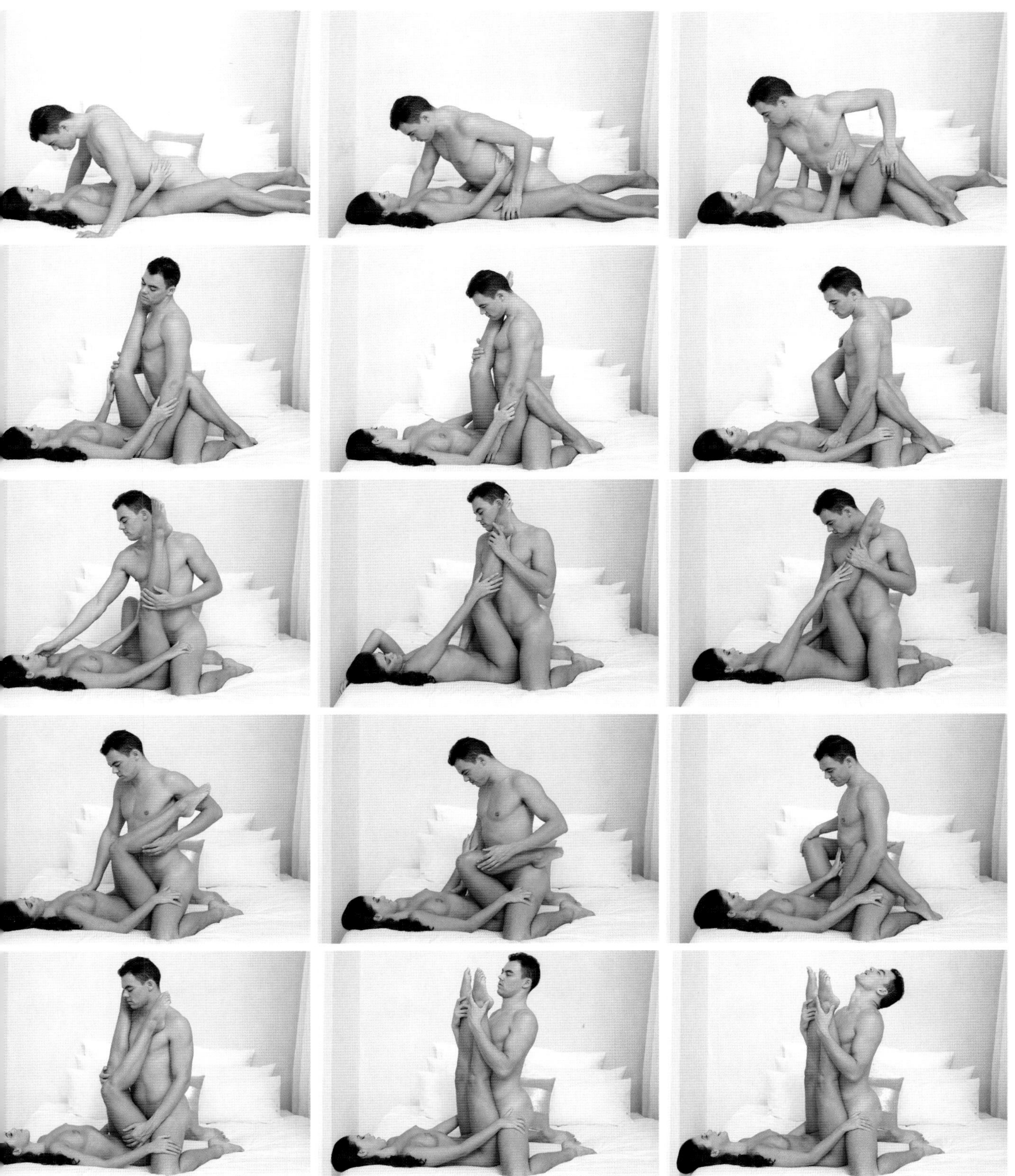

Supported congress

☆☆ Kama sensation rating

This position is made for when you're dancing together at a party and lust overcomes you. You slip off to your host's tiny bathroom/broom closet, and she presses him against the wall. Before you know it, she has her leg around his waist and you're in Supported Congress.

Why it works

– As long as your genitals are height-aligned, he can make a sudden thrilling entrance. If she's a little shorter than him, he can try squatting to compensate.

– Even if he can't penetrate, he can rub his penis against her clitoris.

– Supported Congress is fast and impulsive, and it makes you feel incredibly sexy.

– If you're disturbed in a public place, it's easy to dismount, adjust your clothes, and prepare your excuses or getaway.

– If you're doing it at home, it's an ideal position for role play.

Turn on...

... Use this position to kiss, make out, and writhe. Use it for clandestine, height-of-passion sex. If you have no reason to be clandestine, pretend. Use role play to create naughty scenarios.

Turn off...

... Don't expect an easy or quick orgasm in Supported Congress. This position is about pressing close and savouring the connection.

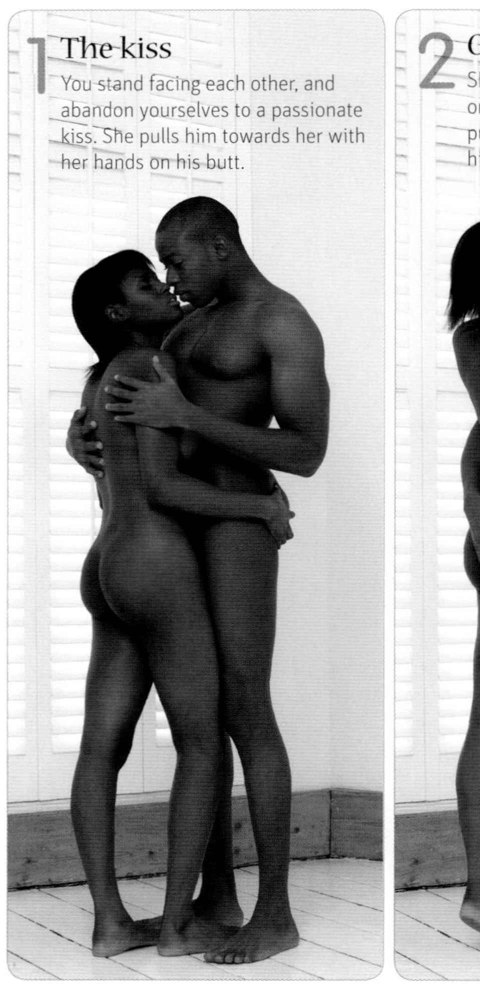

1 The kiss

You stand facing each other, and abandon yourselves to a passionate kiss. She pulls him towards her with her hands on his butt.

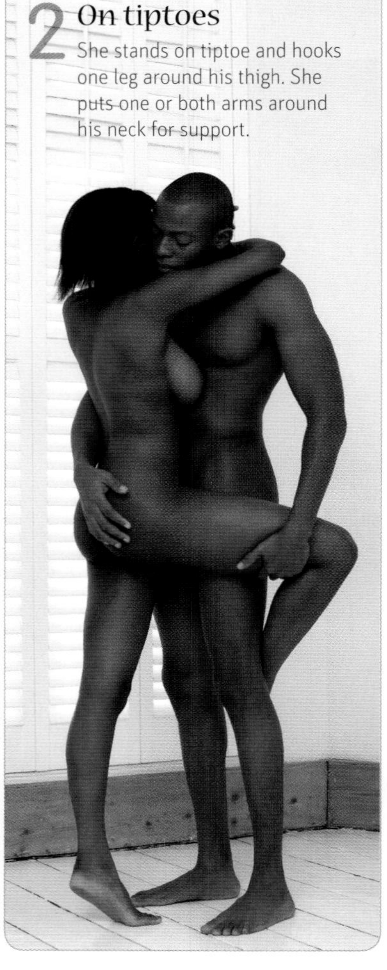

2 On tiptoes

She stands on tiptoe and hooks one leg around his thigh. She puts one or both arms around his neck for support.

"A man should gather from the actions of the woman of what disposition she is, and in what way she likes to be enjoyed." KAMA SUTRA

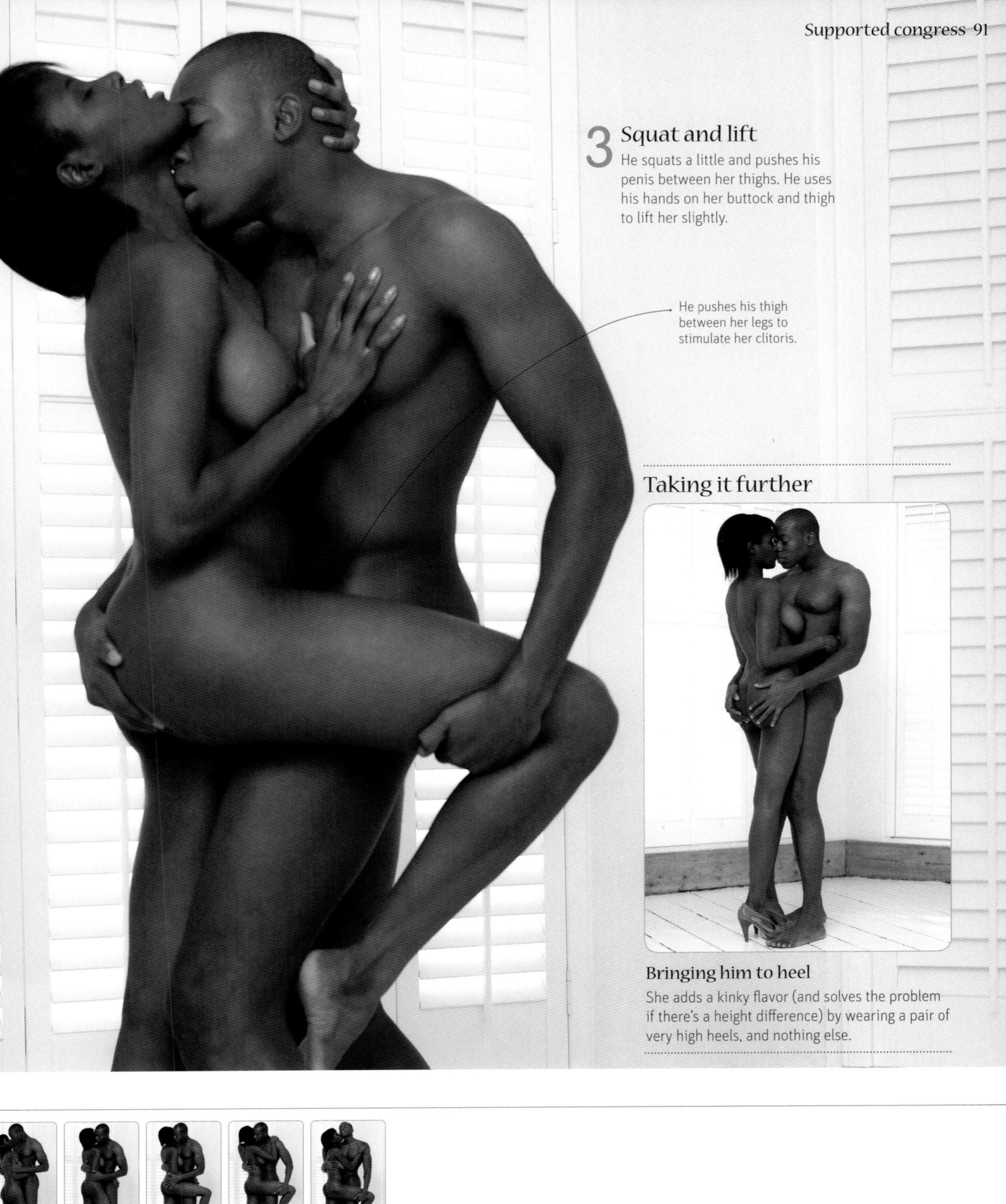

3 Squat and lift

He squats a little and pushes his penis between her thighs. He uses his hands on her buttock and thigh to lift her slightly.

He pushes his thigh between her legs to stimulate her clitoris.

Taking it further

Bringing him to heel

She adds a kinky flavor (and solves the problem if there's a height difference) by wearing a pair of very high heels, and nothing else.

The stopperage

☆☆☆☆ Kama sensation rating

Next time you have sex, grab some cushions from the sofa and slip them under her ass. This will raise her pelvis high and produce sublime sensations for both of you. In fact, after The Stopperage, you'll look at cushions in a whole new light.

Why it works

– Her pelvis is raised by one or more cushions, so it's easy for him to slide into her, and the angle of penetration is a winner.

– Her vagina is contracted because her knees are drawn up to her chest. This creates a fantastically tight fit between the two of you.

– She can slip her fingers between her legs if she wants extra clitoral stimulation.

– Although you don't have full body contact, you can enjoy plenty of face-to-face intimacy.

– You get romance combined with intense erotic sensation.

1 Cushion support

She lies back on the bed and lifts her hips so that he can slide a cushion under her ass.

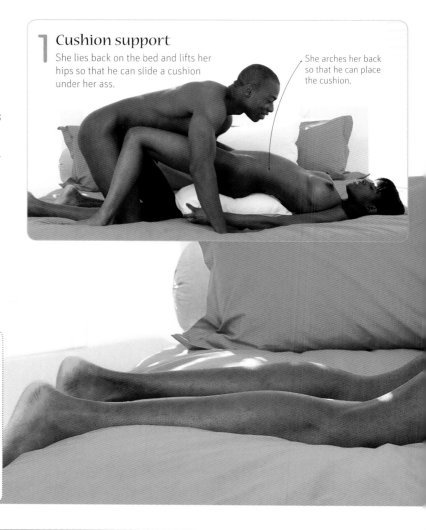

She arches her back so that he can place the cushion.

Turn on...

... Spend a few moments positioning the cushions underneath her, to get the right height and angle. Make sure that the cushions go under her ass, not the small of her back, so that her pelvis tilts slightly toward the ceiling.

Turn off...

... Don't penetrate too deeply until she's fully aroused. As the *The Perfumed Garden* points out, this position can be painful for the woman.

"Introduce your member and draw her toward you at the moment of ejaculation." THE PERFUMED GARDEN

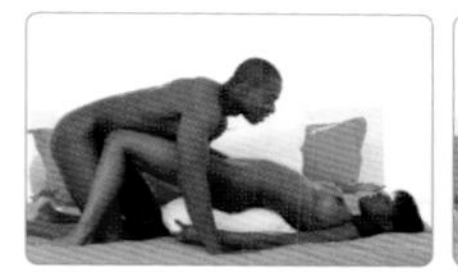

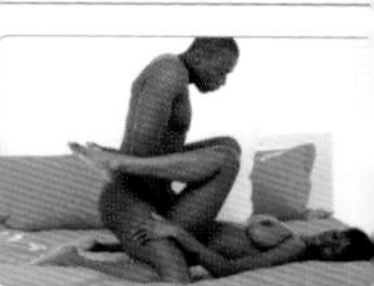

2 Knees to chest

She bends her legs and pulls her knees up toward her chest as he penetrates gently.

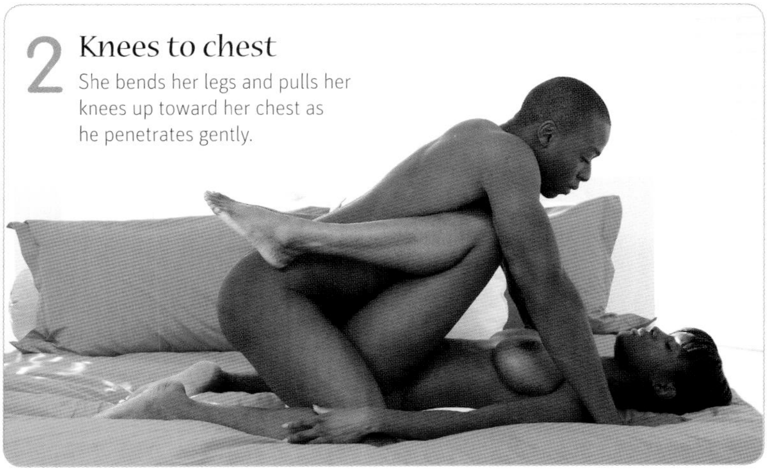

Taking it further

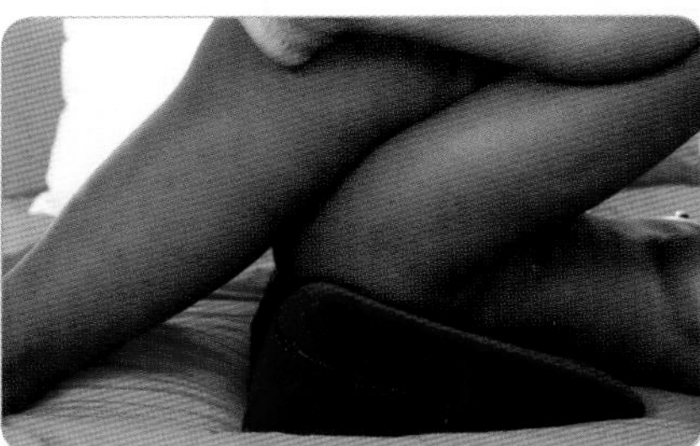

The perfect angle

She puts a "sex wedge" under her hips so that he can enter at the perfect angle. (You can find then in online sex stores under "sex furniture".)

3 Going deeper

He leans over her body and puts his hands on either side of her. He thrusts deeply as you both relax into the position.

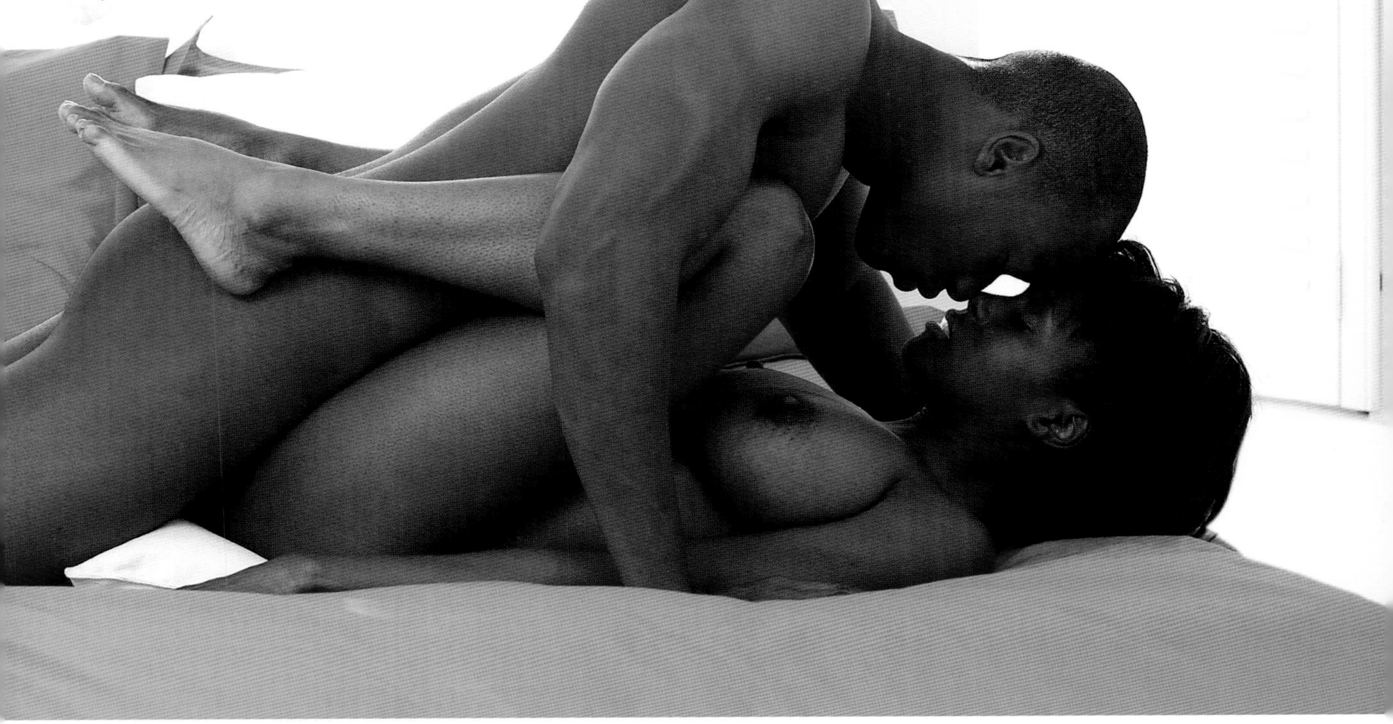

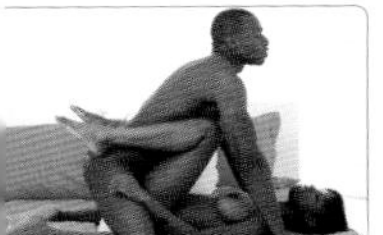

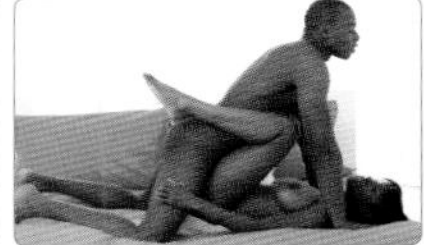

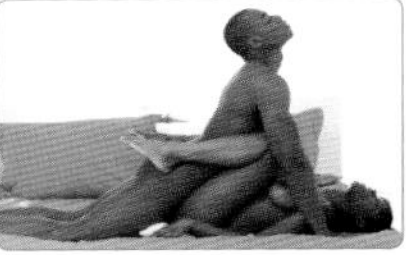

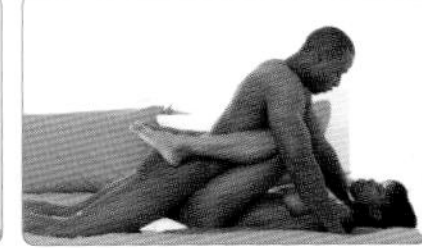

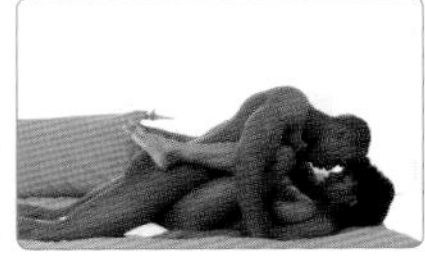

Cat and mouse sharing a hole

☆☆☆☆☆ Kama sensation rating

This is a perennial favorite for both men and women. She loves it because the freedom of movement often guarantees her an orgasm. He loves it because he gets to witness her enjoyment close-up. Plus his penis benefits from all the good work she's doing on top.

Why it works

– She can angle herself for maximum pleasure: if the head of his penis hits the front wall of her vagina, it massages her G-spot; if it rubs against the back wall, it stimulates her PS-spot (PS stands for "perinial sponge," a sensitive area just beneath her perineum).

– Sustained friction between her clitoris and his pubic bone (or his abs, if he's been working out) can help to make this position super-climactic for her.

– It's tender at first, building to a hot crescendo.

– He can satisfy his lust by grabbing her ass and moving her in tight circles on top of him.

Turn on...

... Keep your hands busy on her body. Pull her closer. Stroke her back, buttocks, and thighs. Fondle her breasts if there's space.

Turn off...

... Don't try any fancy massage strokes when she's on the home stretch to orgasm. Any handwork at this point (however sensual) could distract her from the crucial sensations down below.

1 The drape

You both kiss as he lies on his back. She lies beside him, her body partly draped over his.

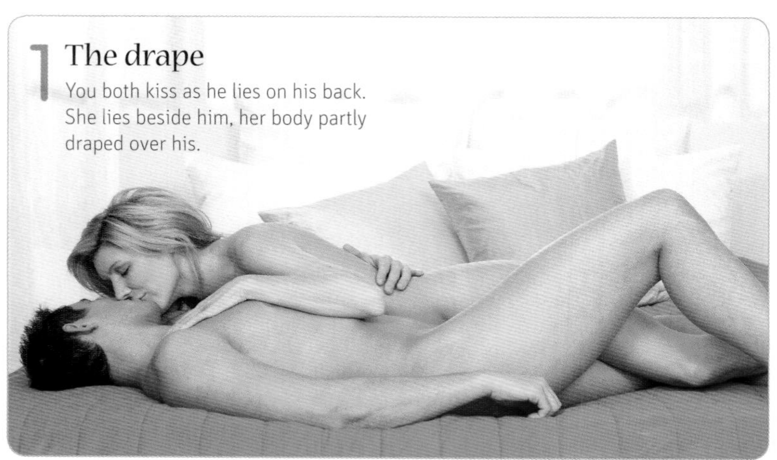

2 Face-to-face cuddle

She slowly eases herself on top of his body as things get hotter. She guides him into her and lies on top of him in a face-to-face cuddle.

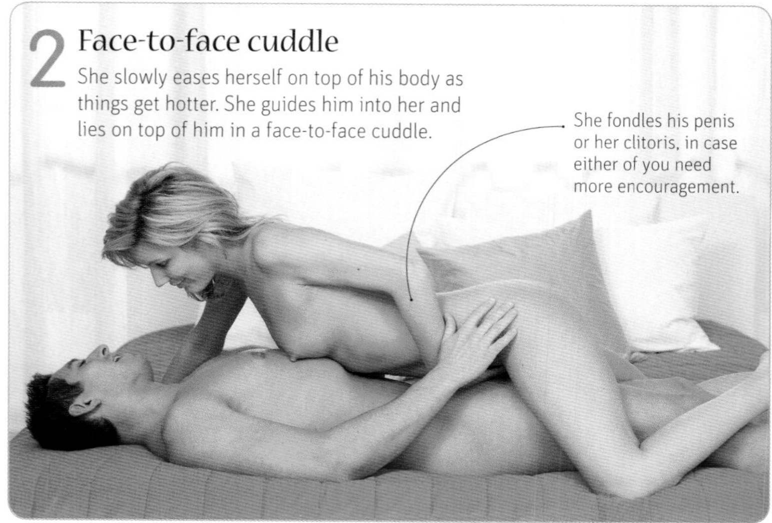

She fondles his penis or her clitoris, in case either of you need more encouragement.

"A man can learn everything about a woman—her personality and what she likes sexually—from the ways she moves when she's on top." KAMA SUTRA

Taking it further

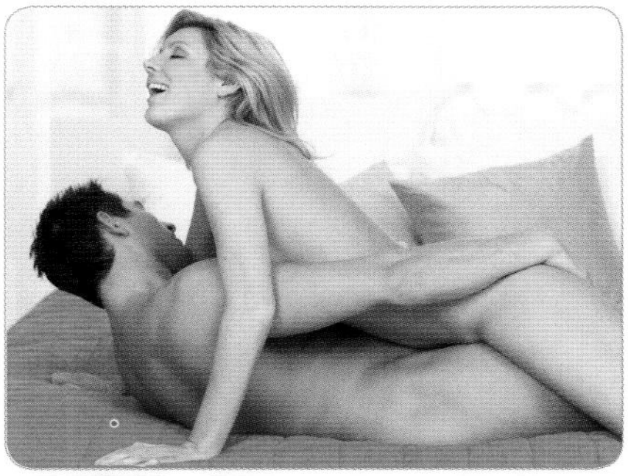

Rear stimulation

He smoothes his palms over the curves of her buttocks and strokes her perineum with his fingertips to tip her over the edge.

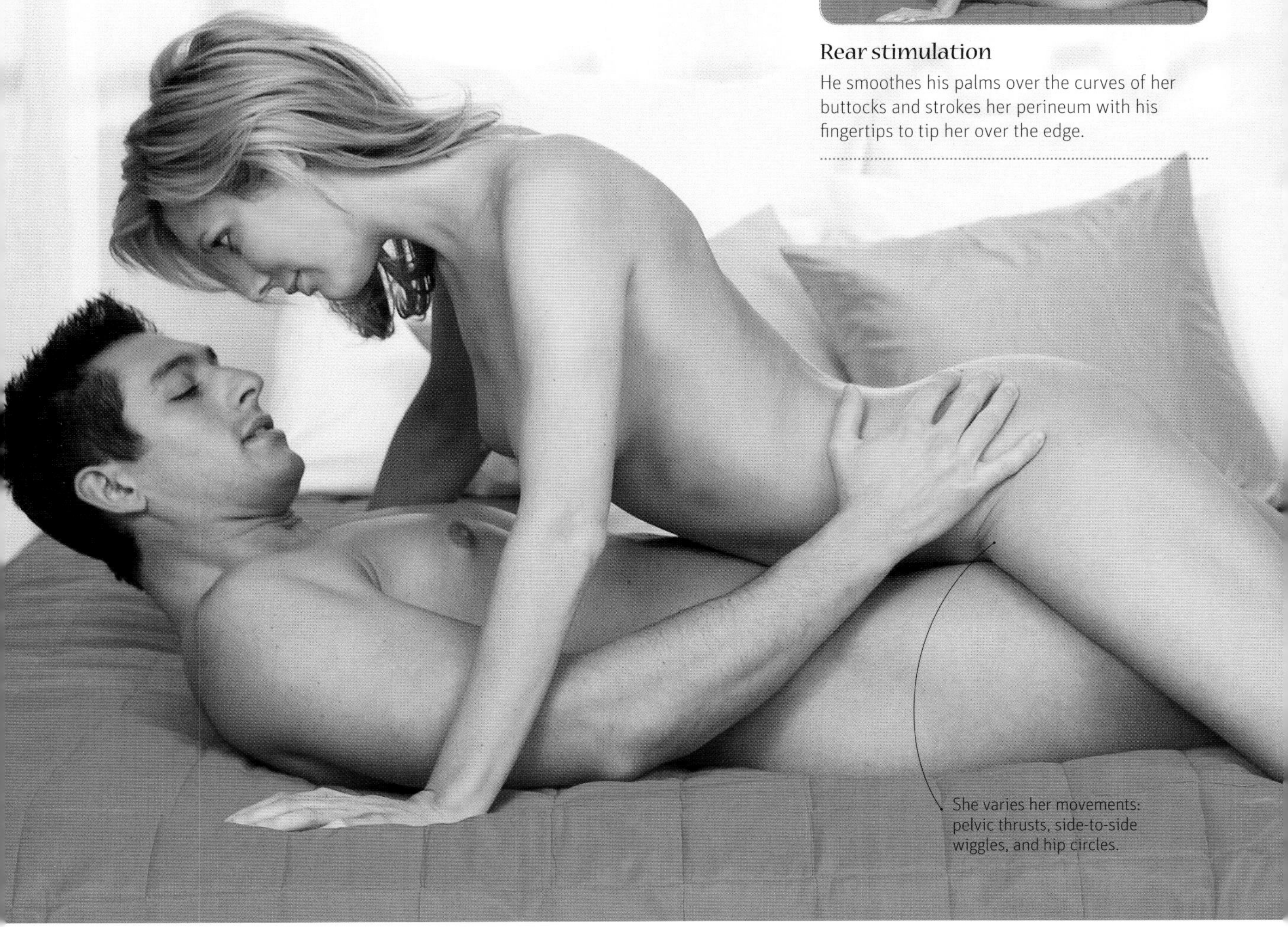

3 Chest raise

She lifts her head and chest so that he can see her breasts and she can move freely. She keeps her thighs outside his.

She varies her movements: pelvic thrusts, side-to-side wiggles, and hip circles.

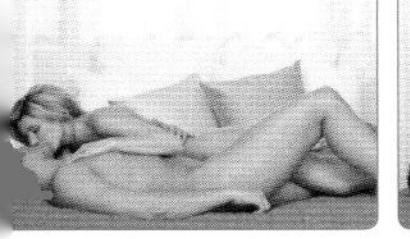
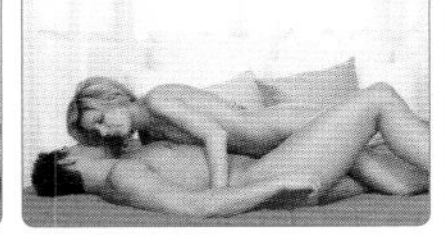
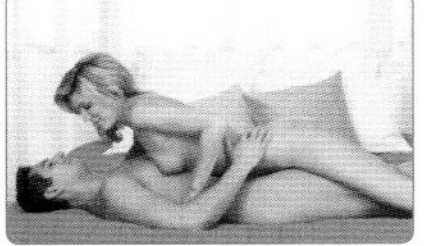
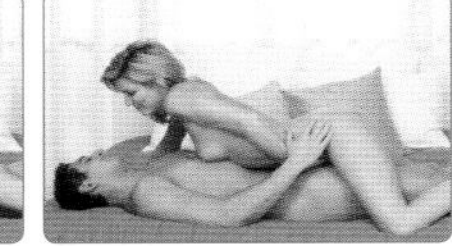
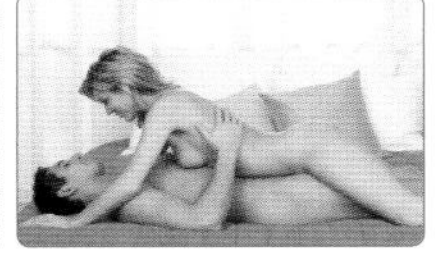
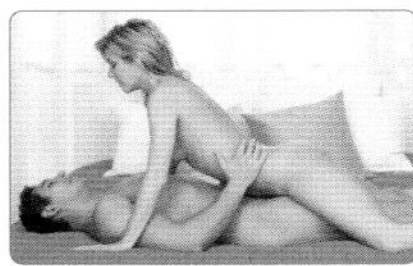

Coitus from behind

☆☆☆☆ Kama sensation rating

This rear-entry position has the same lush sensuality, intimacy, and skin-to-skin contact that you'd get if you were facing each other, but the fact that you're not makes it a touch naughtier. As always with rear-entry sex, the sense of anonymity can be thrilling.

Why it works

– The front wall of her vagina gets nudged on each thrust, so her G-spot is thoroughly stimulated every time he moves.

– He experiences the joy of deep penetration plus warm and sensual skin contact along the front of his body.

– She can sink blissfully into the bed as he surrounds her in a loving full-body embrace.

– If you're into role play, she can be the innocent virgin seduced as she lies in her bed.

– This position is ideal for both vaginal and anal sex, and it feels more comfortable than being on all fours.

Turn on…

… Use plenty of lubricant on your penis and on her anus if you're having anal sex. And make your entry smooth and slow, especially if your lover is new to anal penetration.

Turn off…

… Don't follow anal sex with vaginal sex until you've washed thoroughly. This is to avoid spreading bacteria that can cause infection.

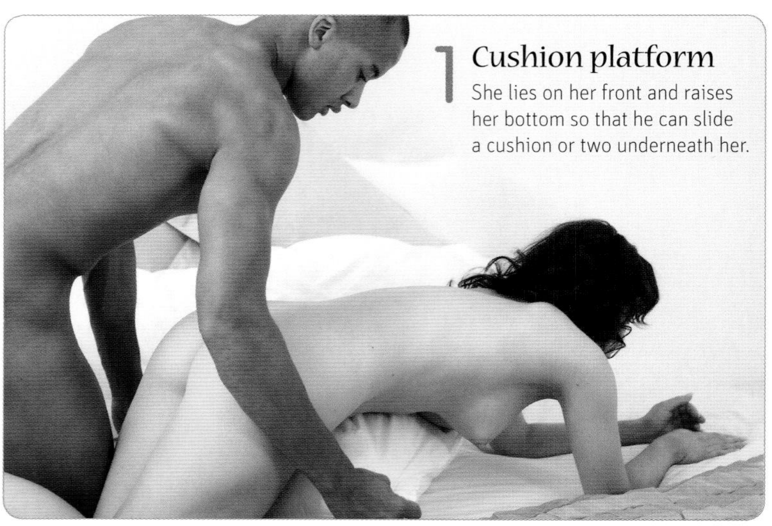

1 Cushion platform
She lies on her front and raises her bottom so that he can slide a cushion or two underneath her.

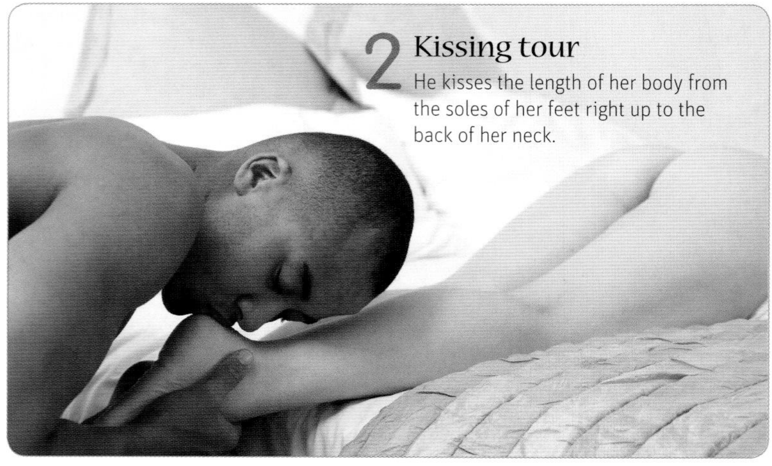

2 Kissing tour
He kisses the length of her body from the soles of her feet right up to the back of her neck.

"The people from the South participate in 'sex below'— penetration of the anus." KAMA SUTRA

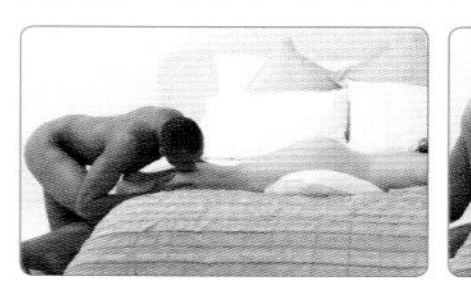

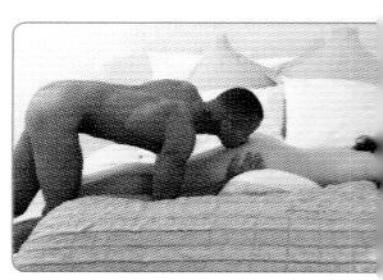

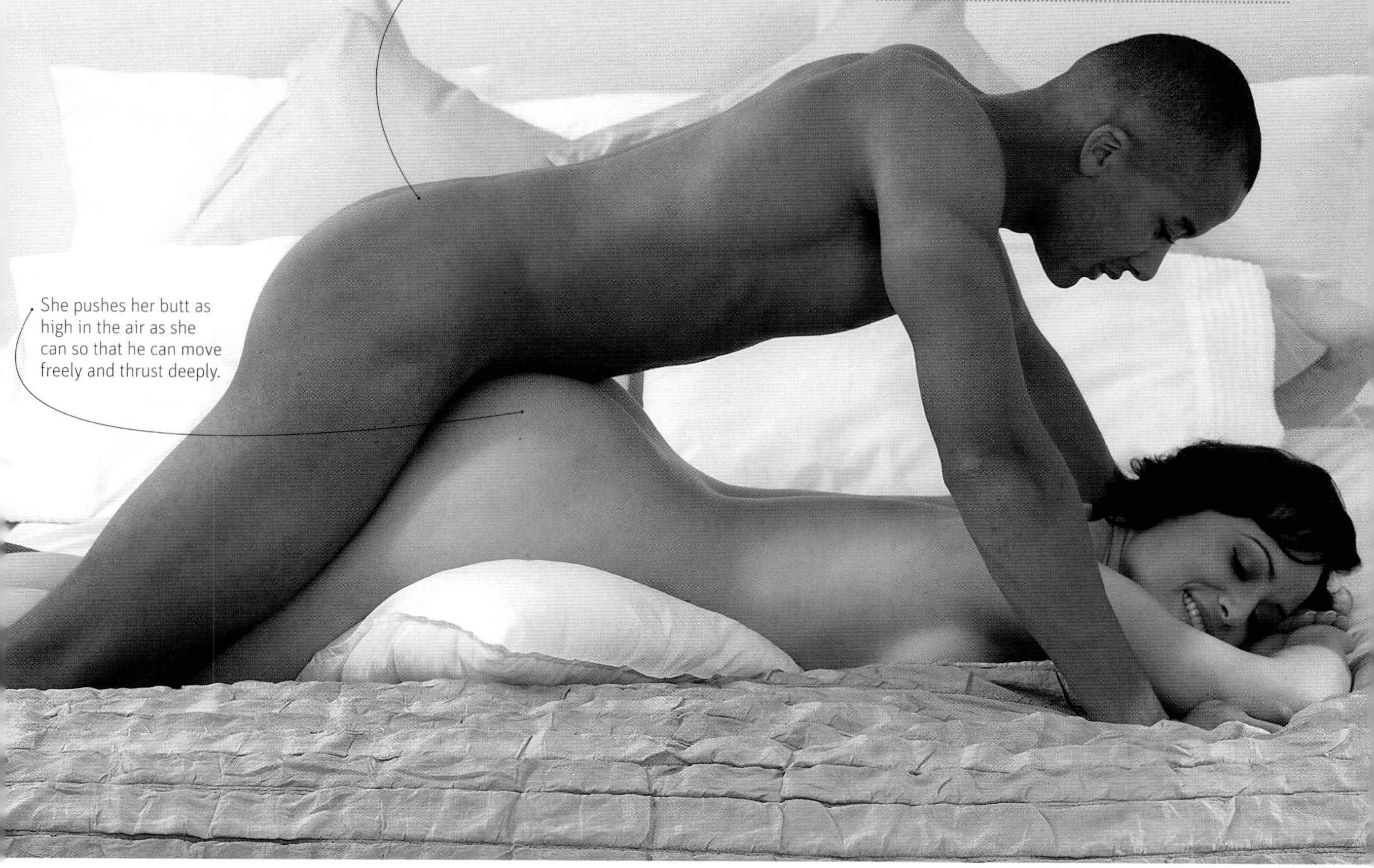

Taking it further

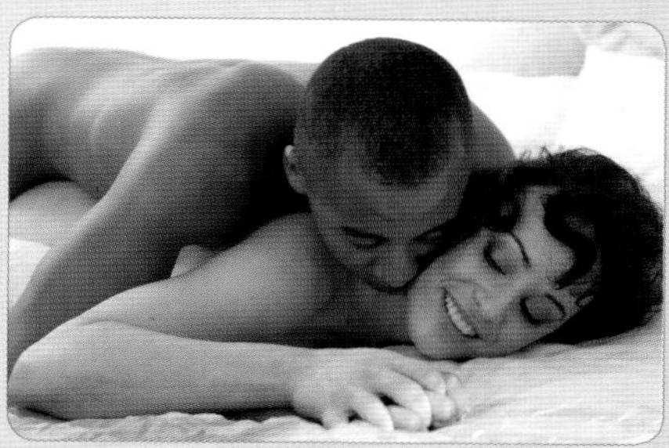

Increasing intimacy

He nestles his face into her neck for maximum sensuality. This introduces a touch of intimacy and tenderness to this rear-entry position.

3 Open and enter

When his head is level with hers, she opens her legs to let him in. He penetrates her deeply.

He pauses for a moment after penetration so that you can both savor the sensations.

She pushes her butt as high in the air as she can so that he can move freely and thrust deeply.

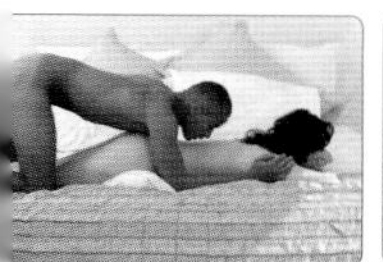 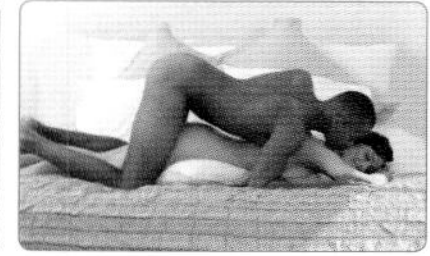 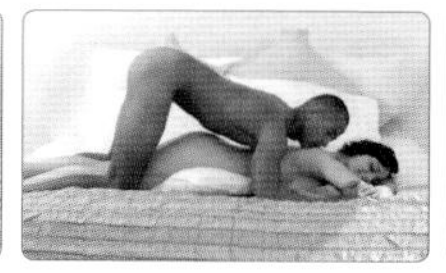 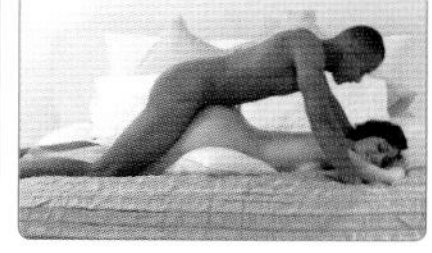 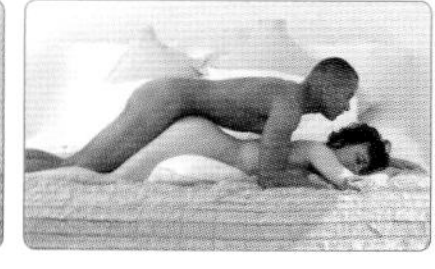 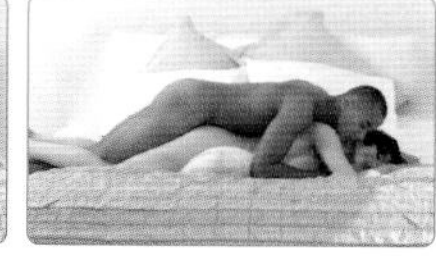

Huge bird above a dark sea

☆☆☆ Kama sensation rating

If she's usually the one to call the sexual shots, try this position in which he's clearly in charge. After some gentle seduction, he fixes her with a wicked glint in his eye, moves in with precision accuracy, and plunges his huge bird into her dark sea.

Why it works

– Her legs are widely open, so he can caress her clitoris with the tip of his penis before making a grand, sweeping entrance.

– She can lie back, let go, and trust him to make the moves.

– You each have opposite roles, which ramps up the sexual tension. She's passive and vulnerable; he's active and predatory.

– He leans over her body, but doesn't crowd her, which is perfect for sustained eye contact right up to orgasm.

– Her hands are free, so she can put them to good use on herself or him.

Turn on...

... Make the position comfortable so that you can stay in it for as long as you want. For example, he can sit on his heels to take the strain off his thighs, and she can dangle her legs over his arms.

Turn off...

... Don't make so many adjustments that you lose the dynamic tension of him hovering over her, which can be a real turn-on for both of you.

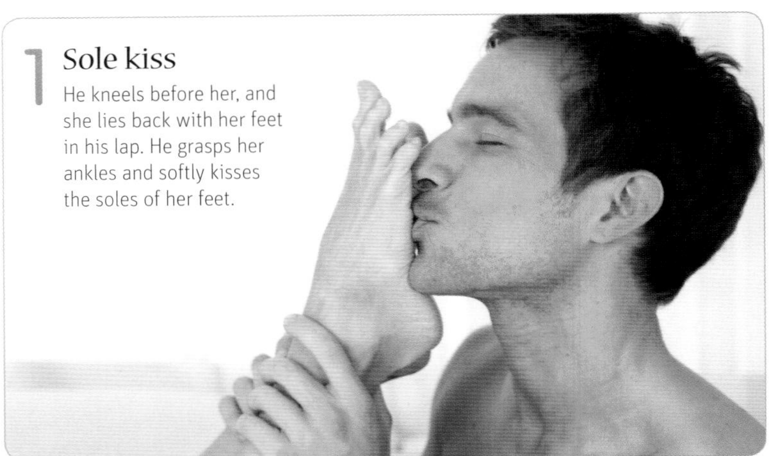

1 Sole kiss
He kneels before her, and she lies back with her feet in his lap. He grasps her ankles and softly kisses the soles of her feet.

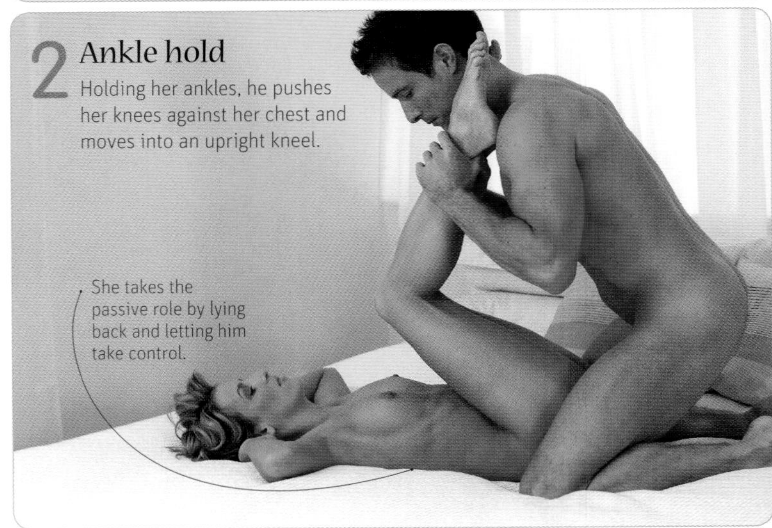

She takes the passive role by lying back and letting him take control.

2 Ankle hold
Holding her ankles, he pushes her knees against her chest and moves into an upright kneel.

"During the first coupling the man's sexual energy is fierce and he lasts only a short duration..." KAMA SUTRA

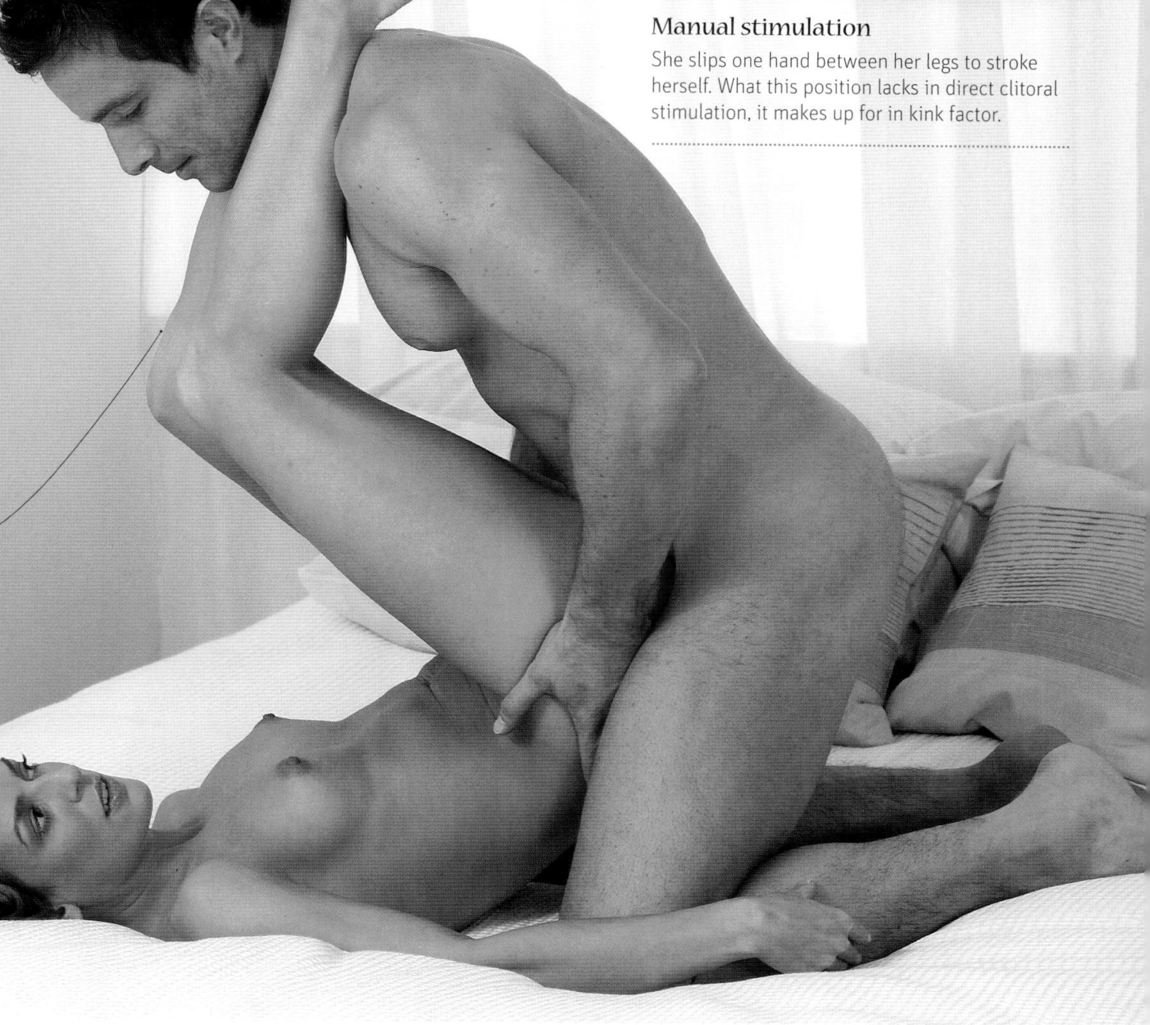

Taking it further

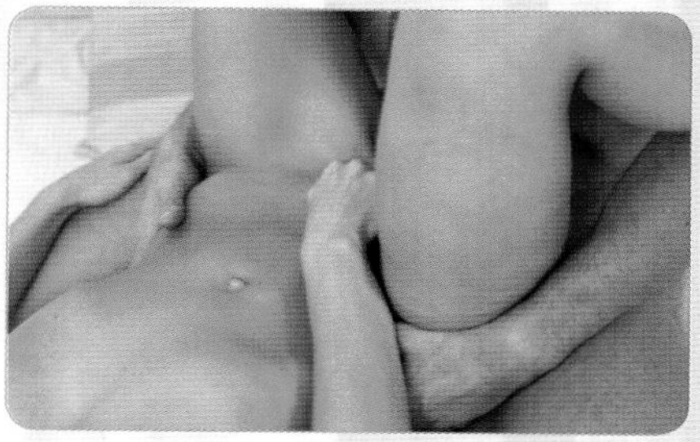

Manual stimulation

She slips one hand between her legs to stroke herself. What this position lacks in direct clitoral stimulation, it makes up for in kink factor.

3 Hands on buttocks

He slides his hands down her legs to firmly grasp her buttocks. He lifts her on to the slope of his thighs and penetrates her.

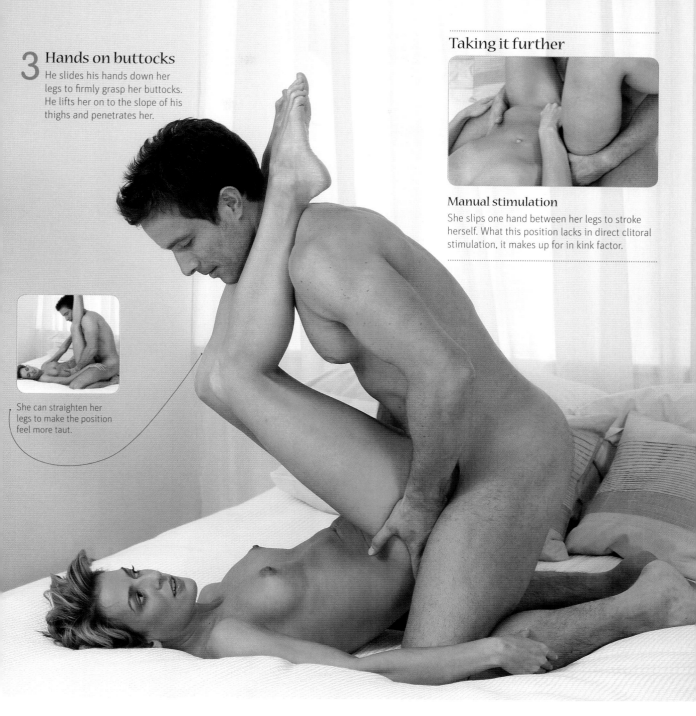

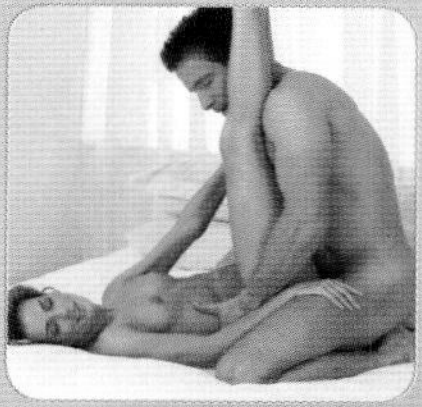

She can straighten her legs to make the position feel more taut.

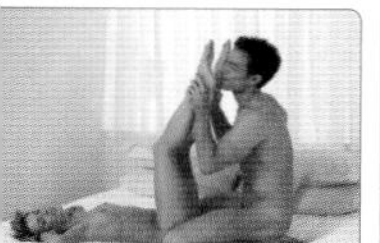
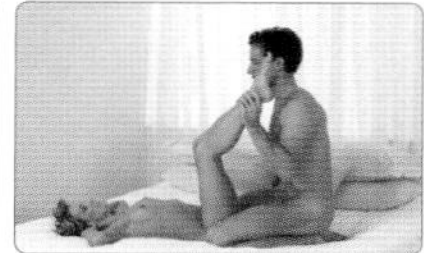
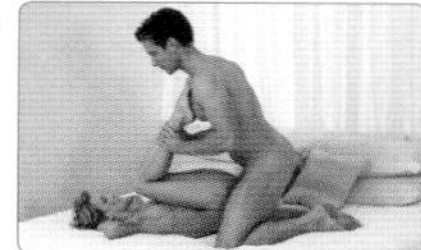
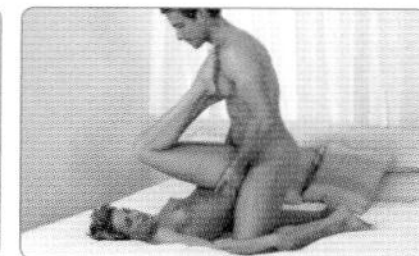
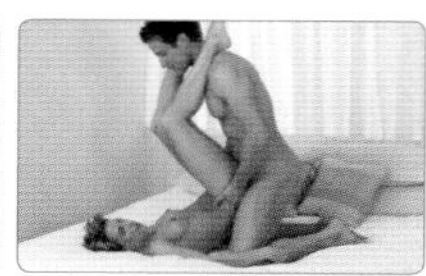

The frog

☆ Kama sensation rating

This is a try-it-and-see position. Depending on your build and flexibility, he may struggle to get close enough to penetrate. If you can't make it work, it's easy for her to get up and straddle him. If it does work: congratulations. You've mastered one of the trickier sex positions of the East.

Why it works

- Because he can't penetrate her effortlessly, you need to liaise closely in achieving the position. This is great for overcoming shyness and getting to know each other (if you didn't already).
- Because you can't thrust in and out, you'll have the sexy task of experimenting to find novel ways of moving.
- It's warm and tactile; you have no choice but to hang on tight to each other.
- It's compact, so you can do it in spaces where sex would otherwise be impossible (the closet/the bathroom/the car).

Turn on...

... Use it as a chance to explore each other's bits with your hands if you can't actually penetrate. Sitting opposite each other with your legs apart is the perfect position for looking and touching.

Turn off...

... Don't spend ages trying to assume the position. If you're in the mood for sitting-up sex, try straddling him while he sits on a chair instead.

1 Intimate stroking

You sit opposite each other on the bed or floor, touching and stroking each other's hot spots.

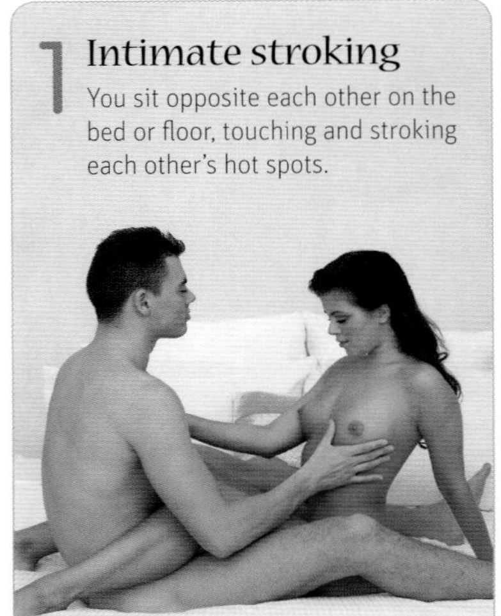

2 Enclosed embrace

He bends his knees and puts his feet flat on the bed or floor. He encloses her between his legs.

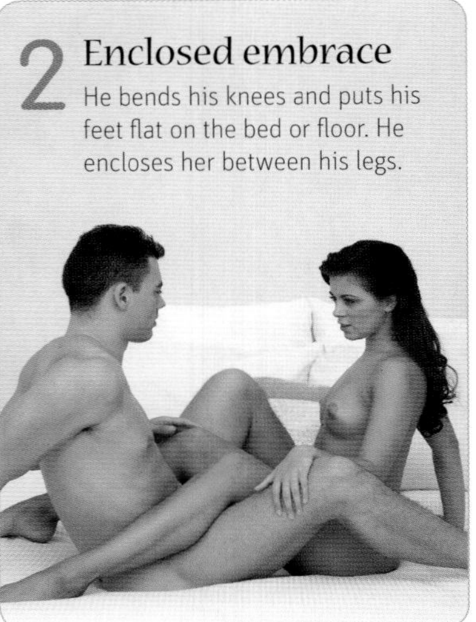

3 Cheek to cheek

She bends her knees and draws them close to her chest. She presses her ass close to his.

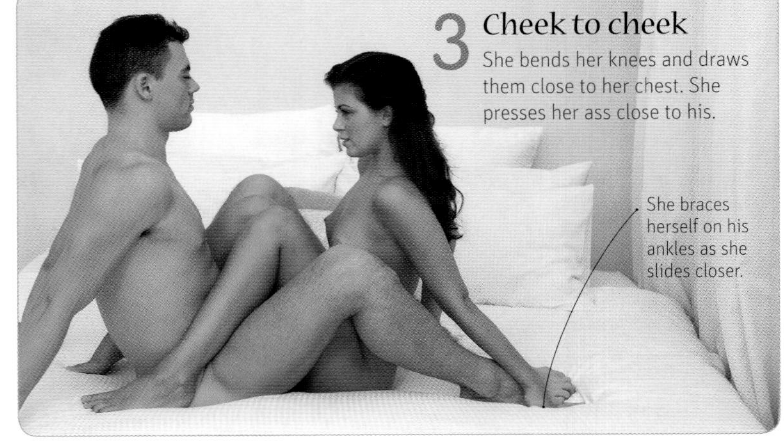

She braces herself on his ankles as she slides closer.

"Her passions being thoroughly aroused, she finds the orgasm more violent, and then she is thoroughly contented." ANANGA RANGA

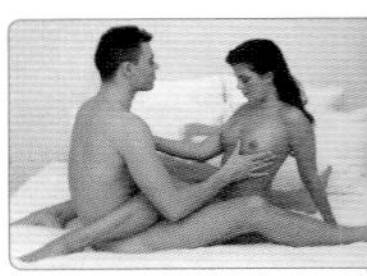

4 Wiggle and penetrate

You both wiggle into a position where he can penetrate her, she leans back, and he moves her back and forth with his hands on her shoulders.

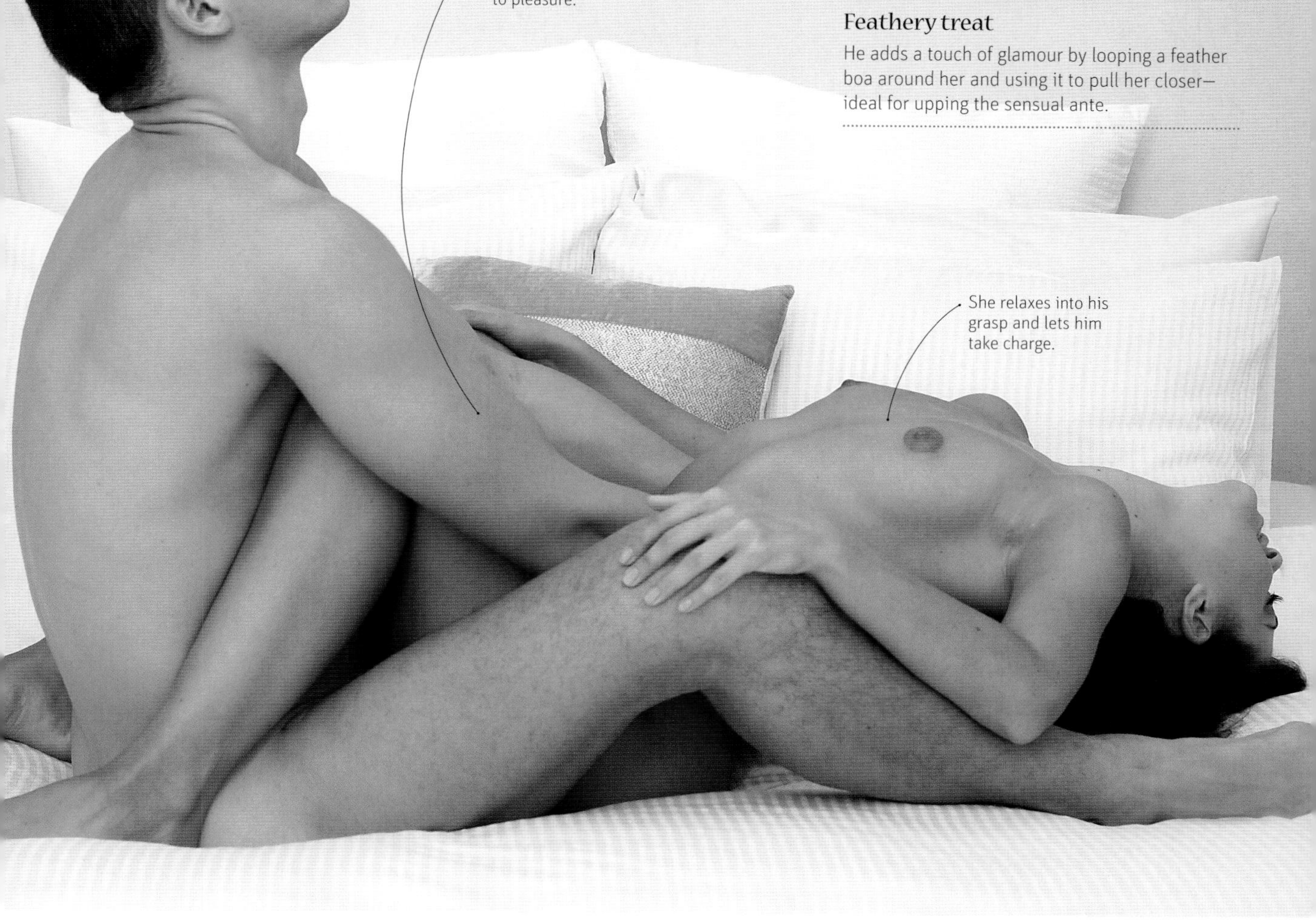

He holds her firmly so that she can lean back and abandon herself to pleasure.

She relaxes into his grasp and lets him take charge.

Taking it further

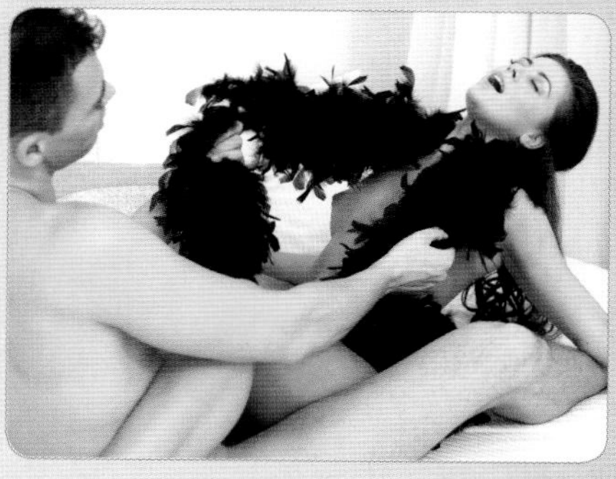

Feathery treat

He adds a touch of glamour by looping a feather boa around her and using it to pull her closer—ideal for upping the sensual ante.

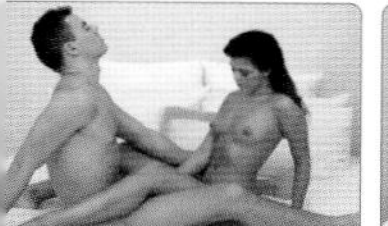
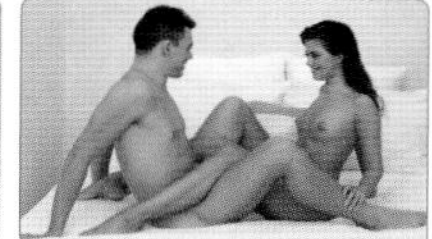
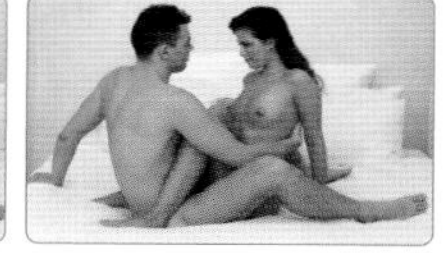
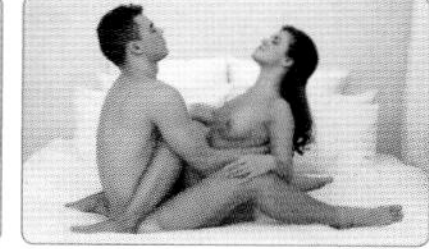
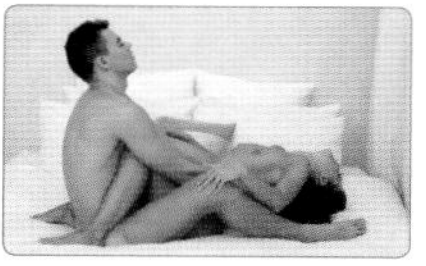

The congress of the elephant

☆☆☆☆ Kama sensation rating

Two mating elephants may not be your idea of erotic heaven, but this animal-inspired position is surprisingly sexy, and can deliver tingling G-spot sensations for her. Try it when she feels submissive, and he wants to play the dominant role.

Why it works

- His penis hits her G-spot squarely on each stroke. This increases her chance of having an explosive vaginal orgasm.
- He can look down and get the porn-style thrill of seeing his penis pumping in and out.
- She enjoys the erotic vulnerability of being taken from behind. He gets a kick out of doing the taking.
- He can move freely because his thrusts are cushioned by her buttocks.
- You can't see each other's faces, so it's easy to abandon your inhibitions and concentrate on pure pleasure.

Turn on...

... Focus on the G-spot sensations on the front wall of your vagina. Some women have vaginal orgasms or even ejaculate from G-spot massage.

Turn off...

... Don't worry if it feels uncomfortable. The G-spot is near the urethra, so you may feel like you need to pee. It's often possible to break through this initial discomfort into a whole new world of pleasure. But don't get stressed if you can't.

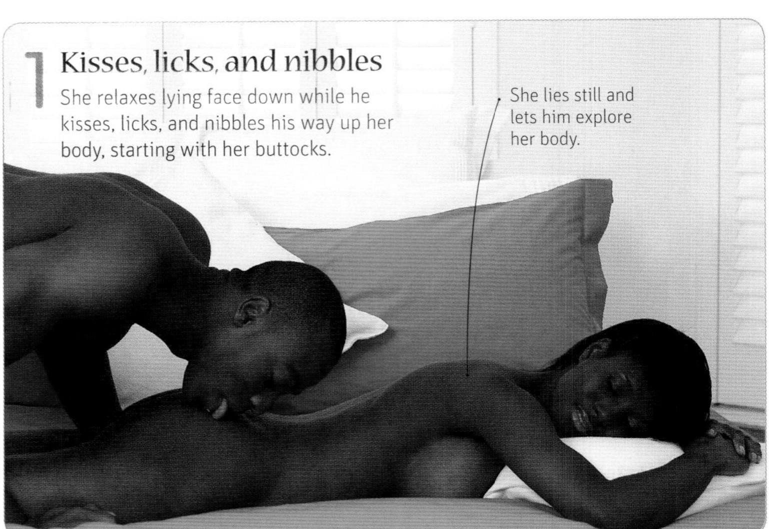
She lies still and
lets him explore
her body.

1 Kisses, licks, and nibbles
She relaxes lying face down while he kisses, licks, and nibbles his way up her body, starting with her buttocks.

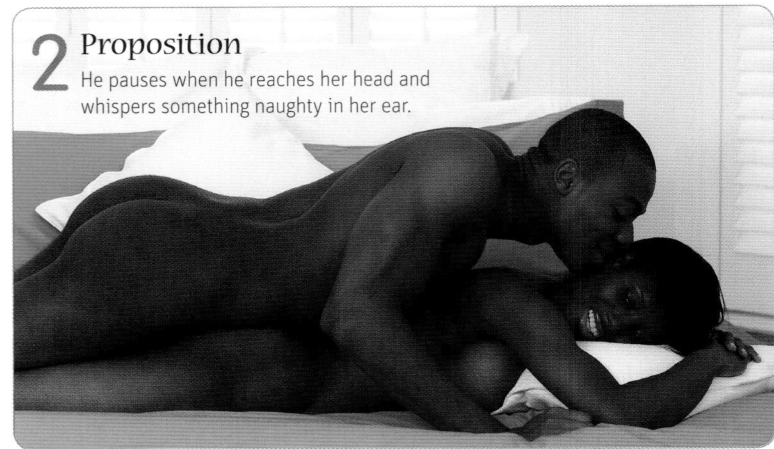

2 Proposition
He pauses when he reaches her head and whispers something naughty in her ear.

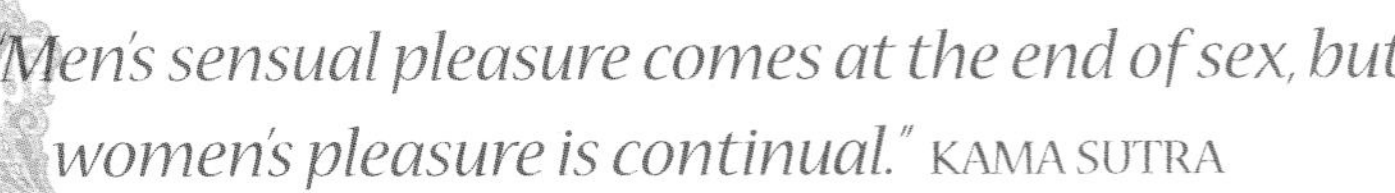

"Men's sensual pleasure comes at the end of sex, but women's pleasure is continual." KAMA SUTRA

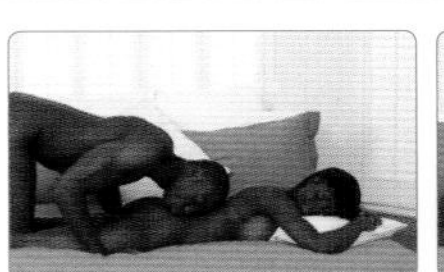

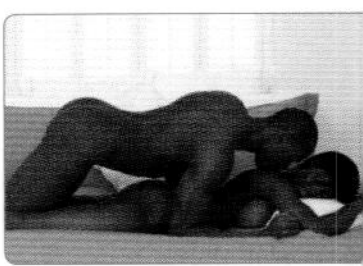

Taking it further

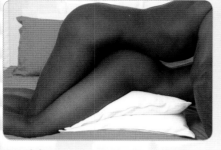

Butt lift

He gets better access if she pops some cushions under her hips to raise her butt in the air. This also improves the angle for G-spot stimulation.

He can take a break to lie close to her body and kiss the side of her face before he begins act two.

3 Penetration

He supports himself on his hands in a half push-up position and guides his penis into her.

She contributes to the movements by writhing against him.

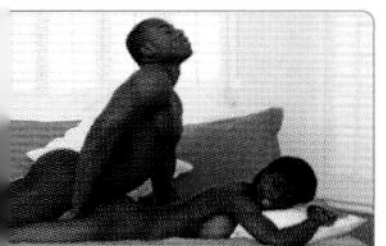
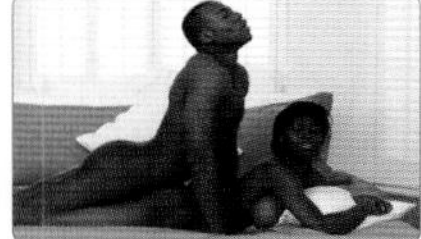
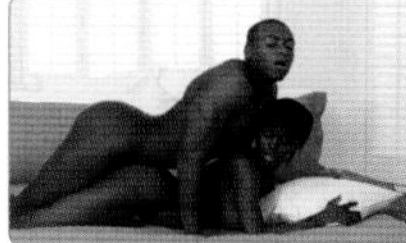
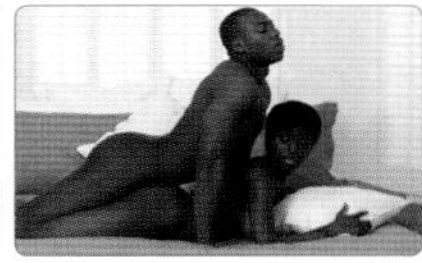
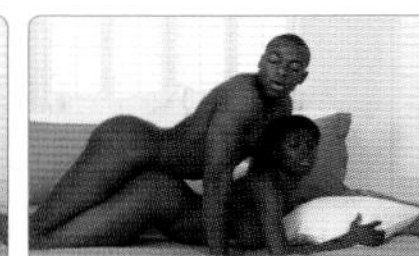
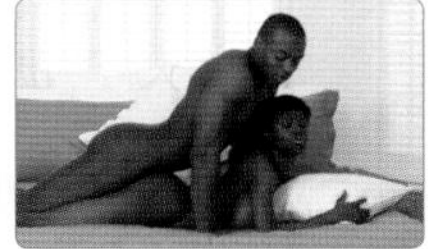

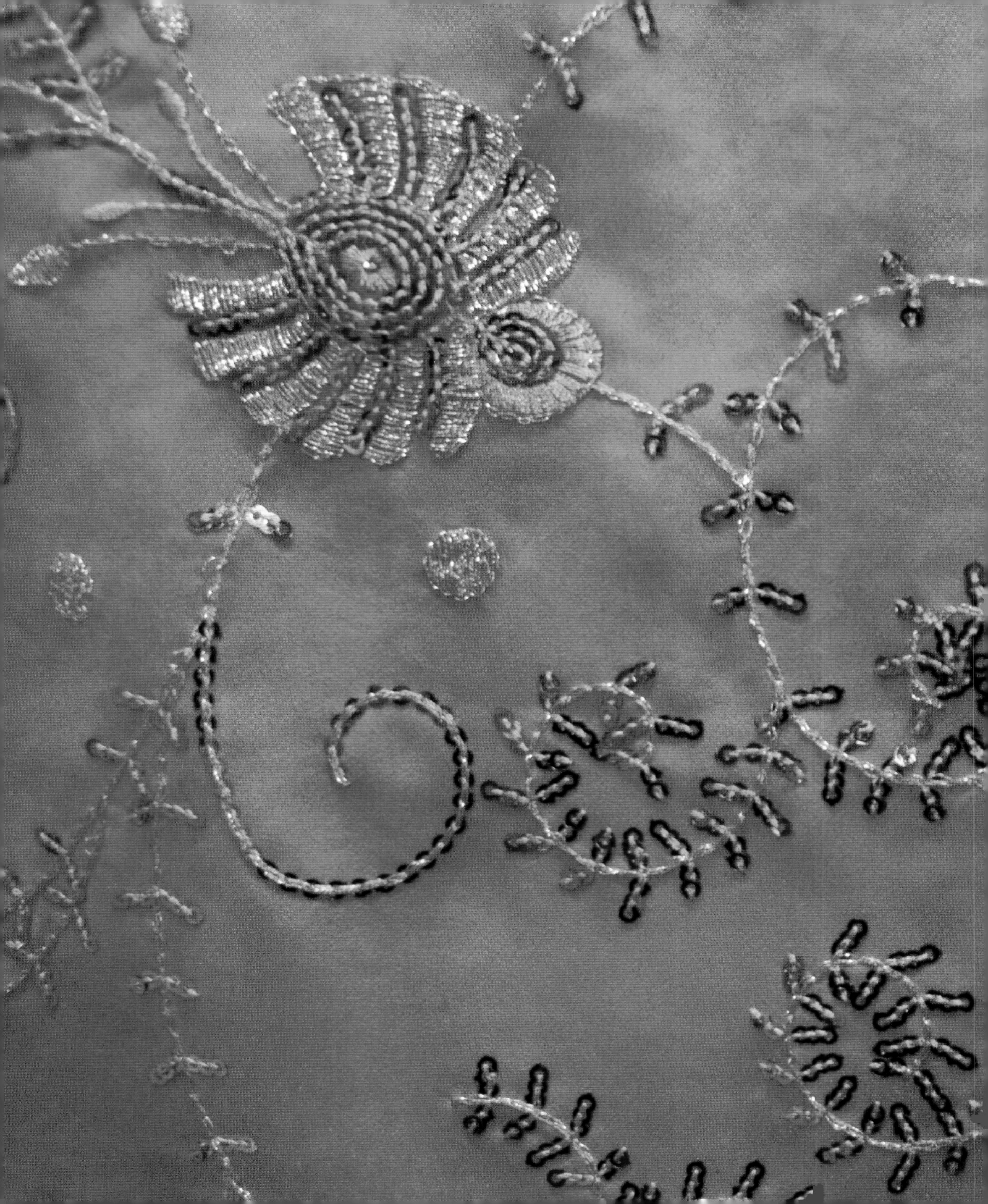

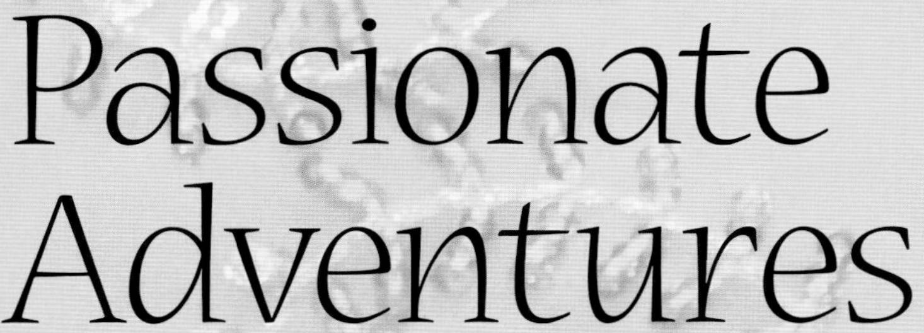

Passionate Adventures

If your lust is bucking like a wild horse, you're in the right place; these positions are intended to gallop you and your lover straight to the finishing line. Try positions such as the Tiger Step and Late Spring Donkey when you're super-hot and insatiable. Forget the rules about foreplay; throw each other on the bed and get on with it.

Sprinkled throughout the chapter are some more sedate positions, which are equally intense but not so demanding on the genitals, hips, and pelvis. When you want to concentrate on sensation without athletics, try postures such as The Lotus Position and Seagulls on the Wing.

Passionate adventures are always best in unfamiliar places, so take your lover's hand, and drag them out of bed and as far away as you can afford. If your budget won't extend to a five-star hotel, go to the nearest B&B, motel, or park bench (deserted, of course). At the very least, make it as far as the bathroom and do it in the shower. For plenty of other ideas on how to keep your passion varied, read on.

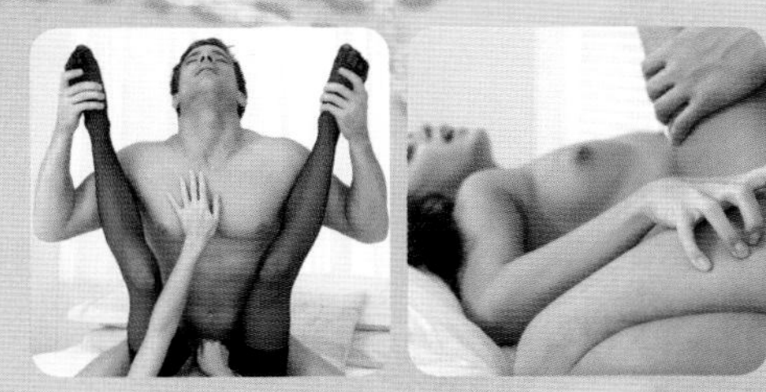

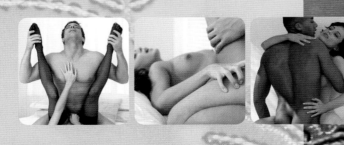

The encircling position

☆☆ Kama sensation rating

The power play of dominance and submission is a major turn-on in this position. She's knotted into position on her back as he bears down on her. The fact that she can't move unless he allows her to can be extremely arousing for both of you.

Why it works

– She gets an exhibitionist thrill of exposing her body as she lies with her knees drawn up to her chest.

– She's in a sexy trap that frees her from responsibility and performance pressure.

– The idea that he's free to "help himself" to her body is an instant arousal booster.

– He gets to see her in a titillating new position and from a new angle.

– It's a mild way of experimenting with bondage sensations. There are no ropes, chains, handcuffs, or knots; if you don't like it, you just unravel from the position.

Turn on...

... Experiment further if you like the idea of power play. Try tying her wrists together above her head to add to her feeling of helplessness.

Turn off...

... Trying this position if you don't have supple leg muscles and flexible hip joints. The idea is to be blissfully crushed beneath your lover, not inwardly screaming, "owwwww."

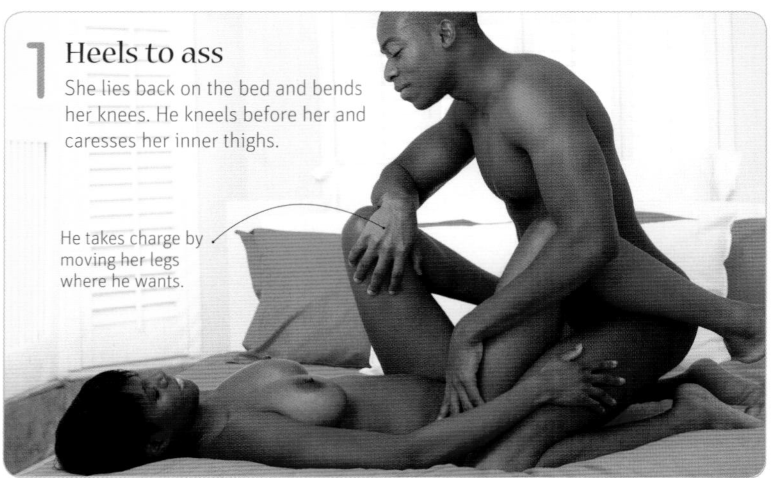
He takes charge by moving her legs where he wants.

1 Heels to ass
She lies back on the bed and bends her knees. He kneels before her and caresses her inner thighs.

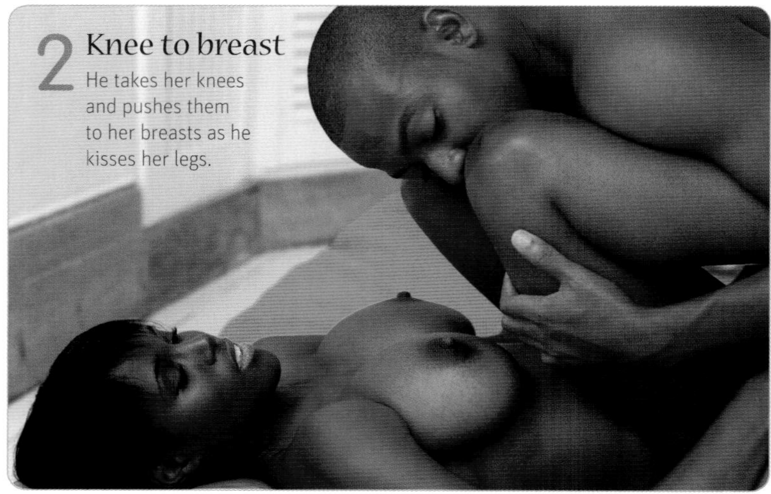

2 Knee to breast
He takes her knees and pushes them to her breasts as he kisses her legs.

"There takes place between them wrestling, intertwinings, a kind of animated conflict." THE PERFUMED GARDEN

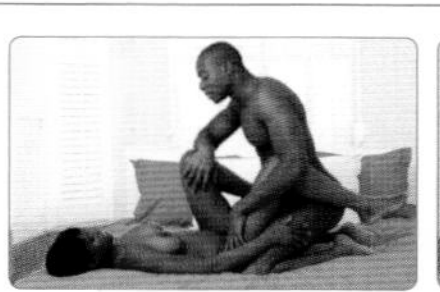

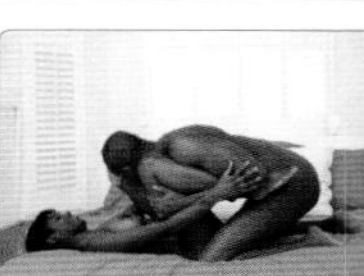

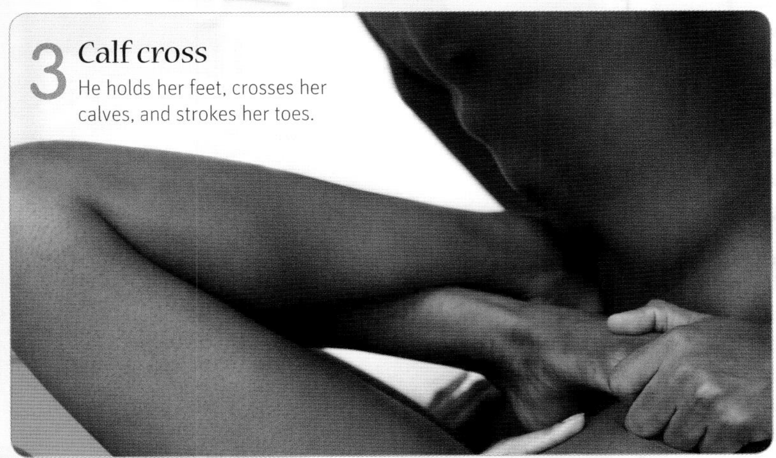

3 Calf cross

He holds her feet, crosses her calves, and strokes her toes.

Taking it further

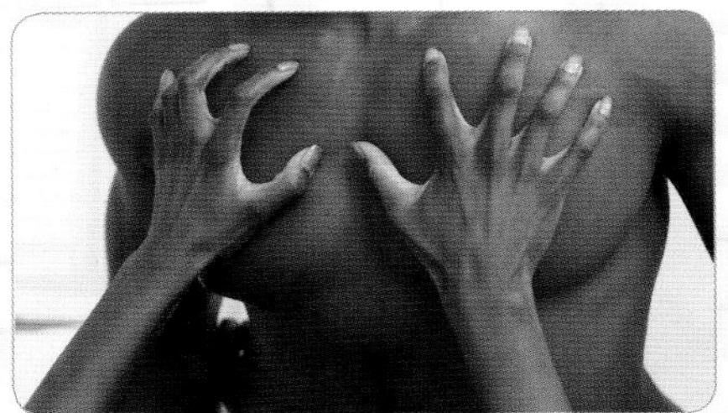

Letting out your inner beast

She gives him an animalistic thrill by raking her fingers over his chest (or her fingernails if she wants to make him squirm).

4 Leg press

He kneels over her body and enters her so that her crossed legs are crushed against her chest.

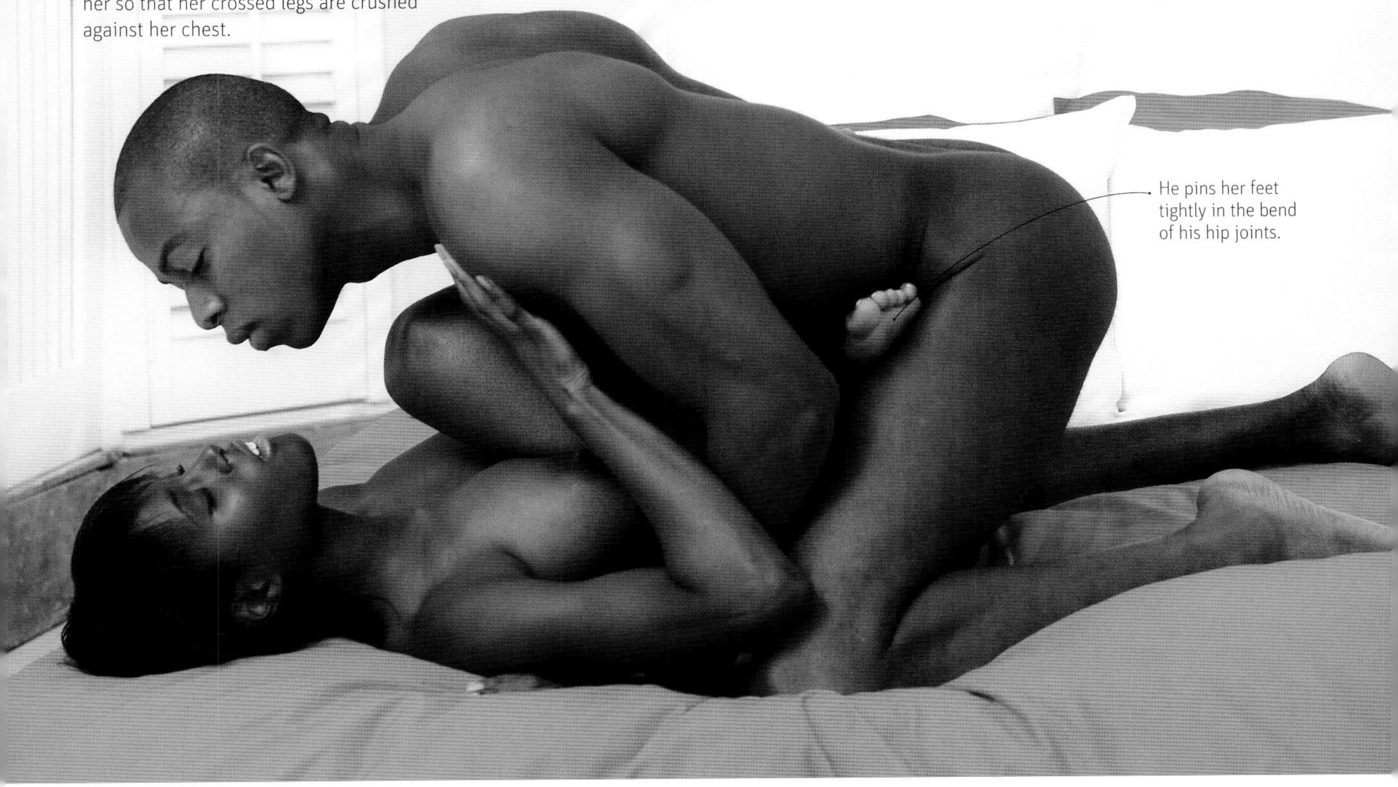

He pins her feet tightly in the bend of his hip joints.

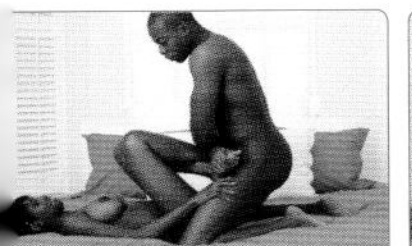
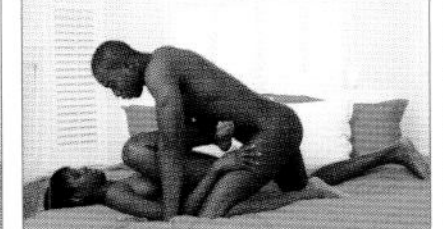
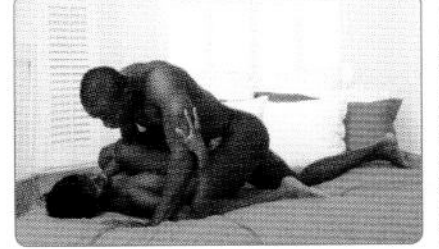
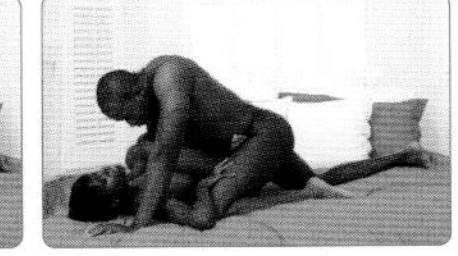
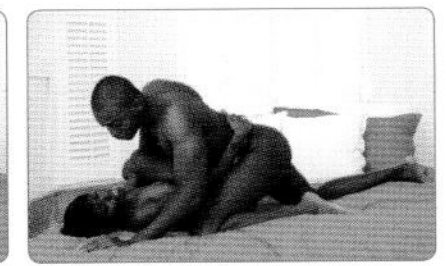
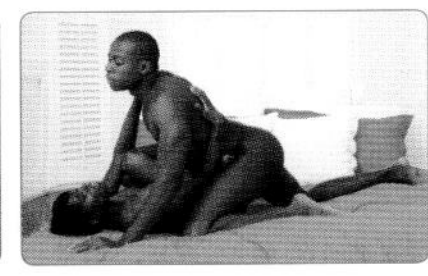

The fourth posture

☆☆☆☆ Kama sensation rating

The front of her body is tantalizingly exposed in this satisfyingly dramatic L-shaped position. This means that both of you can lavish succulent kisses and breathtaking caresses on all of her frontal pleasure zones from nipples to navel, collarbone to clitoris.

Why it works

– He controls her position on his lap, so he can maneuver her to a spot where he can slide easily and deeply into her.

– He gets a fantastic view of her legs, belly, breasts, neck, and face.

– It's highly stimulating for both of you, yet comfortable and restful, so you can use it for loving that's leisurely yet intense.

– It's the perfect position for her to have a blended orgasm. (This is a clitoral and a G-spot orgasm combined.) His penis supplies the G-spot/vaginal stimulation while his/her fingers work on her clitoris. Or either of you can use a vibrator.

Turn on...

... Be vocal. Give her an X-rated description of what you're going to do next. If you're still capable of speech, tell him what you're feeling. If you're not, an ecstatic "mmmmmmm" will do the job.

Turn off...

... Don't keep asking questions such as: "Does that feel good?" Too many questions and requests for reassurance are a notorious passion killer.

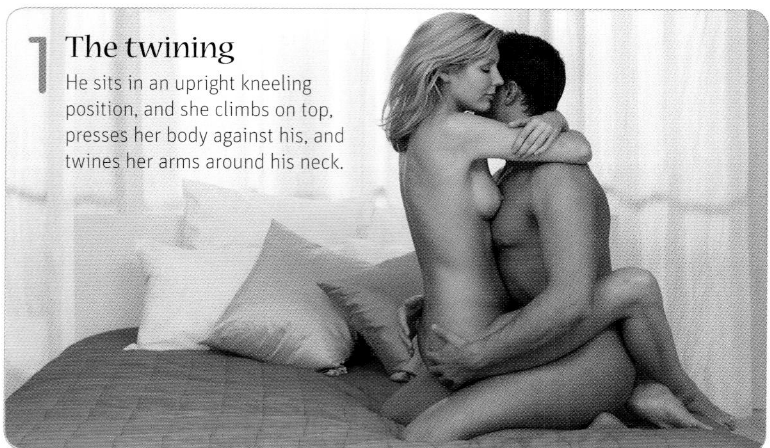

1 The twining
He sits in an upright kneeling position, and she climbs on top, presses her body against his, and twines her arms around his neck.

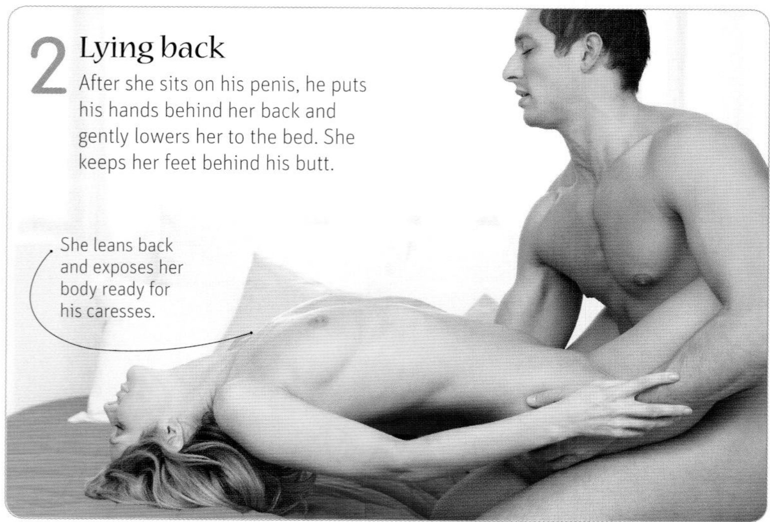

She leans back
and exposes her
body ready for
his caresses.

2 Lying back
After she sits on his penis, he puts his hands behind her back and gently lowers her to the bed. She keeps her feet behind his butt.

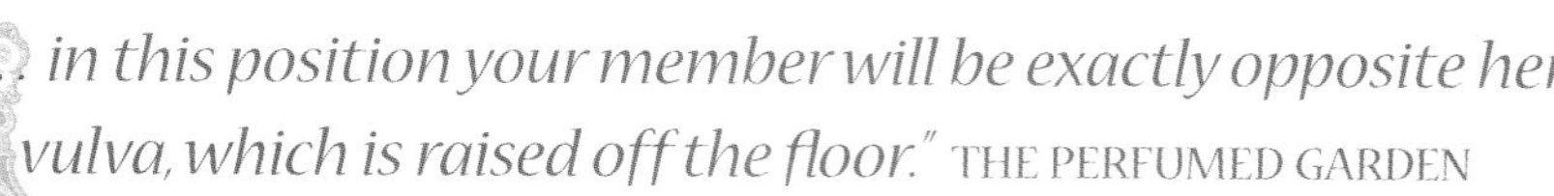

in this position your member will be exactly opposite her vulva, which is raised off the floor." THE PERFUMED GARDEN

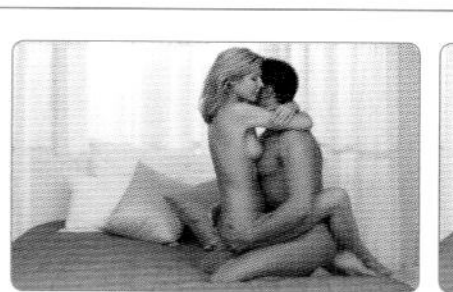

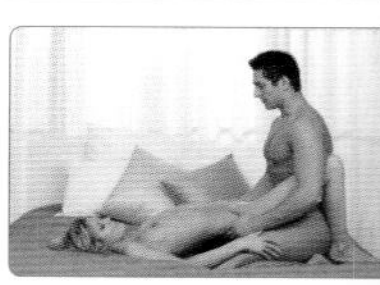

Taking it further

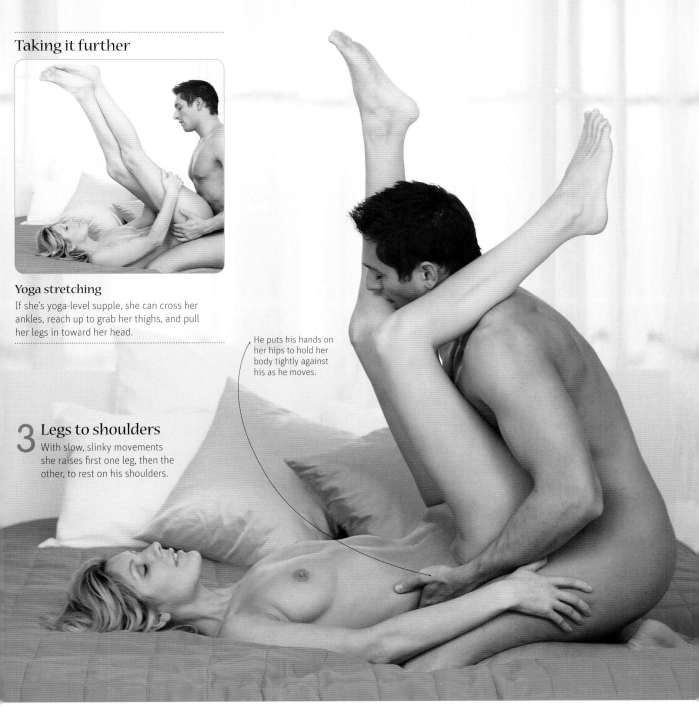

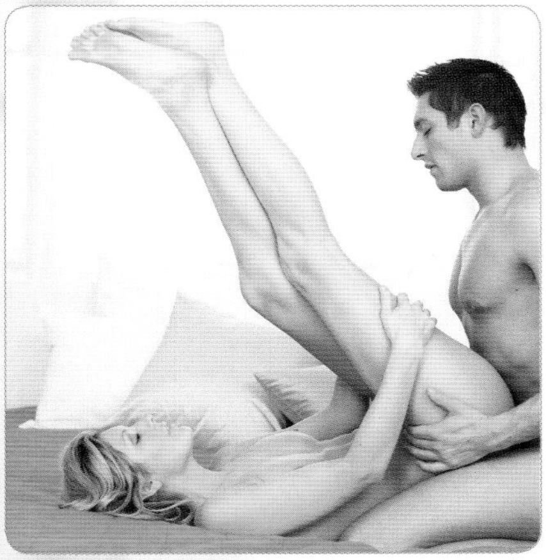

Yoga stretching

If she's yoga-level supple, she can cross her ankles, reach up to grab her thighs, and pull her legs in toward her head.

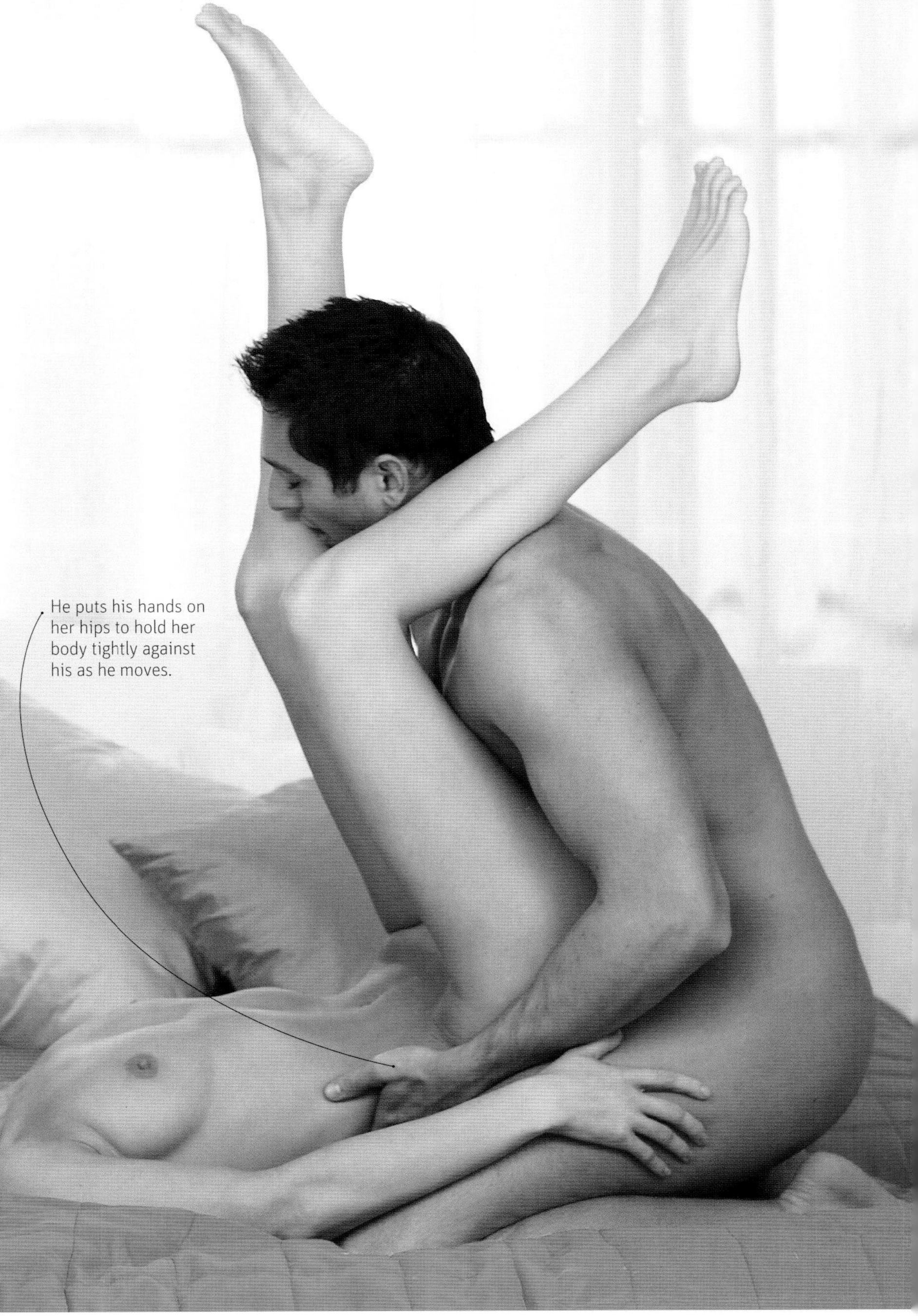

He puts his hands on her hips to hold her body tightly against his as he moves.

3 Legs to shoulders

With slow, slinky movements she raises first one leg, then the other, to rest on his shoulders.

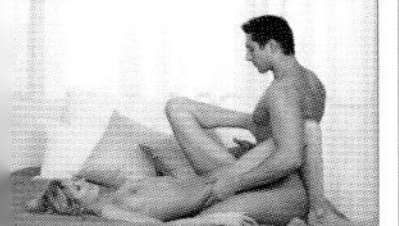
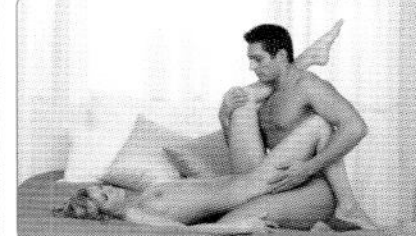
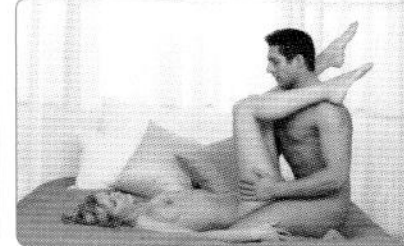
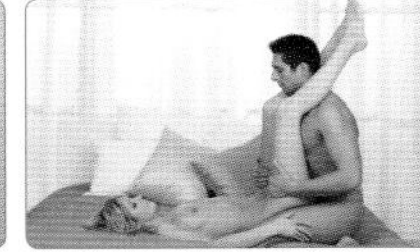
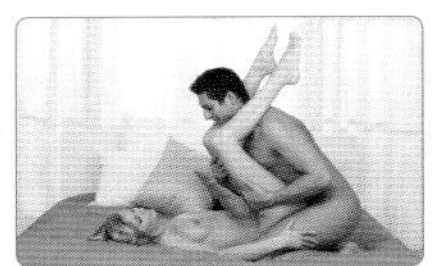
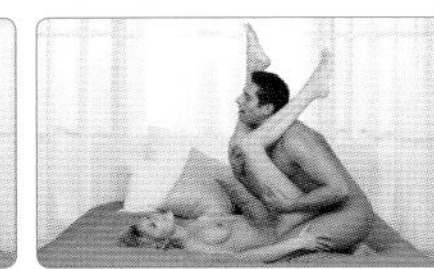

The intact posture

☆☆☆☆ Kama sensation rating

This is compact sex at its raunchiest: she lies on her back with her knees drawn up to her chest, and he gets on top and compresses her with his body. It's a good position for deep thrusting, with a frisson of domination to add extra adventure.

Why it works

– She has very little room to move around. Lying still is a great way to focus her mind on erotic intensity.

– His powerful presence above her is an electric turn-on if she's in a submissive mind-set or wants to let him take the lead.

– The barrier created by her legs delivers an erotic friction that he gets off on.

– He's aroused by being in control and able to move and thrust freely.

– Her hands are free to grip or grab his body as she gets closer to the summit.

Turn on...

... Take complete control in your dominant role. Position her body in the way you want. Give her firm instructions. Be confident and bold. If power play turns you on, take it a step further and build it into a dominant role-play scenario.

Turn off...

... Don't enter into dominant/submissive power play without first agreeing acceptable boundaries (especially if you use any restraining props, such as ropes or handcuffs).

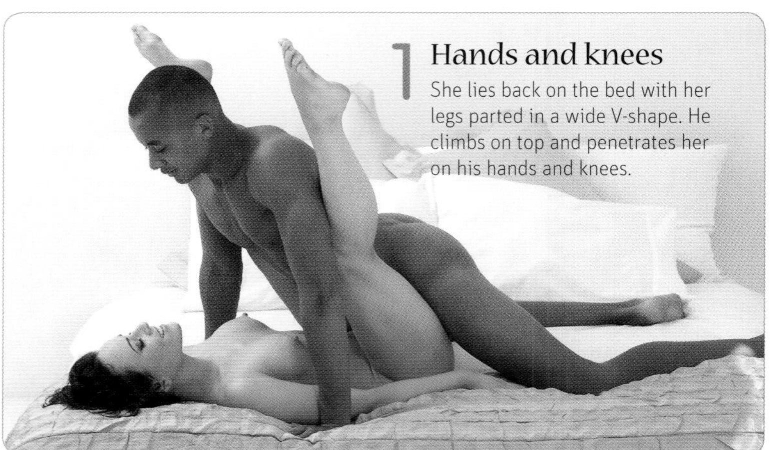

1 Hands and knees

She lies back on the bed with her legs parted in a wide V-shape. He climbs on top and penetrates her on his hands and knees.

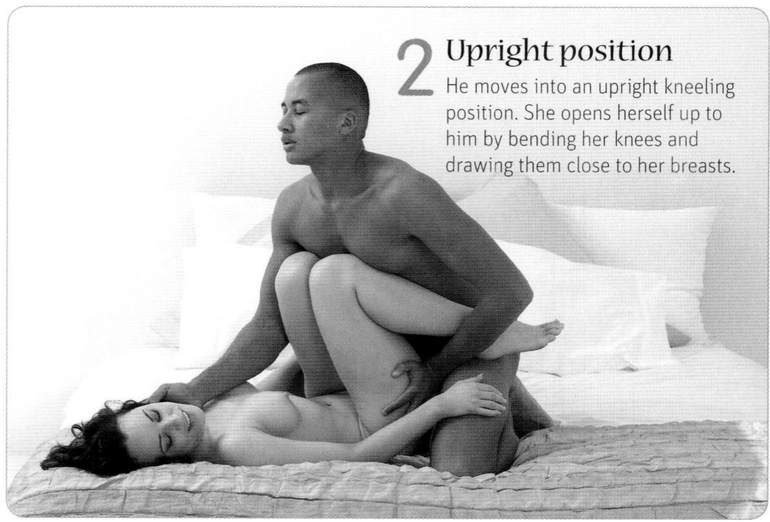

2 Upright position

He moves into an upright kneeling position. She opens herself up to him by bending her knees and drawing them close to her breasts.

"The man is aroused by the thought 'I am taking her', the woman by the thought 'he is taking me'." KAMA SUTRA

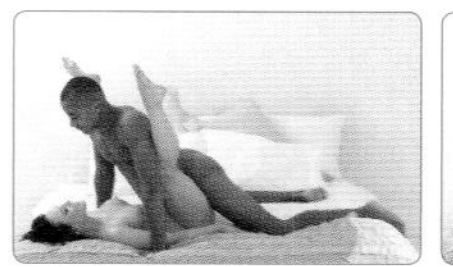

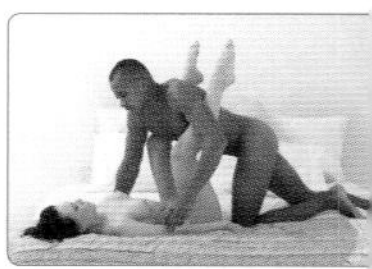

Taking it further

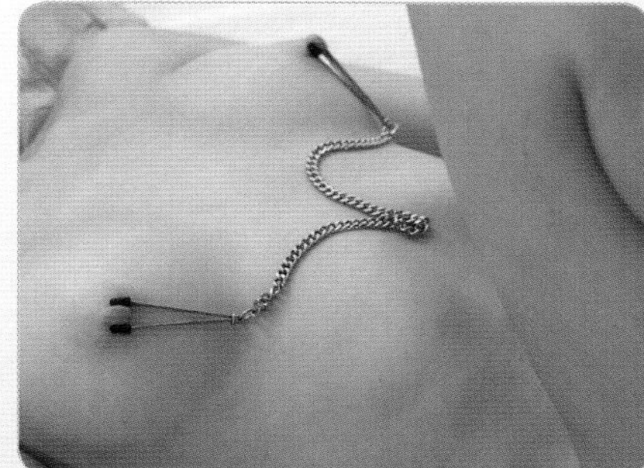

Clamp it up

She gives her nipples a light squeeze with a pair of nipple clamps, which can be a fun and kinky addition to your sex adventures.

3 Bearing down

He bears down upon her so that his chest presses against her knees as he thrusts, and she enjoys his physical power.

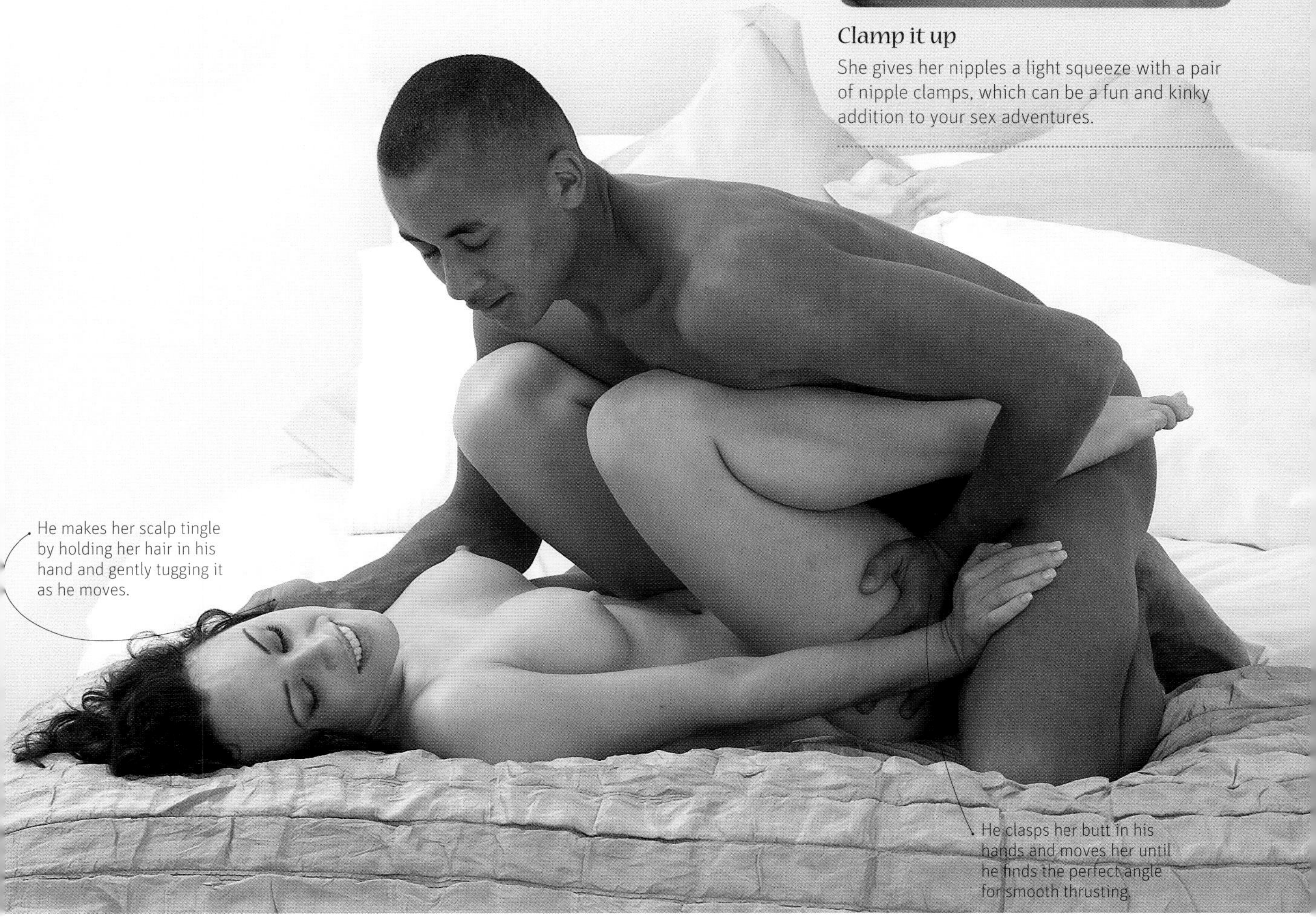

He makes her scalp tingle by holding her hair in his hand and gently tugging it as he moves.

He clasps her butt in his hands and moves her until he finds the perfect angle for smooth thrusting.

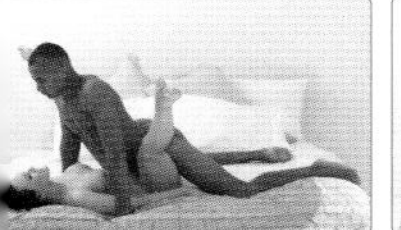 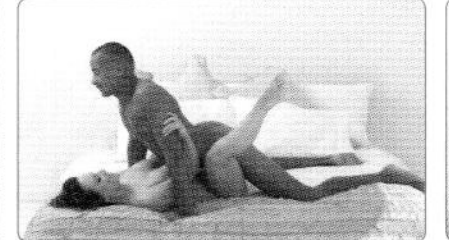 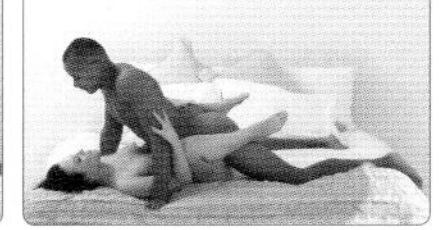 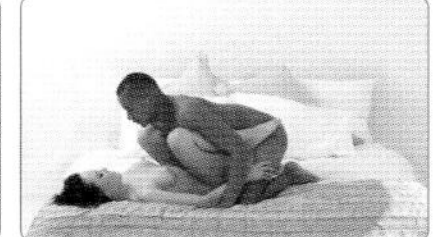 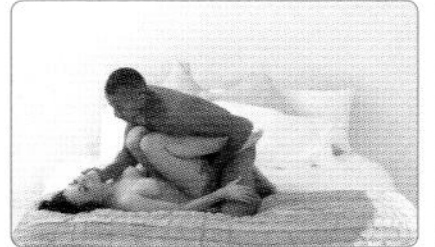 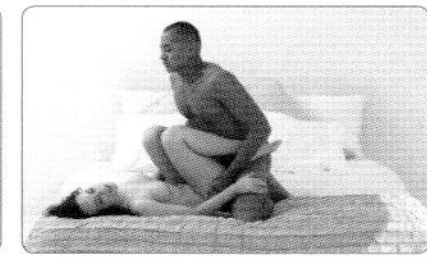

The goat and the tree

☆☆☆☆ Kama sensation rating

If she's stripping or lap dancing for him, this is the ideal finale. She can tease him by gyrating and swirling in front of him, then seductively lower herself on to his lap. Alternatively, he can cut to the chase and just demand that she comes and sits on his knee.

Why it works

– It's the perfect position for a deeply penetrating, satisfying quickie.

– He loves the sheer sexiness of being sat upon.

– If you're discreet, you can do it in public. She simply hitches up her skirt and takes a seat.

– It's one of the best positions for her to have a hand-delivered orgasm.

– He can bite her neck and shoulder as the passion mounts.

– Providing you're not doing it on a park bench, she can give him a practical lesson in how she likes to be touched. He simply rests his hand on top of hers as she masturbates, a technique called "hand-riding."

Turn on...

... Guide her into a standing position with her hands on her thighs if you want to thrust.

Turn off...

... Don't thrust too hard if you're standing. Either restrain yourself, or do the gentlemanly thing and move the chair so that she can lean on it.

1 Exhibitionism

He sits on a chair while she teases him by standing with her back to him and ever-so-slowly bending over.

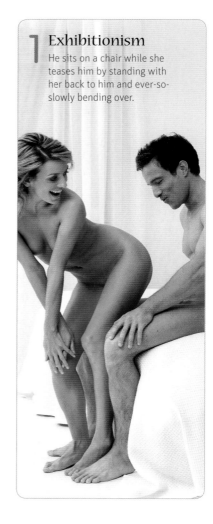

2 Knee perch

She gets one step closer by perching on the end of his knees and giving him a cheeky over-the-shoulder look.

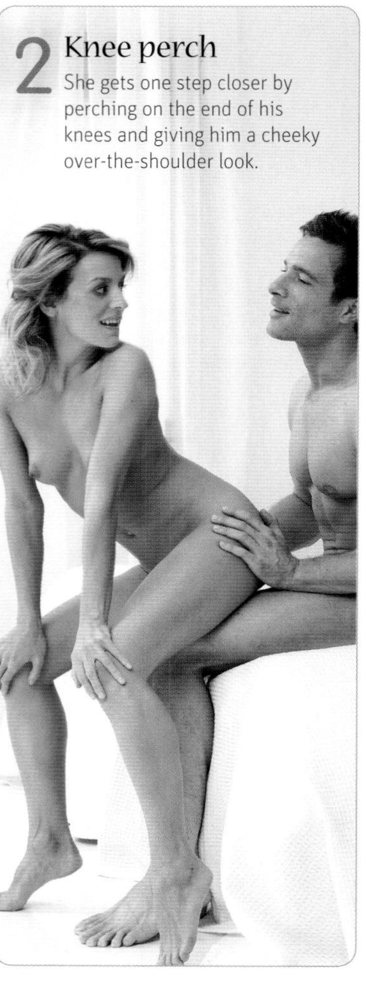

"Even passion demands variety. And through variety, lovers create passion in one another." KAMA SUTRA

3 Legs wide open

She sinks on to his penis with her legs spread wide apart. He slides his arms around her body to embrace her.

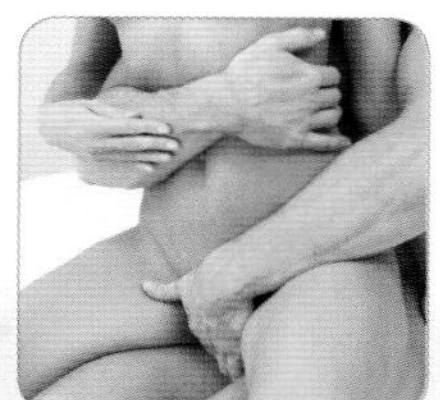

He can bring her to a climax with his fingers working on her clitoris.

She leans forward and rests her hands on her knees as she moves up and down on him.

Taking it further

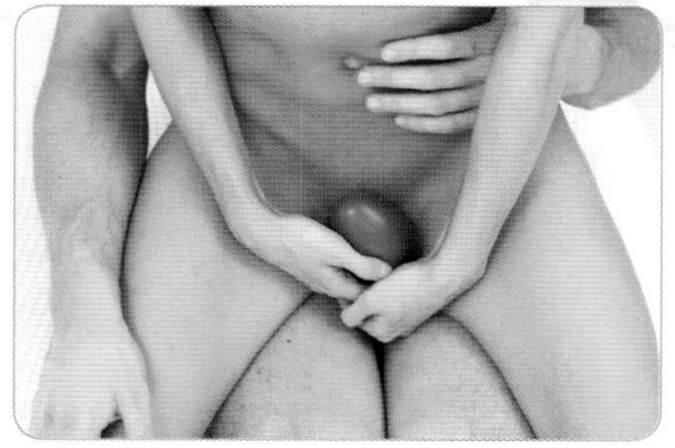

Extra pleasure

This position is made for masturbation; she can hold a pebble-shaped vibrator against her clitoris as she moves on his lap.

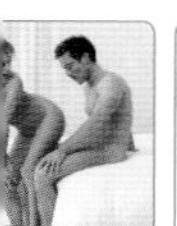
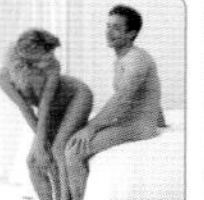
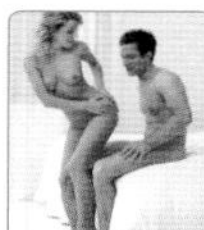
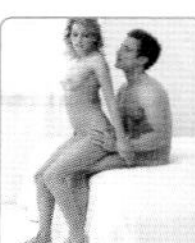
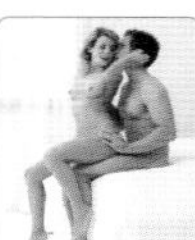
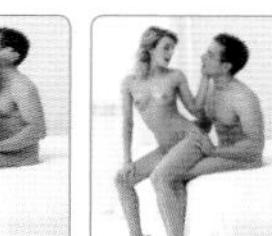
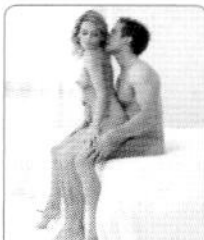
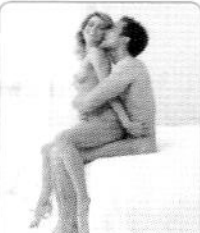
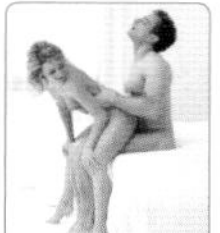
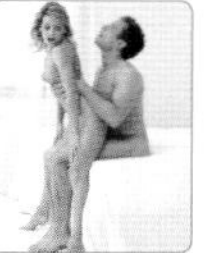

Lotus and Accomplishing positions

☆☆☆ Kama sensation rating

You can move seamlessly between these two positions. The Lotus Position in particular is a favorite position for tantric sex. Try it when you're in the mood for slow lovemaking in which erotic sensations build up, then ripple throughout your body.

Why they work

- In both positions you rock your pelvises gently against each other (imagine you're on a rocking horse). You'll feel delicious tingling sensations expanding from your genitals up into your belly.
- He's ideally placed to pay lots of attention to her breasts and nipples.
- Being so closely entwined creates a powerful emotional connection between you.
- The act of stretching out her leg in the Accomplishing Position creates a subtle but sensual change in the fit between his penis and her vagina. *Vive la différence!*

Turn on...

... Synchronize your breathing with your movements. Breathe in as you rock backward, and breathe out as you rock forward, to gain an insight into basic tantric practices.

Turn off...

... Don't worry if his erection wanes. He can always recover it by moving more vigorously in a man-on-top position for a while.

1 Sitting cuddle

He sits cross-legged on the floor; she sits in his lap with her arms and legs around him. You both rock your pelvises backward and forward. This is the Lotus Position.

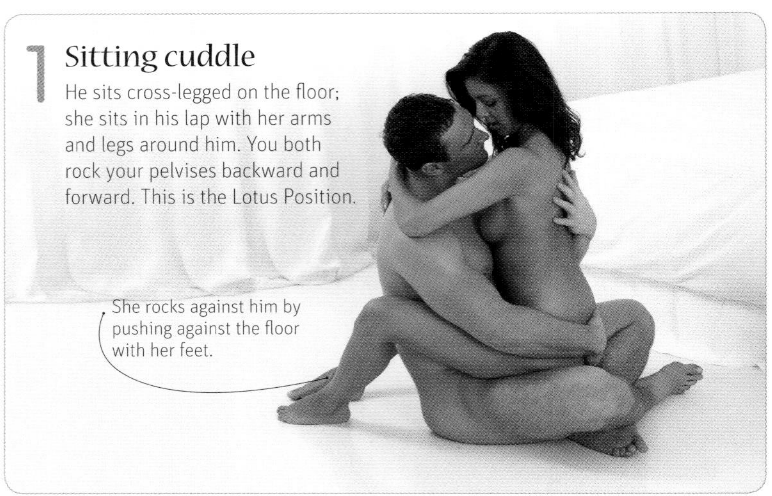

She rocks against him by pushing against the floor with her feet.

2 Vertical lift

She keeps her body pressed tightly to his, and he lifts her up and down with his hands under her armpits or her buttocks.

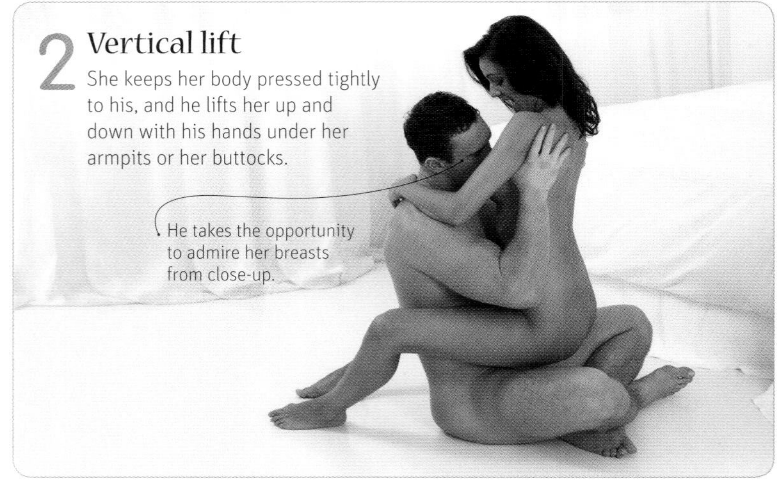

He takes the opportunity to admire her breasts from close-up.

"If a man and woman live together in close harmony, as one soul in one body, they shall be happy in this world and in the next." ANANGA RANGA

Taking it further

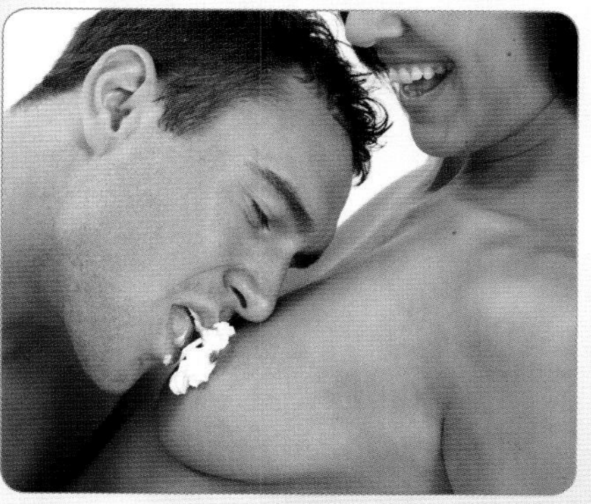

A delicious mess

He licks whipped cream (or anything else from your fridge with a sexy texture) from her skin to make these positions supremely sensual.

3 Thigh trap

She raises one leg so that her knee is near his armpit. He traps her raised thigh under his arm. She leans back on one hand for support. This is the Accomplishing Position. You continue the back-and-forth rocking movement you started in the Lotus Position.

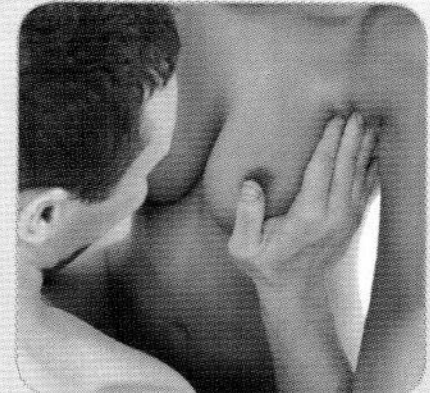

He cups her breasts from the sides and uses his thumbs to brush, flick, and stroke her nipples.

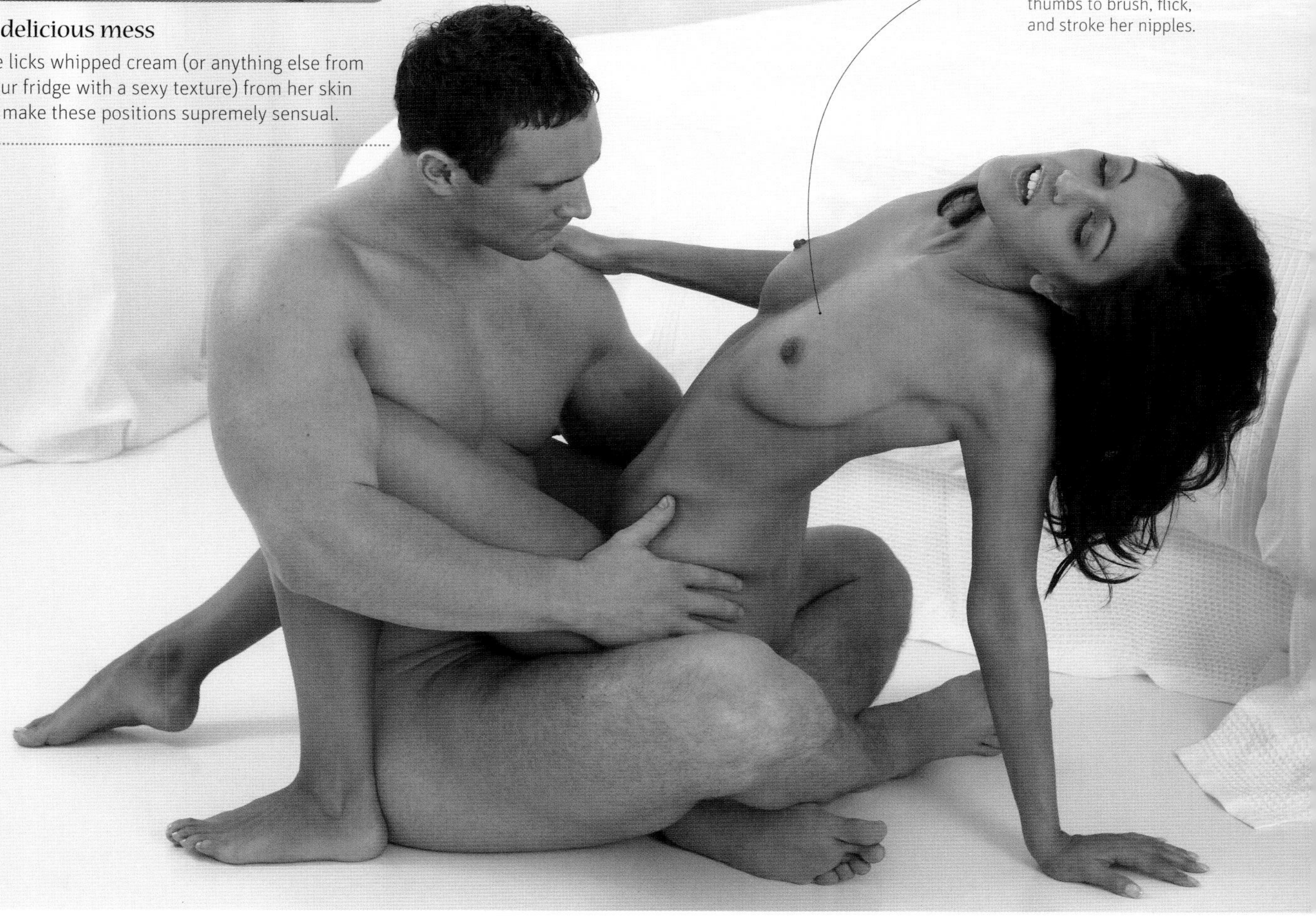

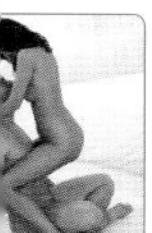
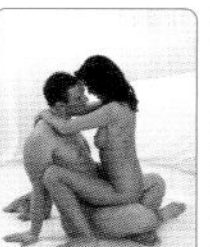
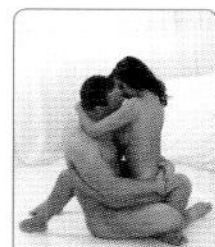
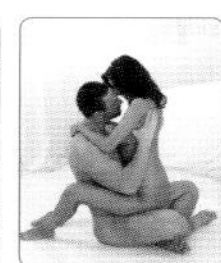
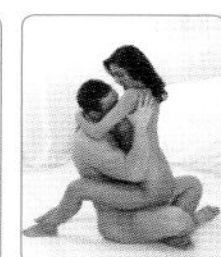
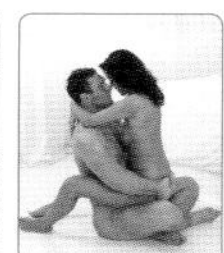
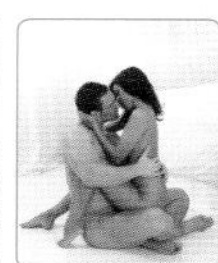
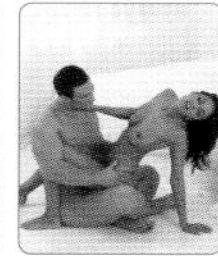

The sixth posture

☆☆☆☆☆ Kama sensation rating

More popularly known as doggie style, this is a classic sex position that couples often fall into when they're hungry for simple, sensational sex, without frills or romance. It's sex at its most raw, basic, and animalistic, which is exactly why people love doing it.

Why it works

– There are no barriers so he can thrust deeply.

– Her vaginal entrance points directly backward because she's on her knees and elbows, making this one of the most easily accessible positions for penetration.

– He not only gets a titillating view of her buttocks and vulva as he penetrates, but also enjoys the thrill of watching himself push in and pull out.

– His hands are free to caress her back, knead her buttocks, or stroke her anus.

– It feels naughty, free, and dirty, which is what mind-blowing sex is often about.

Turn on...

... Try it in front of a mirror, so both of you can experience the exhibitionist thrill that comes with admiring your performance.

Turn off...

... Don't thrust too deeply if you have a big penis. This is one of the positions where it helps to start slow and build up gradually. Applying plenty of lube also helps to ensure a smooth passage.

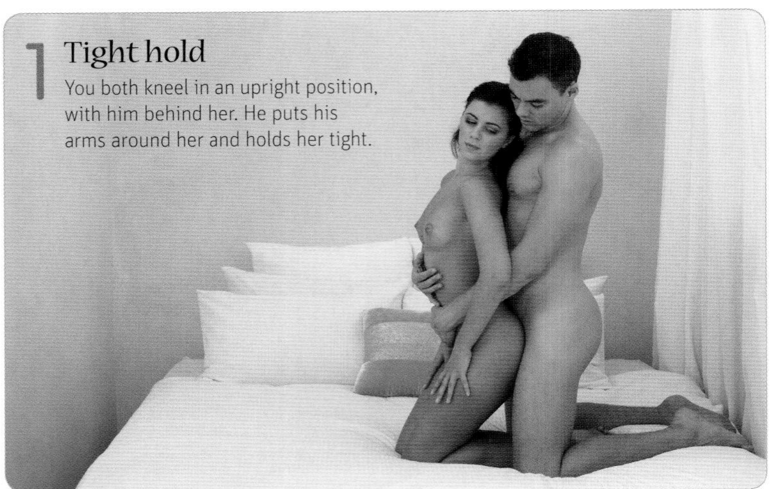

1 Tight hold
You both kneel in an upright position, with him behind her. He puts his arms around her and holds her tight.

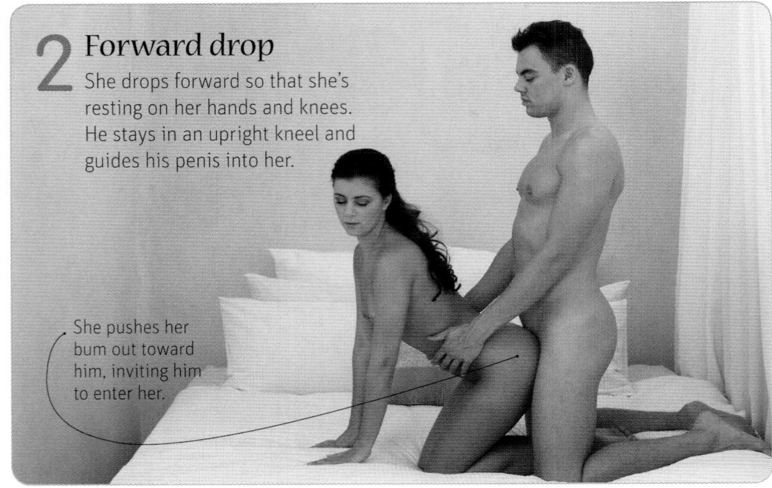

She pushes her bum out toward him, inviting him to enter her.

2 Forward drop
She drops forward so that she's resting on her hands and knees. He stays in an upright kneel and guides his penis into her.

"Unfettered sex occurs between people who trust each other—each does whatever the other enjoys." KAMA SUTRA

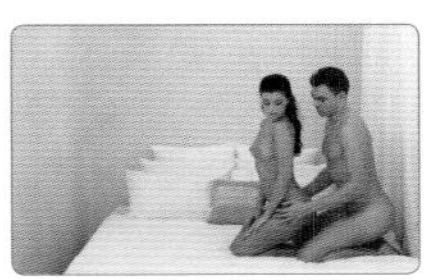

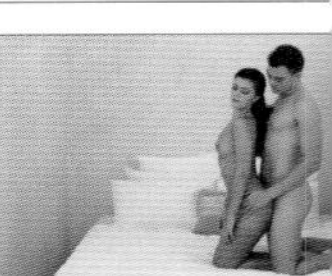

Taking it further

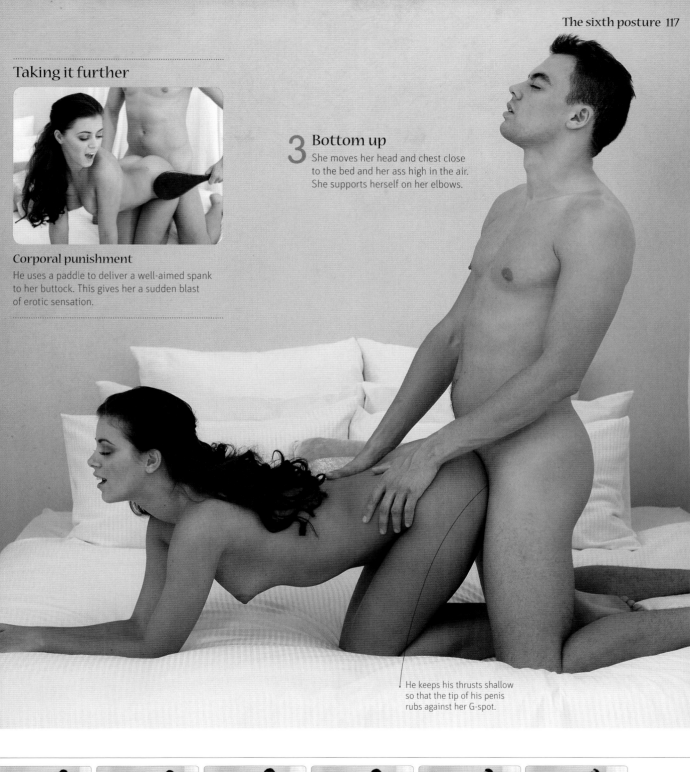

Corporal punishment

He uses a paddle to deliver a well-aimed spank to her buttock. This gives her a sudden blast of erotic sensation.

3 Bottom up

She moves her head and chest close to the bed and her ass high in the air. She supports herself on her elbows.

He keeps his thrusts shallow so that the tip of his penis rubs against her G-spot.

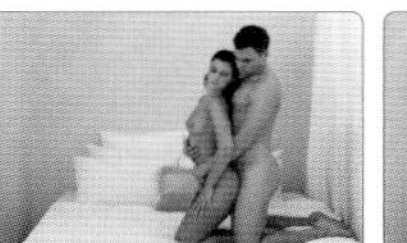
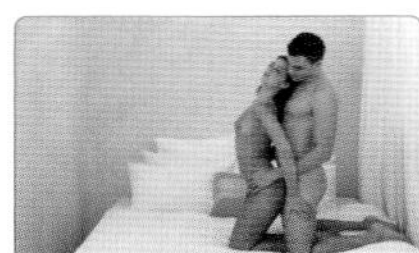
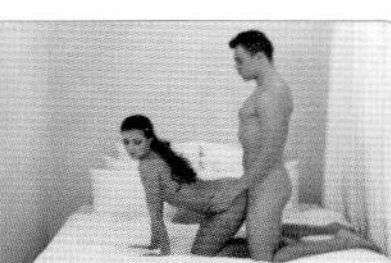
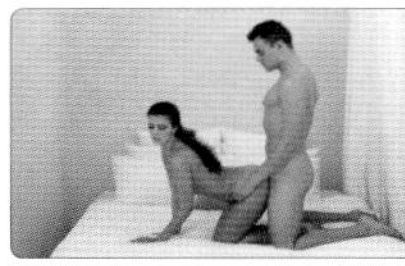
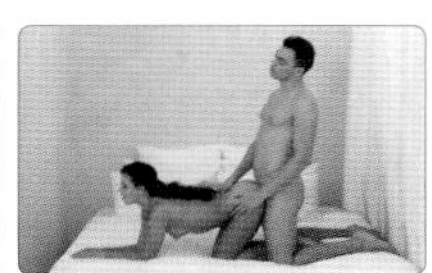
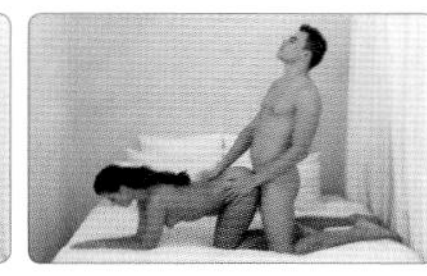

The alternate movement of piercing

☆☆☆ Kama sensation rating

Like the Lotus Position, this is a tantric sex classic. It won't deliver fast and furious pounding, but it generates an intense sexual energy that leads to mind-altering orgasms. Try it when you want to experience tantric bliss in mind, body, and soul.

Why it works

– If you rock against each other, breathe in synchrony, and gaze into each other's eyes, you'll start to get a delicious sense of sexual energy building up in your pelvises.

– Your spines are straight and upright, so sexual energy can travel upward from your hot spots, creating waves of sensual and erotic bliss throughout your bodies.

– According to tantra, she is the goddess (Shakti) and he is the god (Shiva). This position allows you to merge your masculine and feminine essences, and enjoy an ecstatic and soulful sense of union.

Turn on...

... Press your open lips against his open lips to make a seal. When he exhales, take the air straight down into your lungs, then exhale it back to him. Keep passing the same breath back and forth. Imagine that you are merging as you do so.

Turn off...

... Don't do this tantric breathing practice if it feels too difficult (or just breathless). An alternative technique is to blow air toward each other's mouths rather than to make a seal.

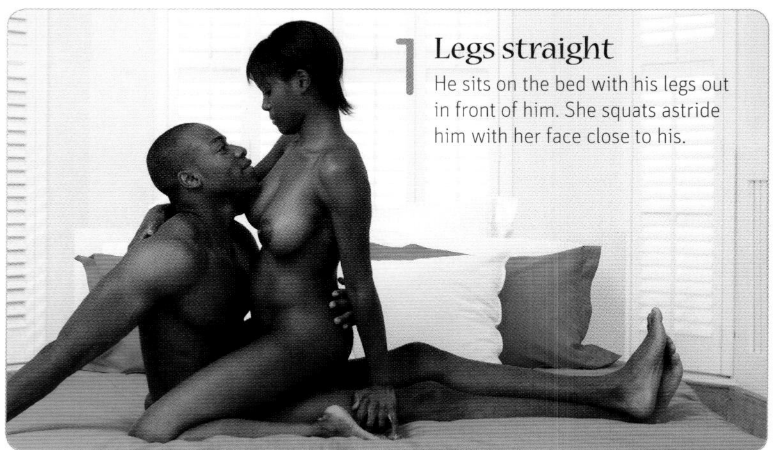

1 Legs straight
He sits on the bed with his legs out in front of him. She squats astride him with her face close to his.

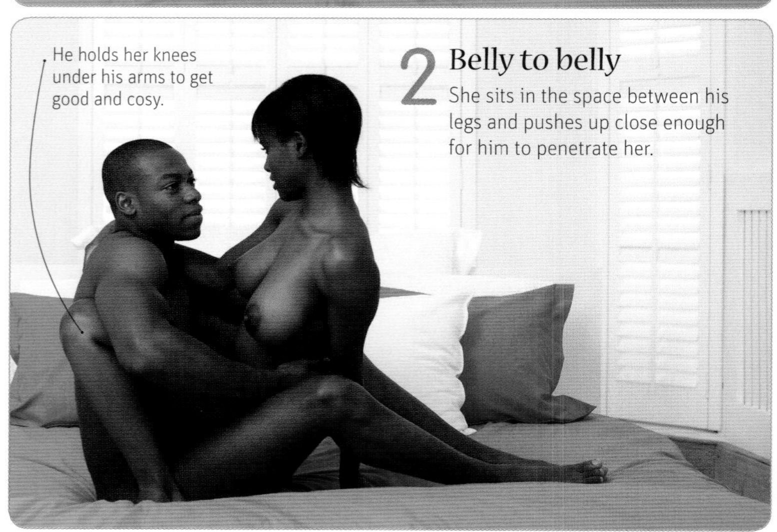

He holds her knees under his arms to get good and cosy.

2 Belly to belly
She sits in the space between his legs and pushes up close enough for him to penetrate her.

"he sends her back and brings her forward again, without ever withdrawing his member." THE PERFUMED GARDEN

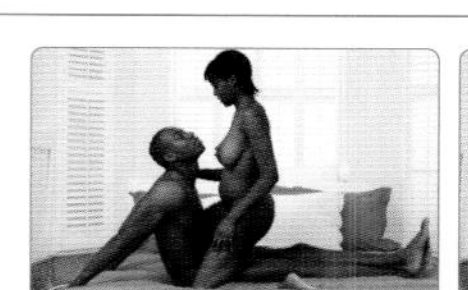

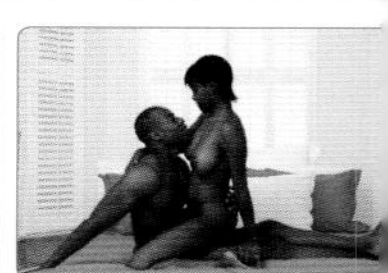

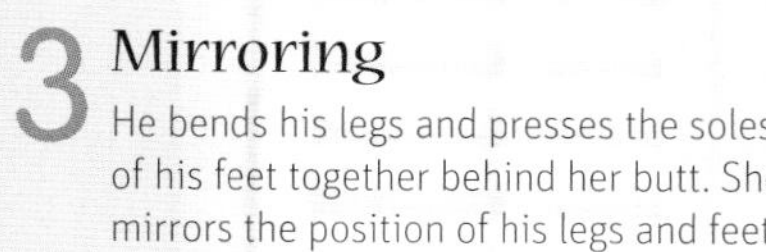

3 Mirroring

He bends his legs and presses the soles of his feet together behind her butt. She mirrors the position of his legs and feet.

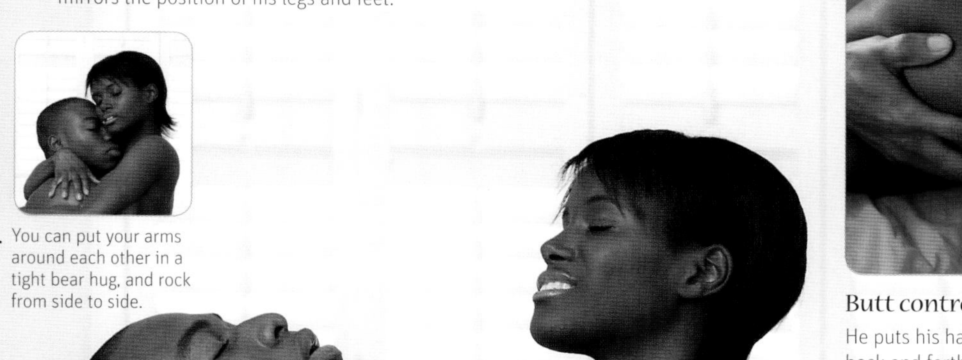

You can put your arms around each other in a tight bear hug, and rock from side to side.

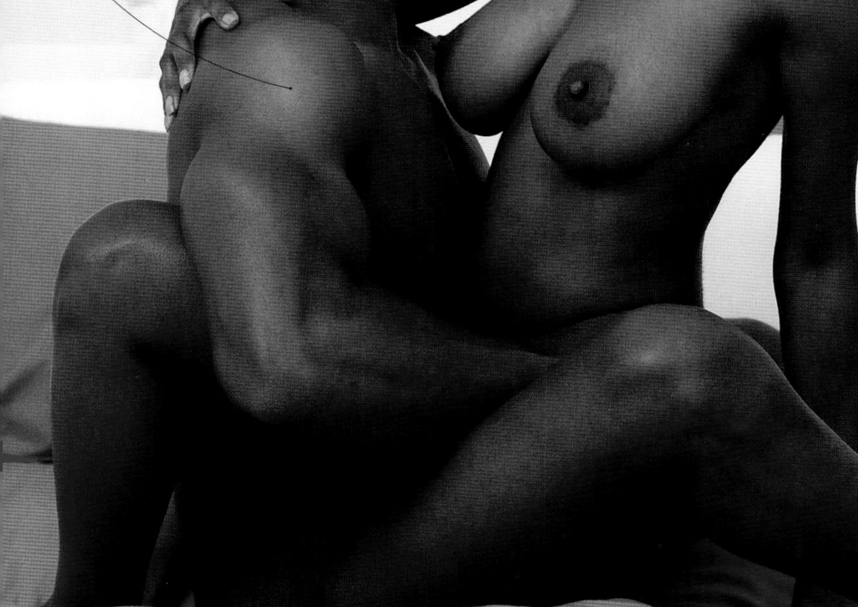

Taking it further

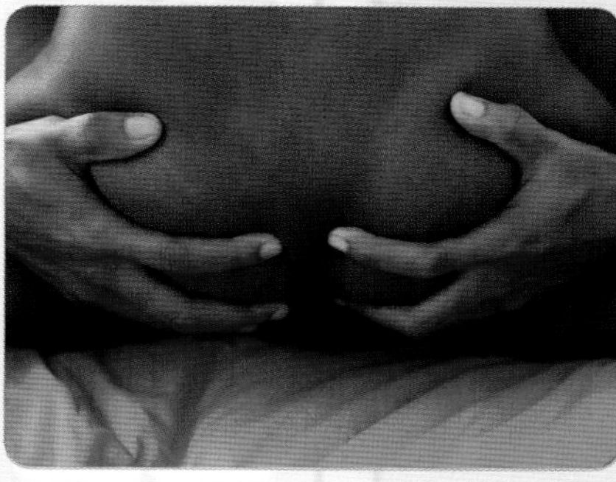

Butt control

He puts his hands under her butt to slide her back and forth, giving her the occasional squeeze to add an erotic surge.

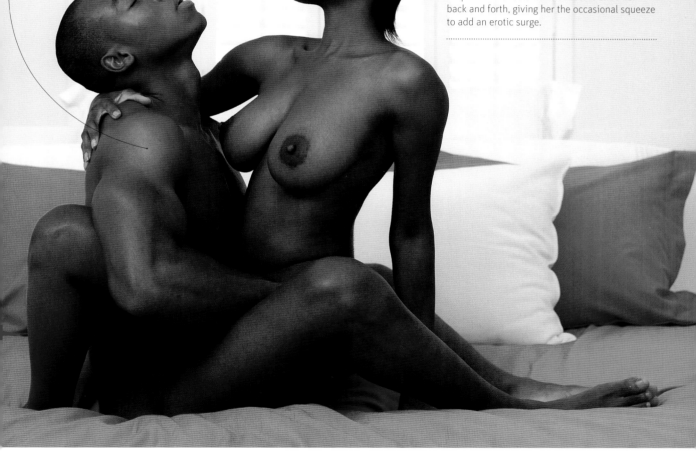

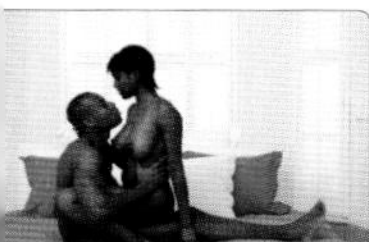
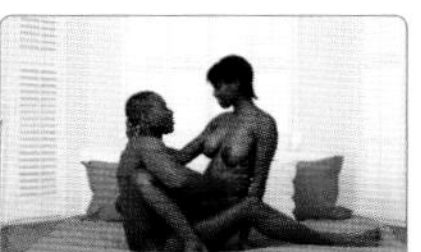
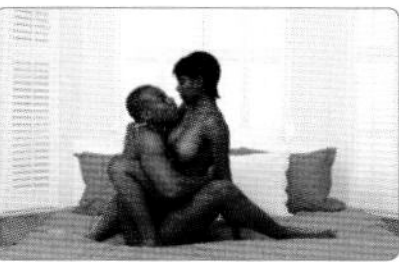
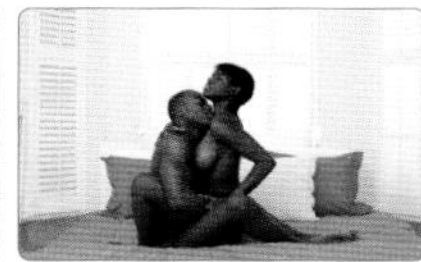
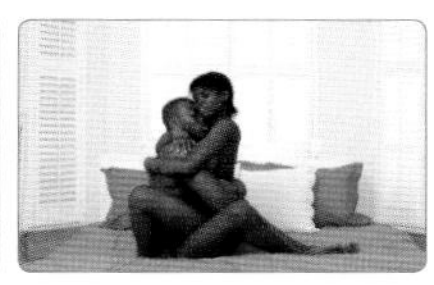

Tiger step

The doggie position with a naughty twist: instead of resting on all fours, in this version she lowers her head to the ground and raises her butt high in the air. Sex positions don't come much more exposed than this so, submission queens, enjoy it. He'll love it in the way he loves all rear-entry poses; it's effortlessly dirty and sexy.

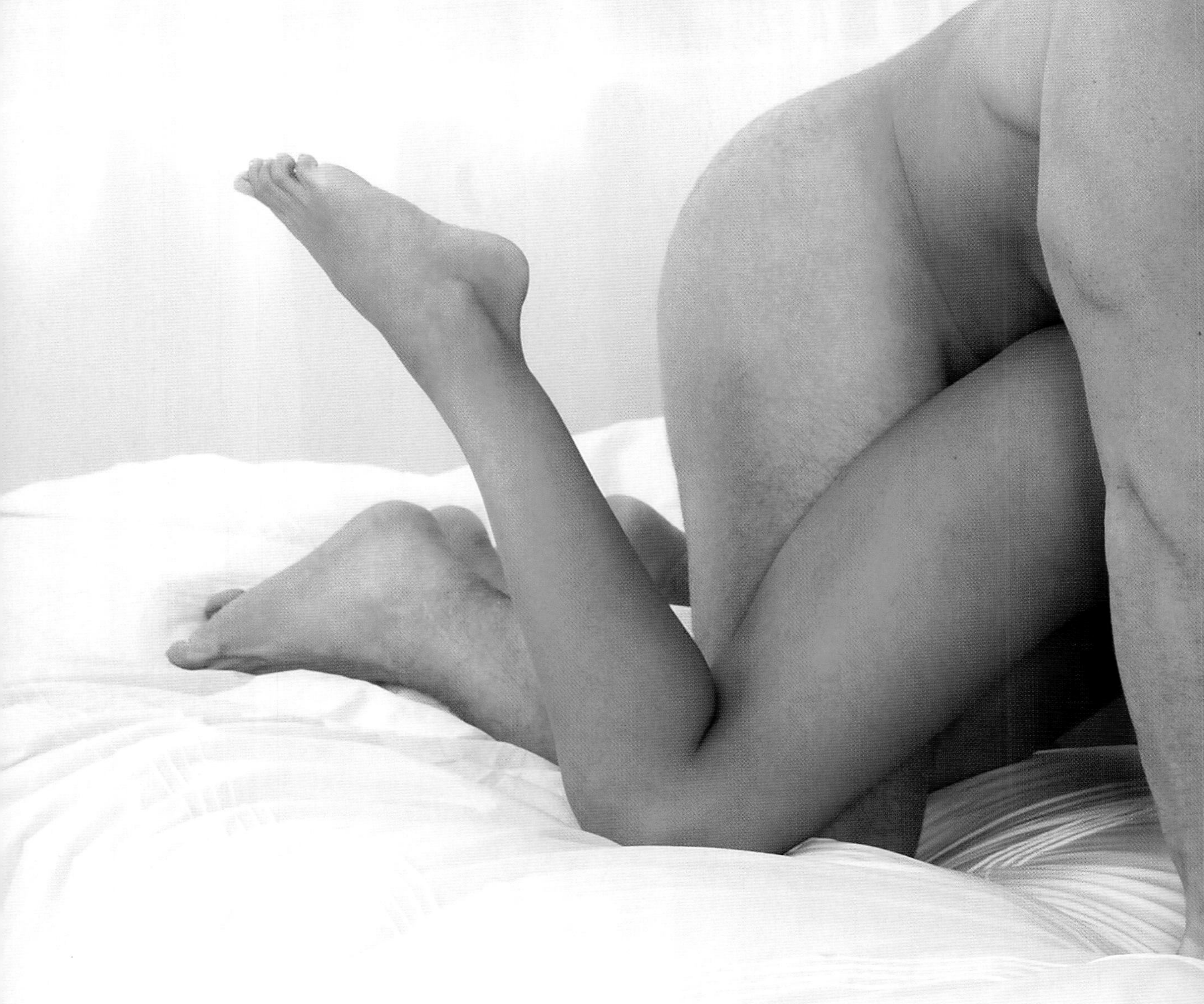

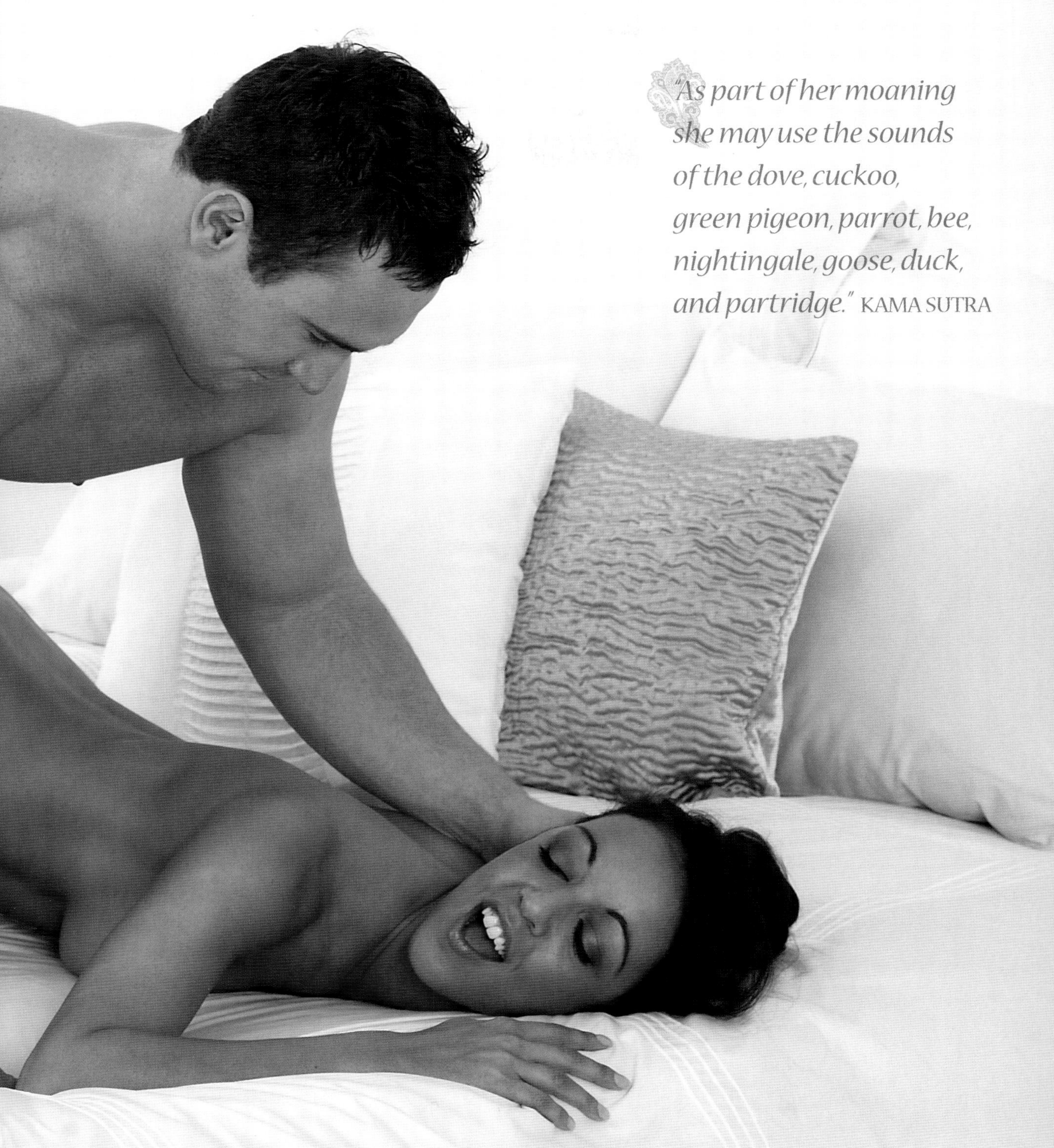

"As part of her moaning she may use the sounds of the dove, cuckoo, green pigeon, parrot, bee, nightingale, goose, duck, and partridge." KAMA SUTRA

Tiger step

☆☆☆☆☆
Kama sensation rating

Why it works

– He can press along the front wall of her vagina with each thrust so that her G-spot gets lots of stimulation.

– He can insert a finger into her anus and move it in and out in time with his thrusts to intensify sensation for her.

– She can put her hand or a vibrator between her legs to stimulate her clitoris.

– If you like rear-entry anal sex, her anus is easily accessible for penetration. Plus, anal sex feels irresistibly filthy in this position. (As always with anal sex, he should enter slowly and use plenty of lube).

– He gets a kick out of her pose of come-and-get-me vulnerability.

– She enjoys relinquishing control and exposing herself to him.

Turn on...

... Reverse roles. If she wants to assume the dominant role, she can penetrate him anally in Tiger Step while wearing a strap-on dildo.

Turn off...

... Don't stay in Tiger Step too long if it's uncomfortable. Make it a brief visit in a whole sequence of positions in which she's on all fours and he's behind her.

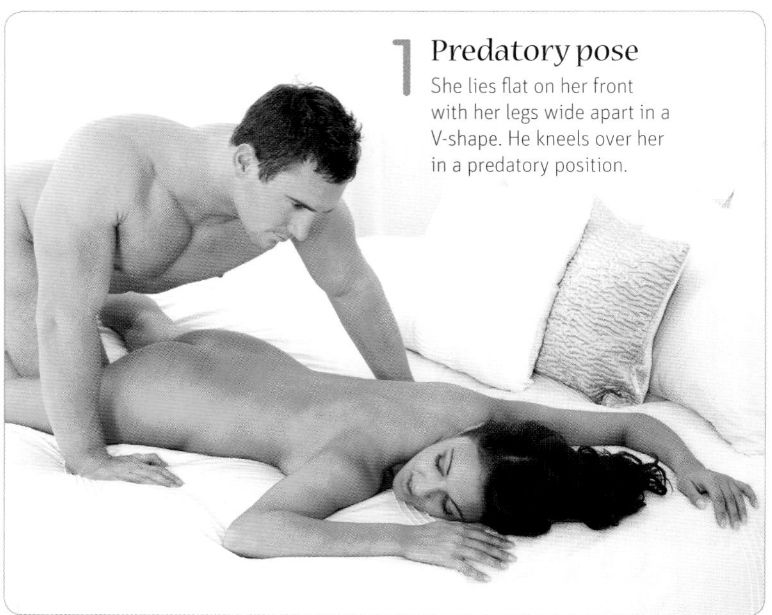

1 Predatory pose
She lies flat on her front with her legs wide apart in a V-shape. He kneels over her in a predatory position.

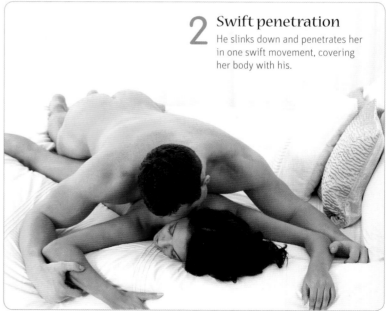

2 Swift penetration
He slinks down and penetrates her in one swift movement, covering her body with his.

"Whenever he gives anything to her or receives anything from her, he invests it with erotic intensity." KAMA SUTRA

3 Rising motion

She pushes her butt in the air so that his body rises with hers, and you both enjoy thrusting.

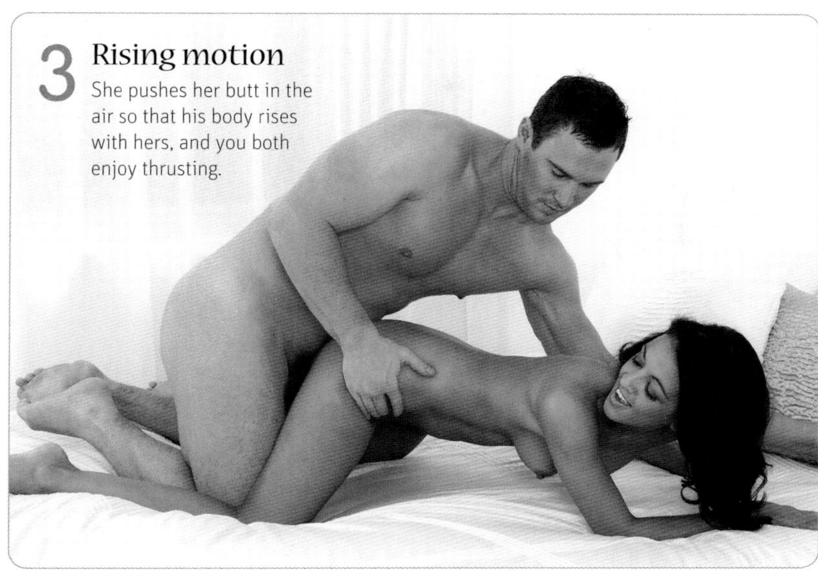

Taking it further

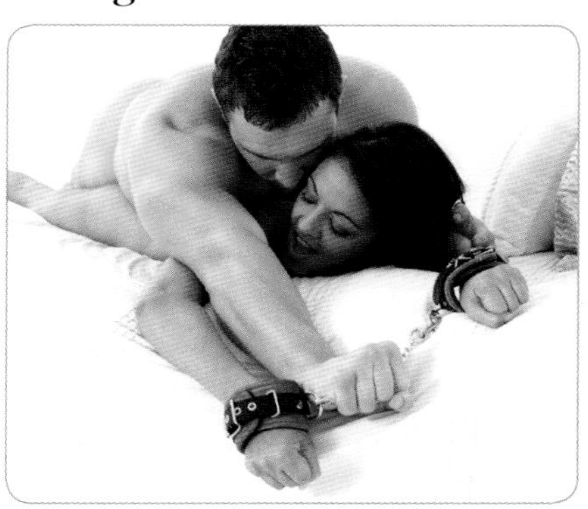

Cuffing up

She wears handcuffs to heighten her trapped and vulnerable sensations. To take her helplessness one step further, he could cuff her to the bed.

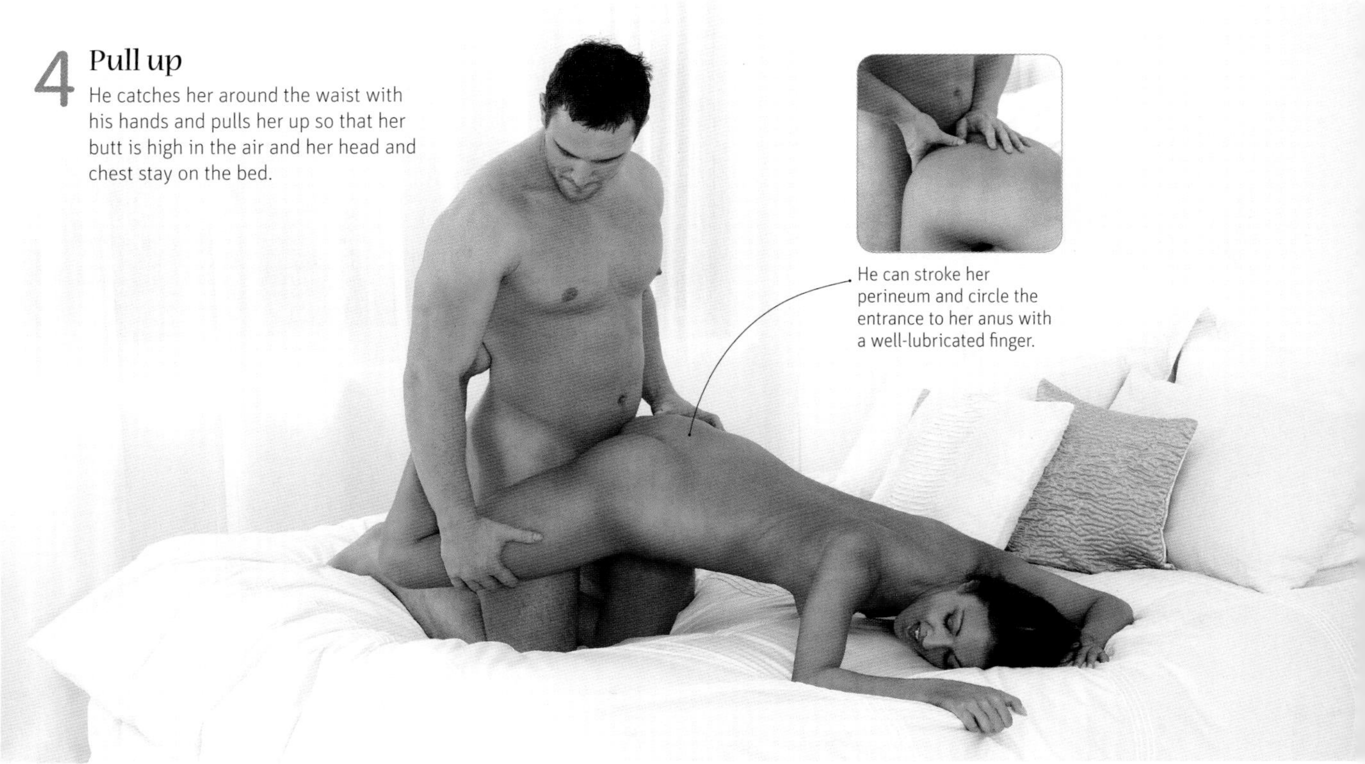

4 Pull up

He catches her around the waist with his hands and pulls her up so that her butt is high in the air and her head and chest stay on the bed.

He can stroke her perineum and circle the entrance to her anus with a well-lubricated finger.

If you liked this, try…

- Another raunchy rear-entry position, The Ninth Posture (see page 134).
- The equally raunchy and more acrobatic Late Spring Donkey (see page 174).

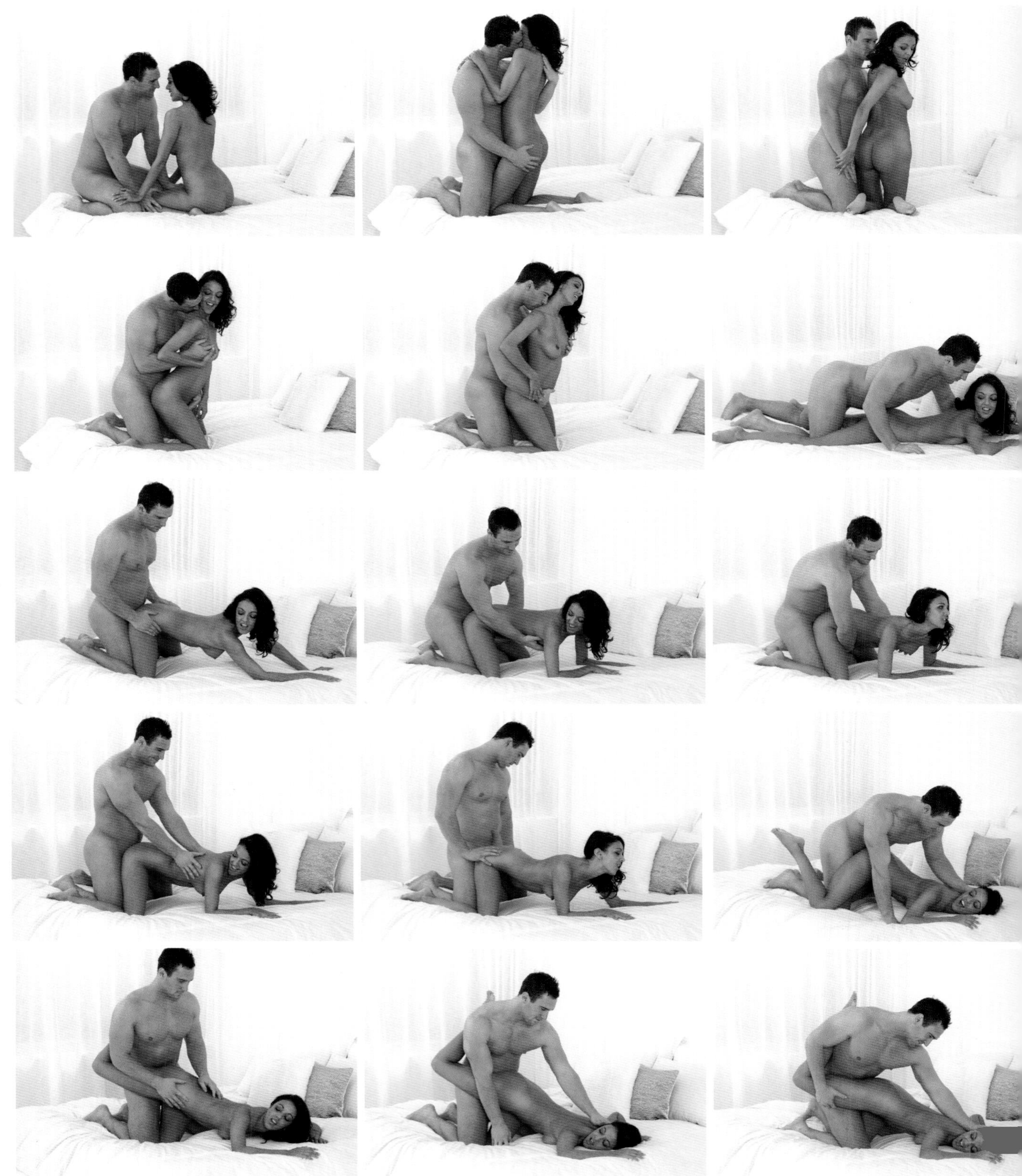

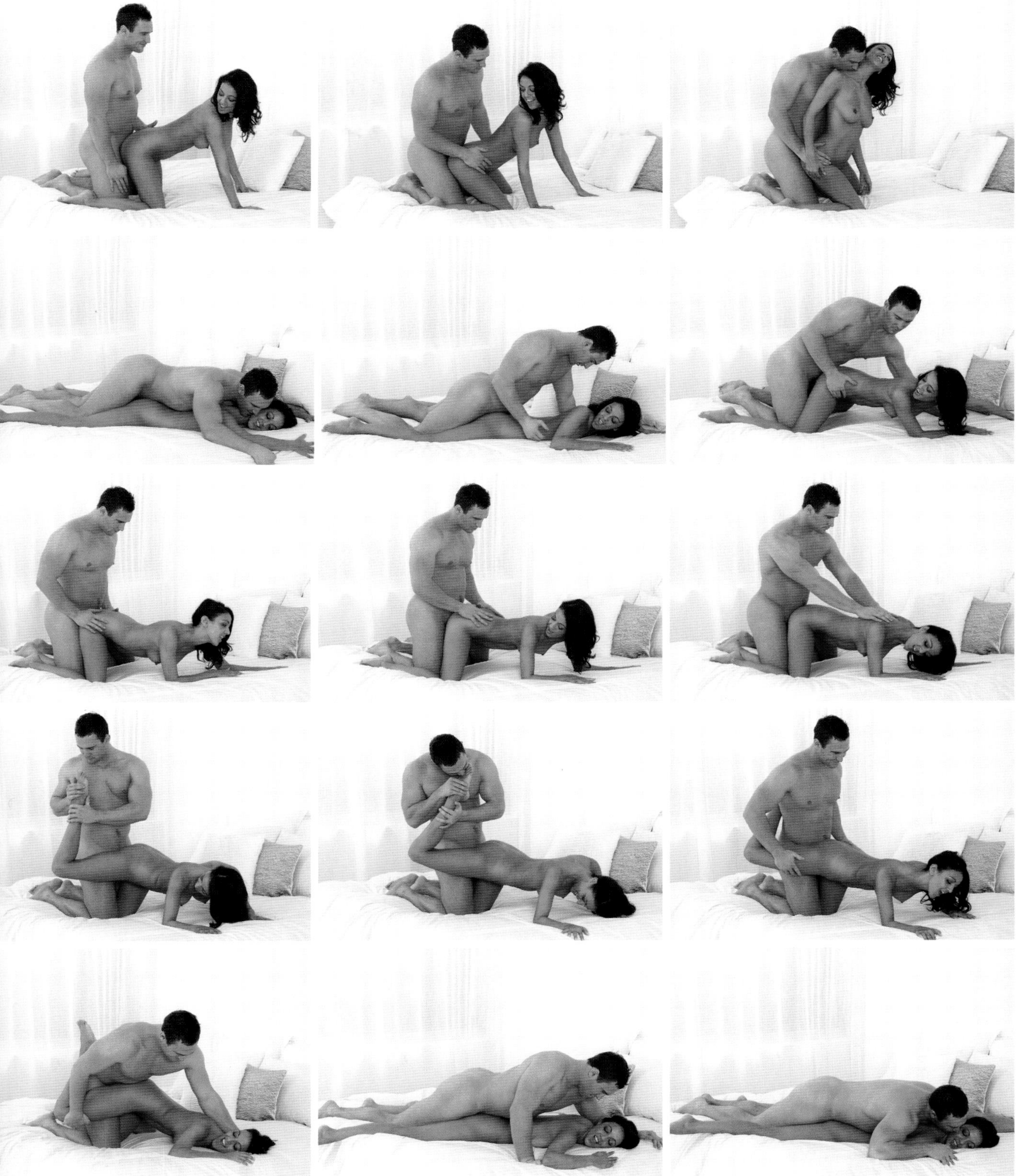

The mare and The swing

☆☆☆ Kama sensation rating

The Mare isn't just a position, it's a technique too. "When the woman forcibly holds the lingam in her yoni, it is called the Mare's Position," says the *Kama Sutra*. Having gripped him hard from inside, she leans into The Swing, one of the hottest rear-entry positions where she's in control.

Why they work

– His penis enters her at an unusual angle. As she leans forward into The Swing, his erection presses strongly against the back wall of her vagina, which stimulates sensitive spots such as the PS-spot (see page 94).

– In The Mare she contracts and relaxes her vaginal muscles around his penis, so he feels tantalizingly squeezed and released.

– He can stroke and fondle her anus, perineum, buttocks, or back.

– The view of her ass in The Swing gets him hot. Plus he can watch his penis being sexily enclosed by her.

Turn on...

... Practice your Kegel exercises to get a super-toned vagina (these involve repeatedly contracting your pelvic-floor muscles, as though you're trying to stop and start the flow of urine while peeing).

Turn off...

... Don't lean forward too far in The Swing. His penis doesn't usually bend in this direction, so it's essential to move slowly and stop when he's reached "maximum bend."

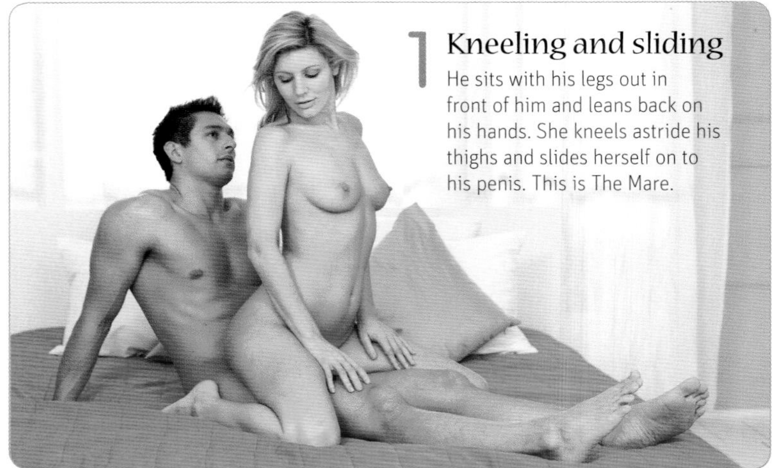

1 Kneeling and sliding
He sits with his legs out in front of him and leans back on his hands. She kneels astride his thighs and slides herself on to his penis. This is The Mare.

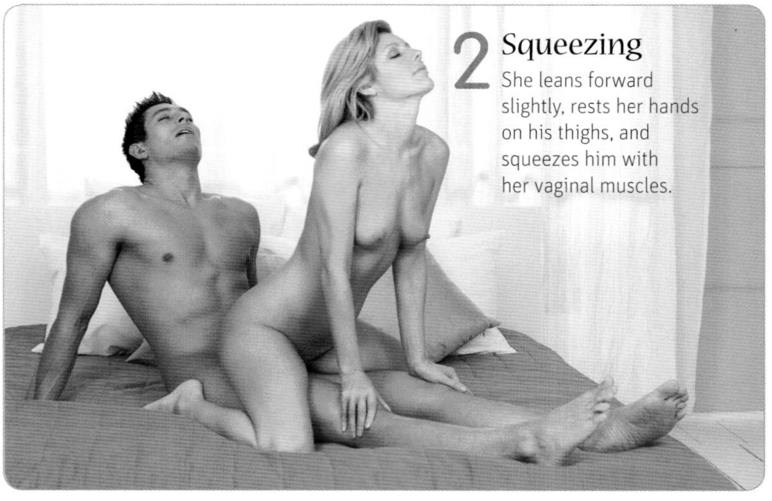

2 Squeezing
She leans forward slightly, rests her hands on his thighs, and squeezes him with her vaginal muscles.

"The Mare's position is learnt by practice only, and is done mainly by women of the Andra country." KAMA SUTRA

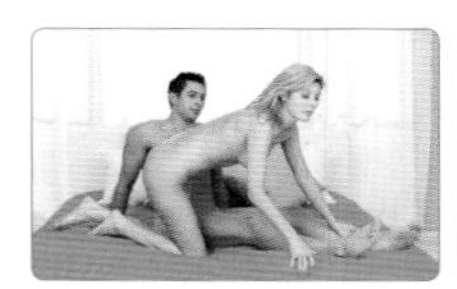

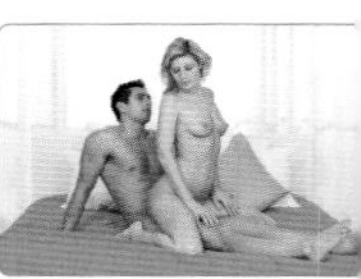

Taking it further

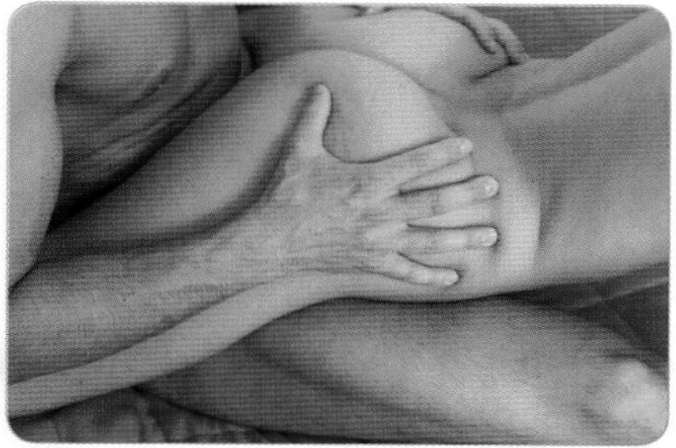

Butt massage

He grabs her buttocks in his hands and moves her in the way he wants, giving her a sexy butt massage at the same time.

3 Getting into The Swing

She walks her hands down his legs tantalizingly slowly. She then puts her hands on either side of his calves so that she's on all fours. This is The Swing.

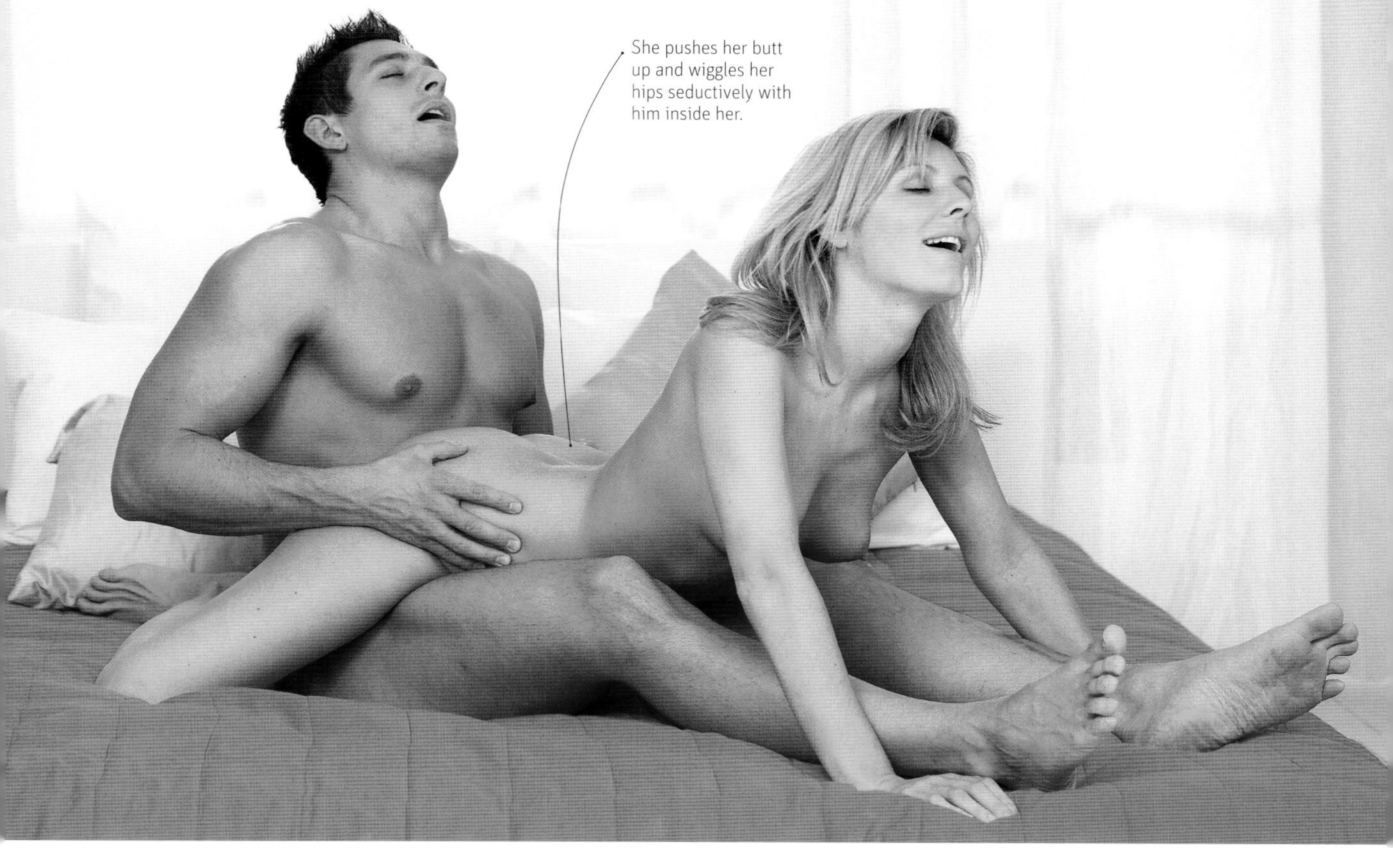

She pushes her butt up and wiggles her hips seductively with him inside her.

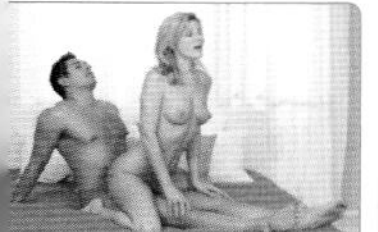
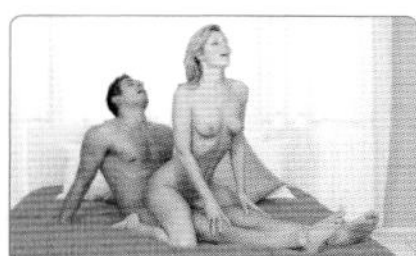
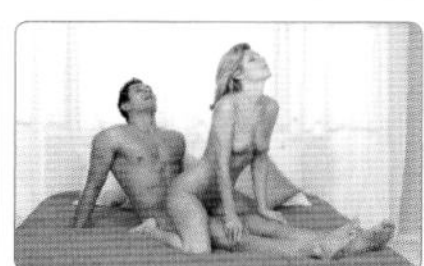
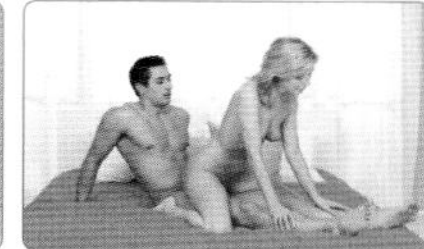
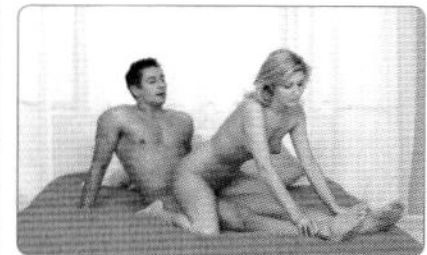
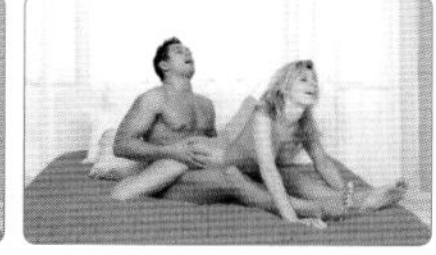

Getting the perfect fit

Many of the positions in the *Kama Sutra* are intended to create the best possible sexual fit between a couple. Strange as it may sound, the best sexual couplings are those between stallions and elephants, bulls and mares, and hares and does.

The *Kama Sutra* divides men into three categories of penis: small (hares), medium (bulls), and large (stallions). Women aren't exempt from Vatsyayana's measuring tape: those with small, medium, and large vaginas are respectively described as does, mares, and elephants.

An equal match The best sex, according to Vatsyayana, is between an "equal" couple, for example, a bull and a mare. In such cases, pretty much anything goes. But when the union is unequal, Vatsyayana instructs couples to get into more elaborate positions to improve the sexual fit and make sex as satisfying as possible.

Low union In a low union, she is bigger than him. Low union combos are a hare man and a mare woman, or a hare or bull man coupled with an elephant woman. The problem with lowest union is lack of sensation for both of you. She won't feel full, and he won't feel gripped.

Vatsyayana's very sensible advice is to have sex in The Mare's position (see page 126), which is as much technique as position: she contracts her vaginal muscles around his penis, having been working overtime on her Kegel exercises. Vatsyayana also recommends that "sex tools may be used"; more than enough permission to whip out a vibrator or dildo from your bedside drawer.

Other positions that help in low union are those in which she draws her knees to her chest (to contract her vagina), such as Phoenix Playing in a Red Cave (see page 148).

High union If a woman with a small vagina has sex with a well-endowed man, this is known as "high union." It sounds appealing, but can actually pose problems in that his penis can sometimes feel too big for comfort. Vatsyayana comes to the rescue with three sex positions that will "widen the yoni": Widely Opened Position (see page 28), Yawning Position (see page 130), and The Wife of Indra (see page 204). Thanks to modern knowledge about female anatomy however, we know that some of these positions may have the opposite effect. If a woman draws her knees up to her chest (as in The Wife of Indra), this contracts her vagina, making it shorter.

An alternative way of managing the potential discomfort of high union is to make sure that a woman is super-aroused and wet before penetration. In practical terms, this means as much foreplay as she wants and indulging her in some of her favorite turn-ons, whether they be cunnilingus, intense kissing, or watching him play the guitar dressed in cowboy hat and chaps. Once she's thoroughly turned on (wait until she gets to the panting, sighing, writhing stage), she should be slick with her natural lubrication, and even the largest penis should slide in with ease.

A new angle Another way of successfully achieving high union is to choose sex positions that minimize the length of his penis or prevent him penetrating her fully. Anything that involves his penis pointing back through his thighs is good, for example, Race of the Member (see page 218). Side-by-side positions work well too, for example, Transverse Lute (see page 54) or The Fifth Posture (see page 58).

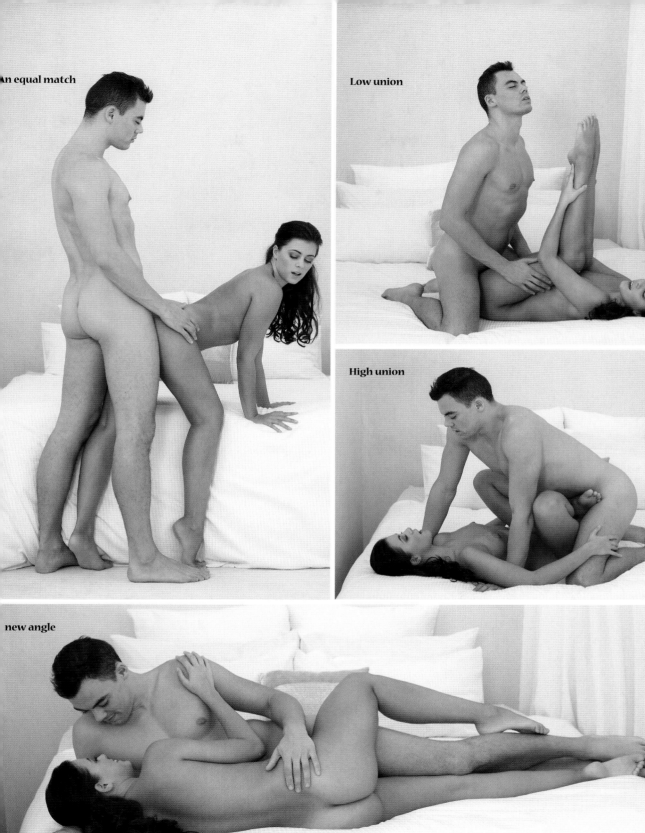

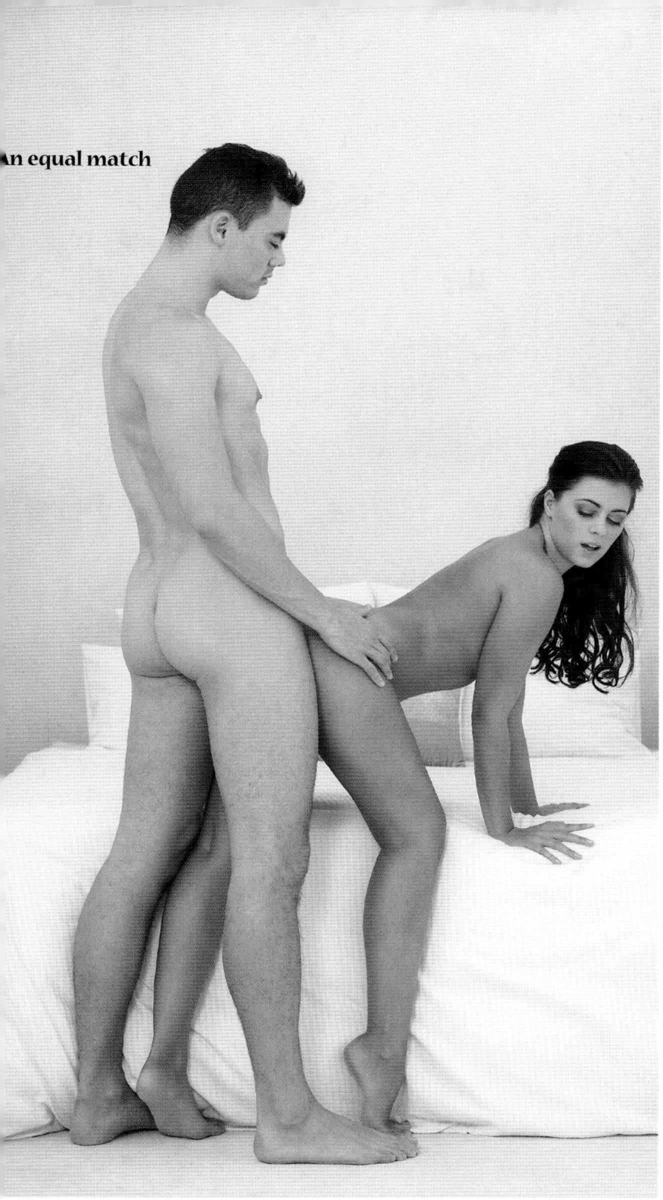

An equal match

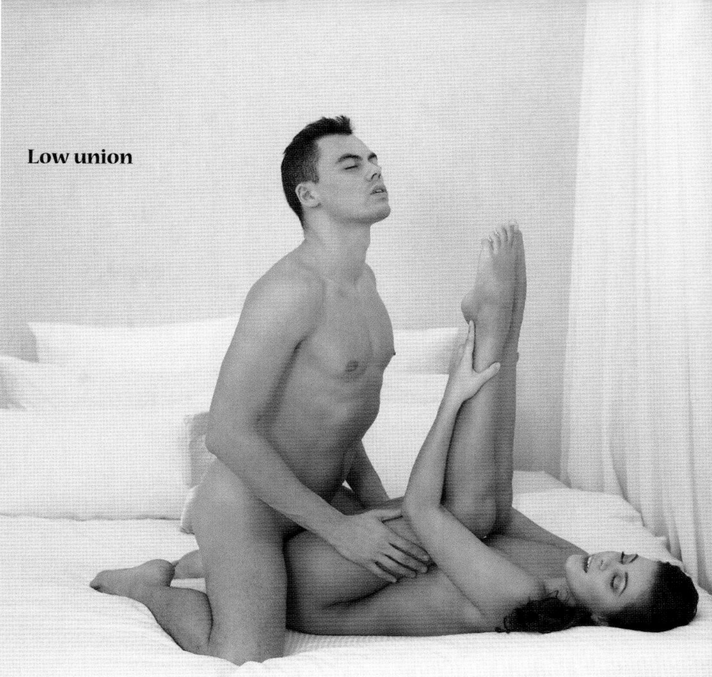

Low union

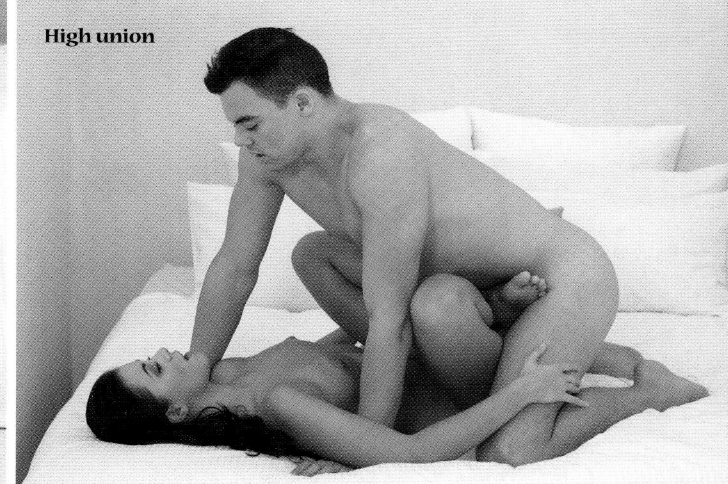

High union

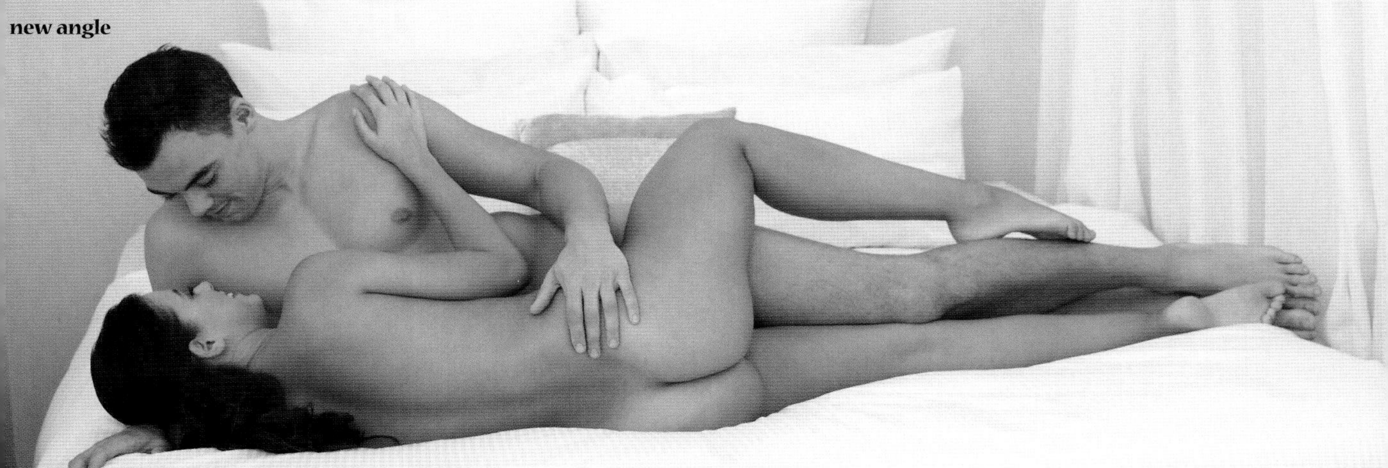

new angle

Yawning position

☆☆☆ Kama sensation rating

Also known as Legs of Victory, this position falls into the hot-enough-to-photograph category. If you fancy yourselves as porn stars, try videoing yourselves in Yawning Position (heels and stockings will complete the look). If you don't, just enjoy it for its dramatic sexiness.

Why it works

- He can stimulate himself (and her) with fast hip flicks so that his shaft pumps in and out at high speed.

- It makes her look and feel strong, supple, and super-sexy, and it's a great chance for her to show off smooth and gorgeous legs, with or without stockings.

- He feels like a stud as he presses up and down between her legs.

- It's got many of the benefits of the missionary position (being face to face, being able to thrust freely, and so on), but it feels about ten times as raunchy.

Turn on...

... Give your legs a break from time to time by putting your heels on his buttocks. And drop into a conventional missionary position if your legs have reached quivering point.

Turn off...

... Don't thrust inside her at a runaway pace that takes you to the point of no return before you're ready. Alternate between fast and slow strokes to keep a lid on your excitement.

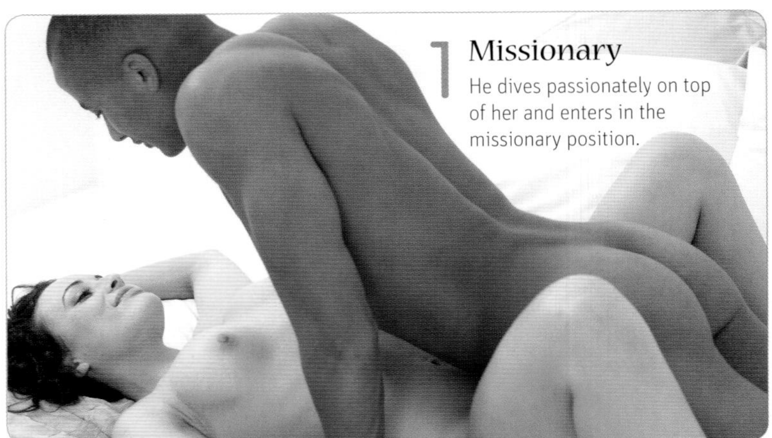

1 Missionary He dives passionately on top of her and enters in the missionary position.

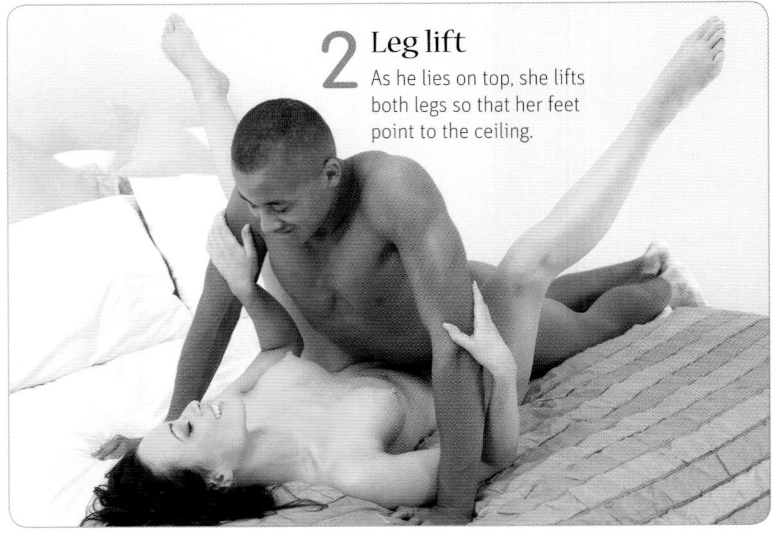

2 Leg lift As he lies on top, she lifts both legs so that her feet point to the ceiling.

"When he pulls out a long way and then plunges down hard and fast, this is called 'the blast of wind'." KAMA SUTRA

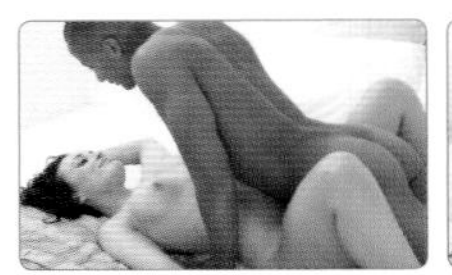

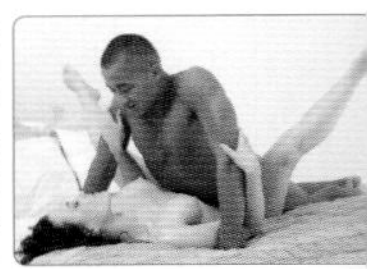

Taking it further

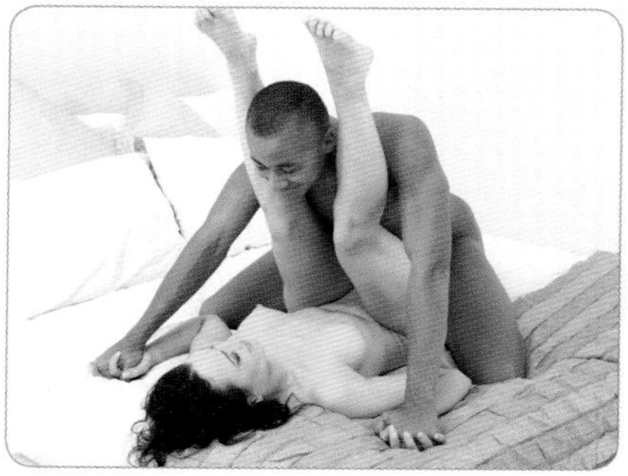

Leg shift

To penetrate her more deeply, he rests his hands on the bed and she rests her legs along the front of his body. (This also gives her legs a break.)

3 Holding hands

He gets into an upright kneeling position, then leans forward and holds her hands for support as he glides in and out.

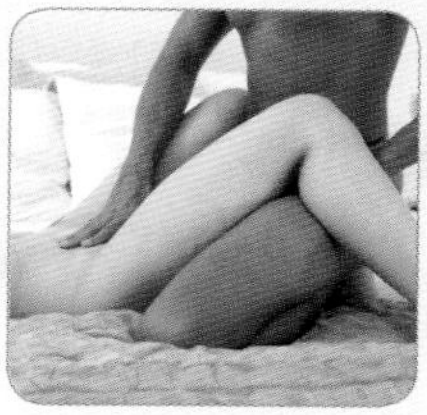

He can take a break to sit back on his heels and give her a clitoral massage.

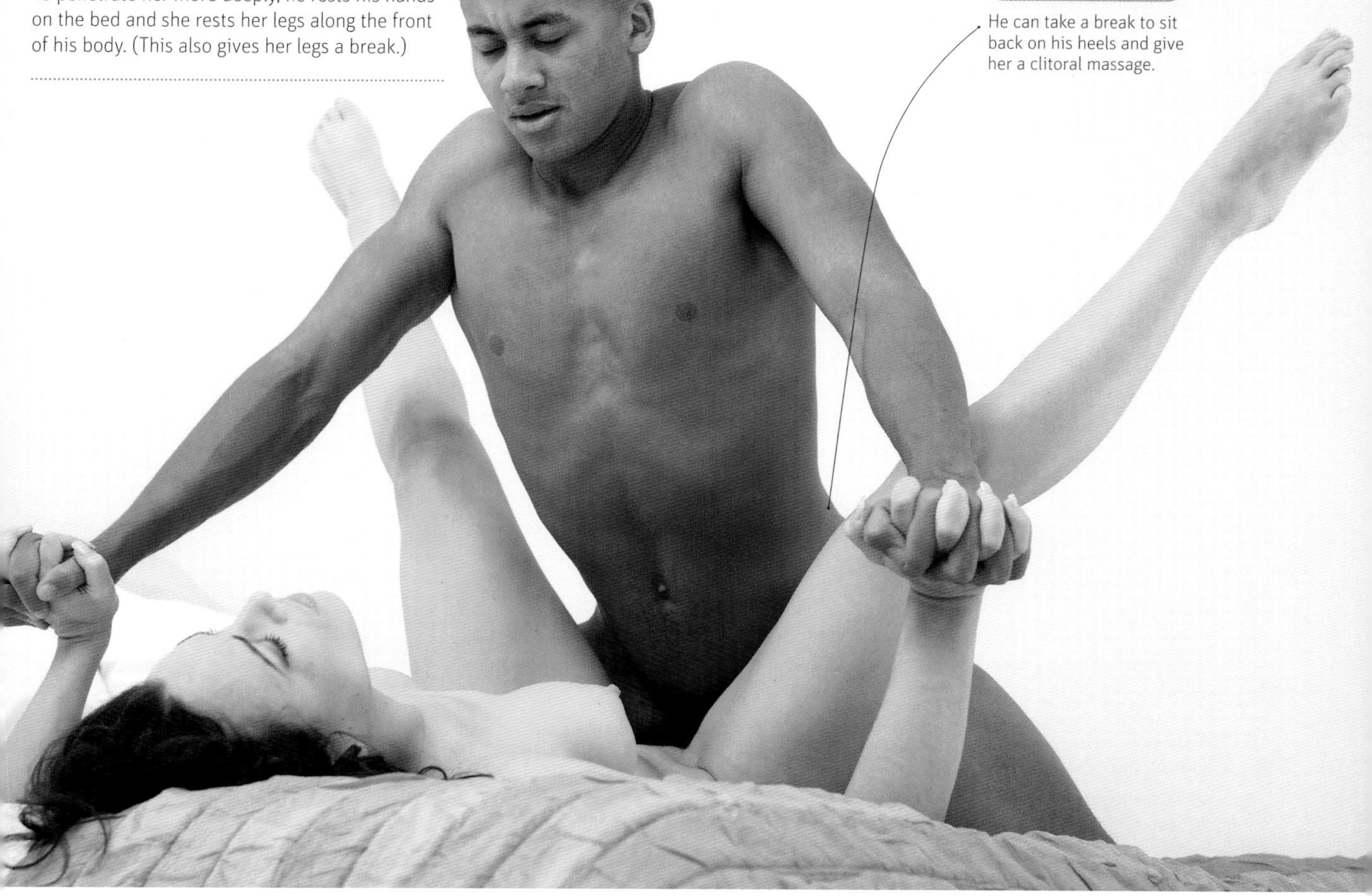

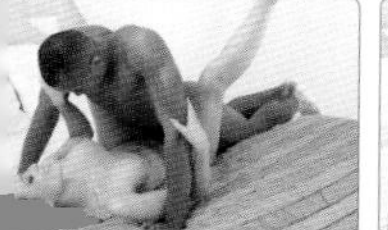
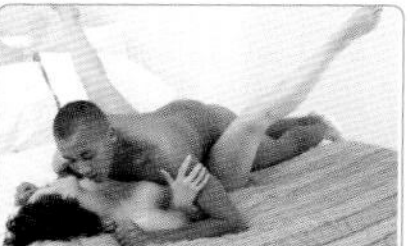
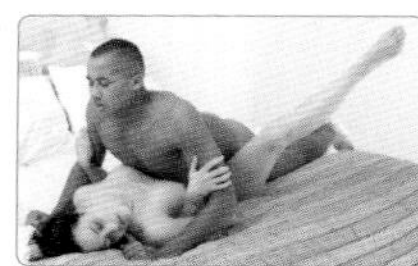
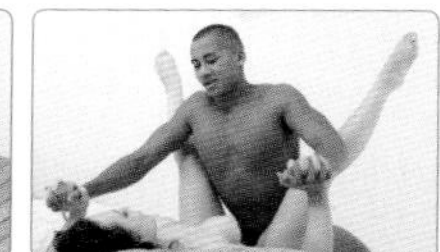
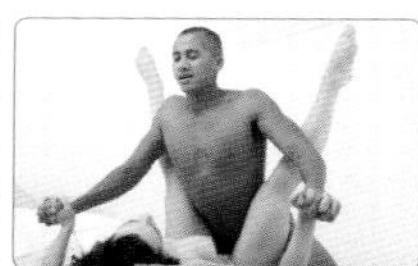

Rising position

☆☆ Kama sensation rating

Although your movements are restricted in this position, it rates highly on erotic tension because you're facing each other, yet her legs prevent him kissing or getting too close. This is also one of the best positions for giving her a pre-coital orgasm.

Why it works

- He can make her come by holding his penis in his hand and circling the tip on her clitoris. He can then make an exciting entrance by penetrating her while she's in the final throes of orgasm, revving her up for the next one.
- He feels the erotic excitement of pushing against the barrier of her raised legs. He can also use her legs to hold onto as he thrusts.
- He has a titillating view of her face, neck, and breasts. It's also easy for him to reach her breasts with his hands.
- You can up the emotional intensity by holding each other's gaze.

Turn on...

... Hold her ankle in your hand, and gently suck her toes to give her electric sensations that run all the way down her leg.

Turn off...

... Don't get hung up on penetrating her all the time. Try thrusting inside her, then pulling out and rubbing your penis against her clitoris, labia, and vaginal entrance; this can actually be more erotic.

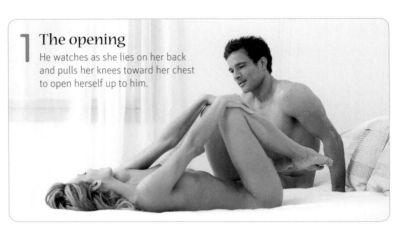

1 The opening

He watches as she lies on her back and pulls her knees toward her chest to open herself up to him.

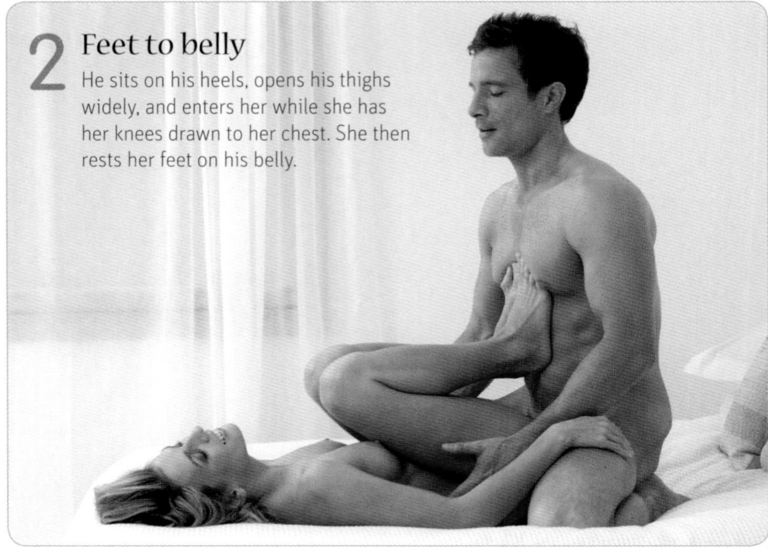

2 Feet to belly

He sits on his heels, opens his thighs widely, and enters her while she has her knees drawn to her chest. She then rests her feet on his belly.

"When he is moving inside her and her eyes roll when he touches particular places, he should make a point of pressing those places." KAMA SUTRA

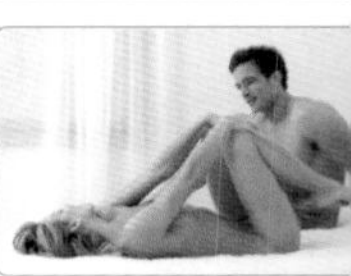

Taking it further

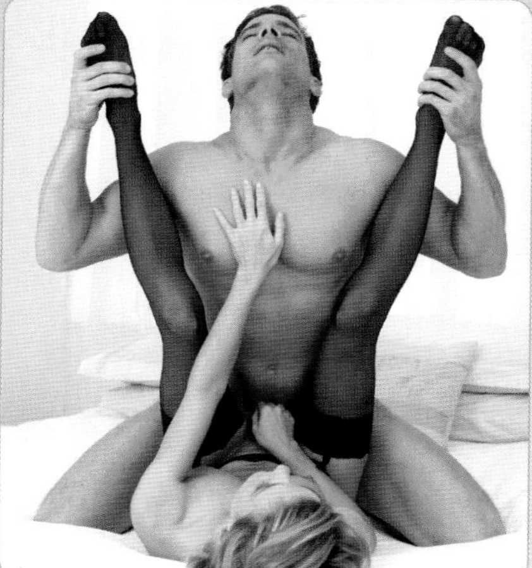

Leg focus

She makes her legs the center of attention by wearing stockings and a garter belt; he won't be able to resist her for another second.

3 Foot walk

She walks her feet slowly up the front of his body from his belly to his chest, then hooks her ankles over his shoulders.

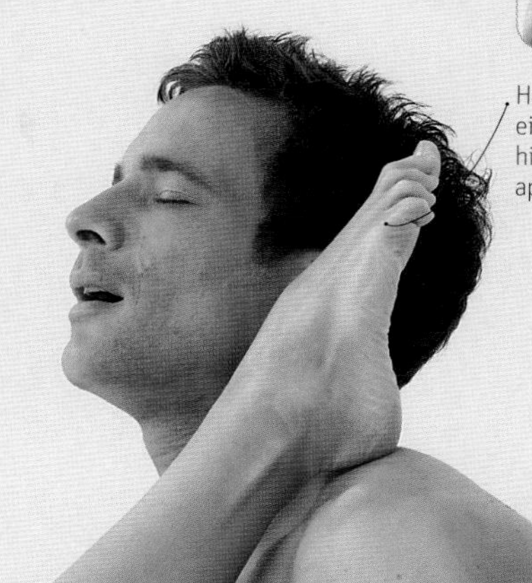

He can hold on to her feet, either squeezing them in his hands or holding them apart as he thrusts.

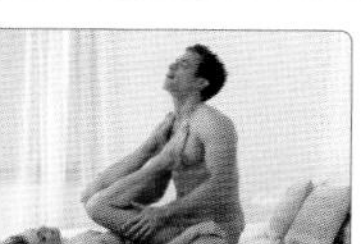
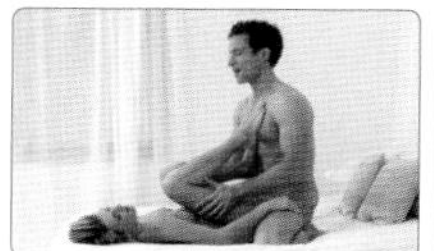
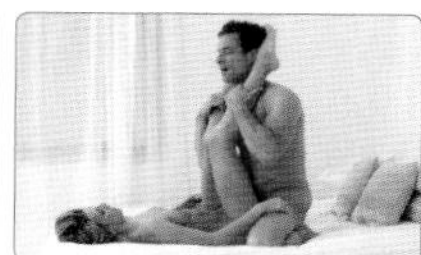
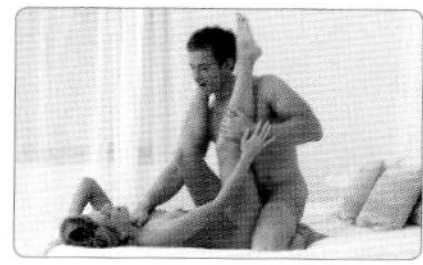
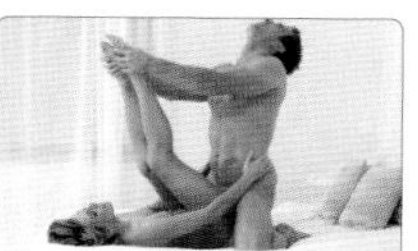
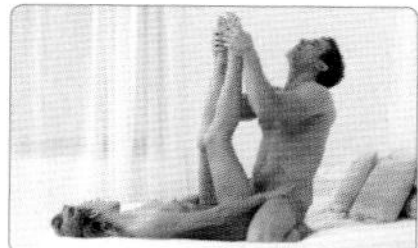

The ninth posture

☆☆☆☆☆ Kama sensation rating

Think of this as the luxury end of the doggie-position market; he kneels upright behind her, and she drapes her top half across a bed or sofa. You're both comfortable, relaxed, and perfectly positioned to give yourselves up to intense pleasure.

Why it works

- He can thrust deeply and freely, and her G-spot receives lots of stimulation as he moves.

- You can make your wildest orgasm face safe in the knowledge that no one can see.

- Unlike other doggie-style positions, she doesn't have to support her body weight on her hands or elbows; this makes for relaxed rear entry, with all the usual eroticism and fantasy potential that doggie offers.

- If he wants to make a back-door entrance, he's ideally poised to do so. And the fact that she's comfortable will help her to relax her anal muscles and let him in.

Turn on...

... Make sure that your penis is roughly parallel with her vaginal entrance; if you need her to be lower, ask her to spread her knees further apart. She can also change the height and angle of entry by tilting her pelvis up or down.

Turn off...

... Don't get friction burns on your knees (unless sex injuries are part of the fun). Lay down a soft blanket or cushions as padding.

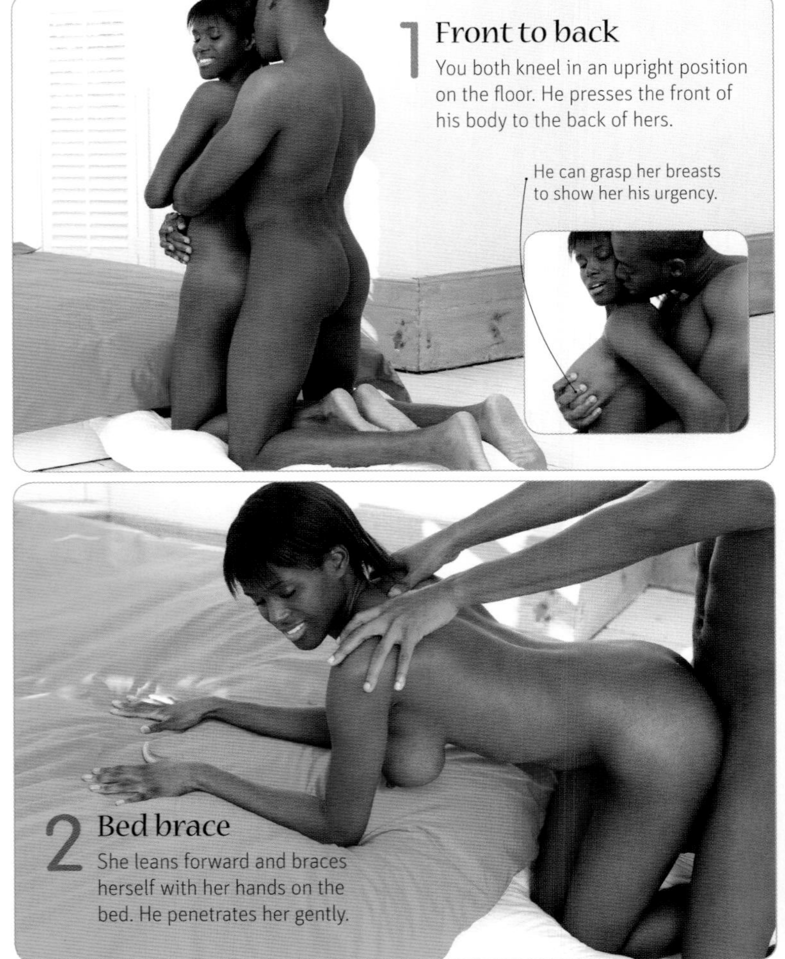

1 Front to back
You both kneel in an upright position on the floor. He presses the front of his body to the back of hers.

He can grasp her breasts to show her his urgency.

2 Bed brace
She leans forward and braces herself with her hands on the bed. He penetrates her gently.

"The things that develop love for the moment of coition are the playful frolics that precede it and the passionate embrace at the climax." THE PERFUMED GARDEN

Taking it further

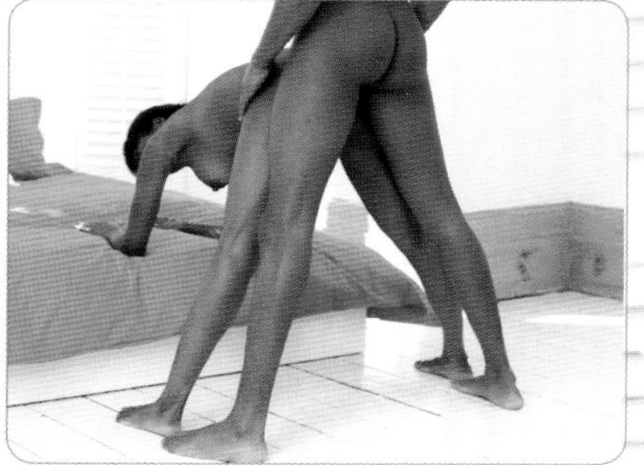

The perfect quickie

For quickie sex that feels both spontaneous and raunchy, he stands up and penetrates her from behind as she bends over, resting on her forearms.

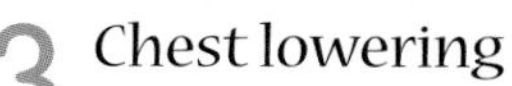

3 Chest lowering

She lowers her chest to the bed and rests on her forearms as he takes her hips in his hands and thrusts.

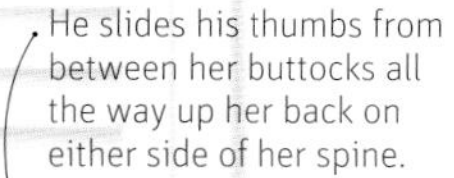

He slides his thumbs from between her buttocks all the way up her back on either side of her spine.

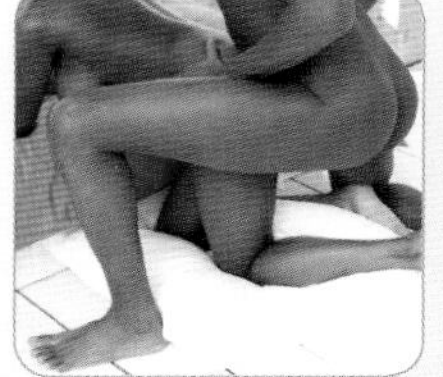

He can try a half-kneeling position with one foot flat on the ground so that he can move more vigorously.

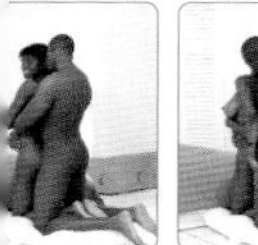
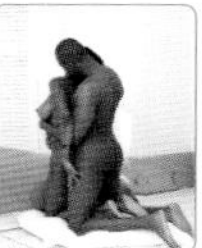
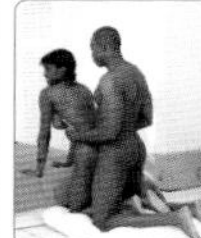
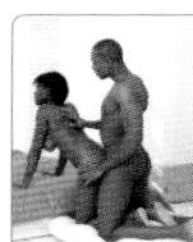
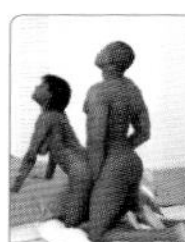
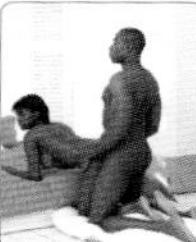
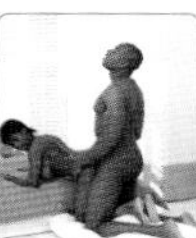
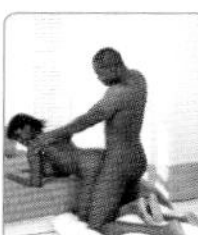
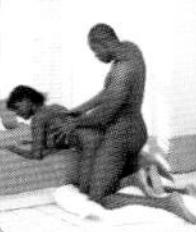
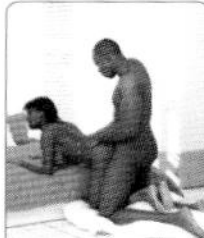
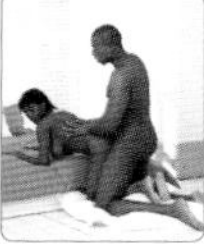

Seagulls on the wing

☆☆☆☆☆ Kama sensation rating

This one will check off lots of boxes for both of you. You don't have to be super-supple or gym-fit, and, providing he's at the right height, the angle of entry produces explosive sensations. You can also put your hands to plenty of good use. In fact, the only thing you can't do is kiss.

Why it works

- Precision entry gives both of you a sharp thrill at the moment of penetration.
- She can have a mid-sex orgasm from some clitoral handwork (self-delivered or from him).
- The freedom to pump, thrust, rub, and gyrate can drive both of you to a fast orgasm.
- You have most of the benefits of a face-to-face, man-on-top position with the bonus that he's quite literally in between her thighs and can sink into her easily and deeply.
- He can grab, stroke, and caress her sides, breasts, and thighs, and she can tweak her nipples and caress her breasts.

Turn on...

... Contribute to the movement by thrusting your pelvis up and down, and back and forth, while he's inside you. Squeeze him tight with your thighs and your vaginal muscles.

Turn off...

... Don't try too hard to climax at the same time. Simultaneous orgasm is an aim that's easy to get hung up on. If it happens, great, but don't worry if it doesn't; don't get too goal-oriented.

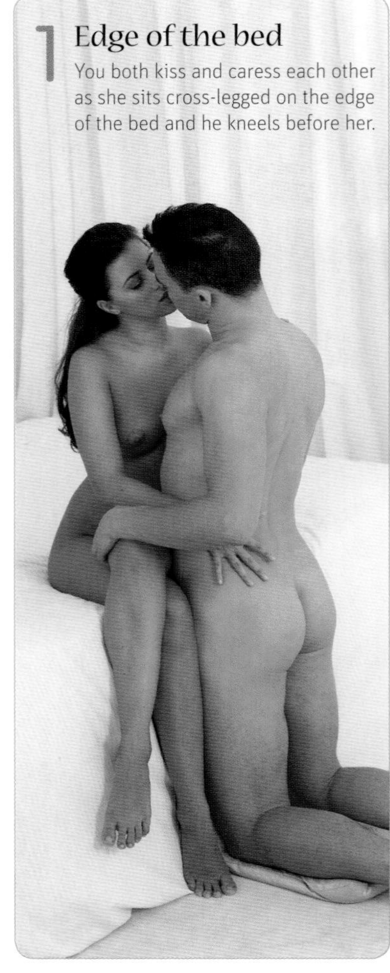

1 Edge of the bed

You both kiss and caress each other as she sits cross-legged on the edge of the bed and he kneels before her.

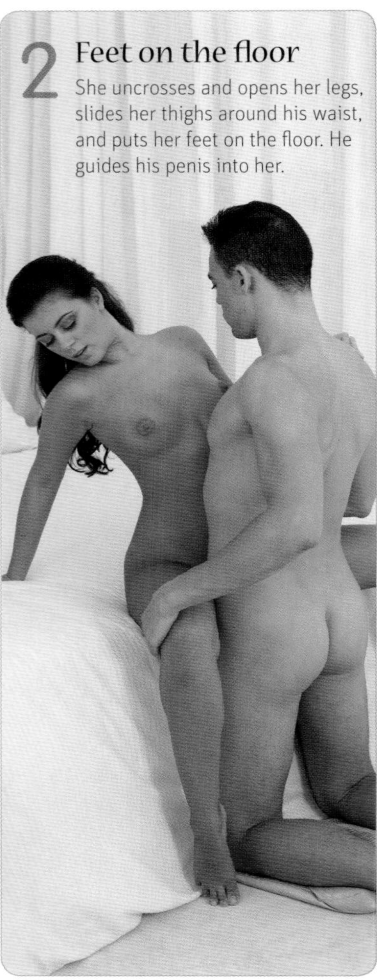

2 Feet on the floor

She uncrosses and opens her legs, slides her thighs around his waist, and puts her feet on the floor. He guides his penis into her.

"Do not unite with a woman until she has been excited by your caresses." THE PERFUMED GARDEN

3 Knees to the side

She lets her whole body relax as her knees fall to the sides and she lies back on the bed and gives in to the sensation.

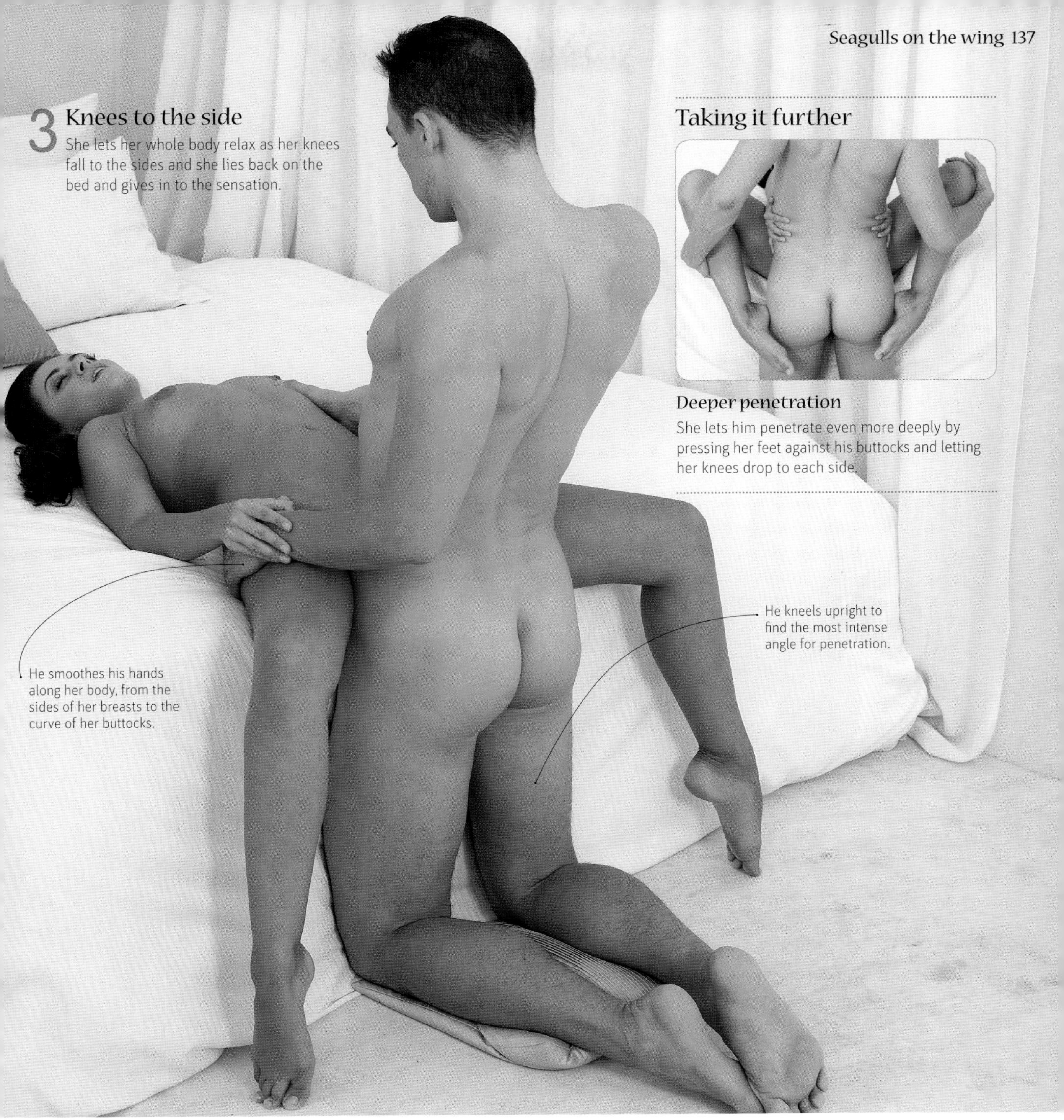

He smoothes his hands along her body, from the sides of her breasts to the curve of her buttocks.

He kneels upright to find the most intense angle for penetration.

Taking it further

Deeper penetration

She lets him penetrate even more deeply by pressing her feet against his buttocks and letting her knees drop to each side.

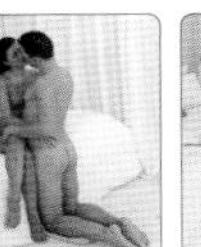
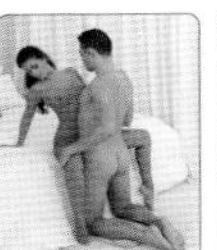
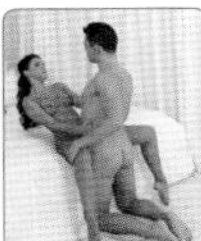
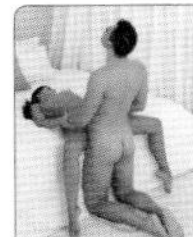
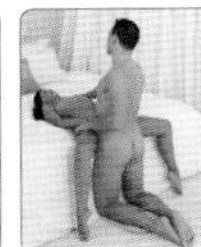
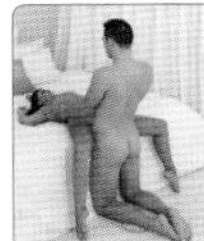
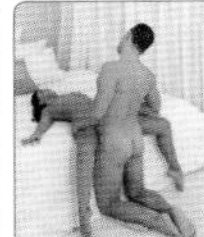
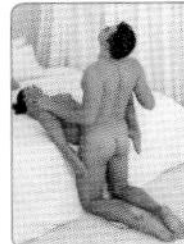
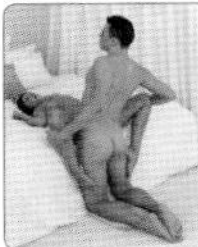
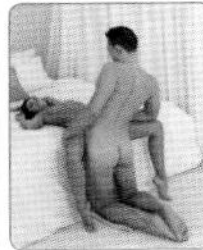

Level feet and Raised feet postures

☆☆☆☆ Kama sensation rating

These two positions come from a category called "uttana-bandha," or "supine posture." The old texts being nothing if not comprehensive, there are nine other variations featured, in which the woman places her legs in different positions.

Why they work

– In the Level Feet Posture you can both caress each other while he moves softly inside her. Your lust increases by the second.

– She stretches out her legs provocatively as the sexual tension increases.

– When you crave more vigorous movement, move into the Raised Feet Posture; because he leans on his hands, he can move more freely and deeply to take you both to the peak.

– If she needs more clitoral stimulation to achieve climax, she can reach through her legs and stroke herself to orgasm.

Turn on...

... Experiment to find out what the other nine subdivisions of leg position are. Find the leg position and angle of entry that presses the most buttons for both of you. For starters, she could try pressing her feet flat against his chest.

Turn off...

... Don't keep your legs in the air if it's frustratingly difficult to reach orgasm. Many women can't orgasm if they don't have their legs in a specific position; for example, flat on the bed and pressed together.

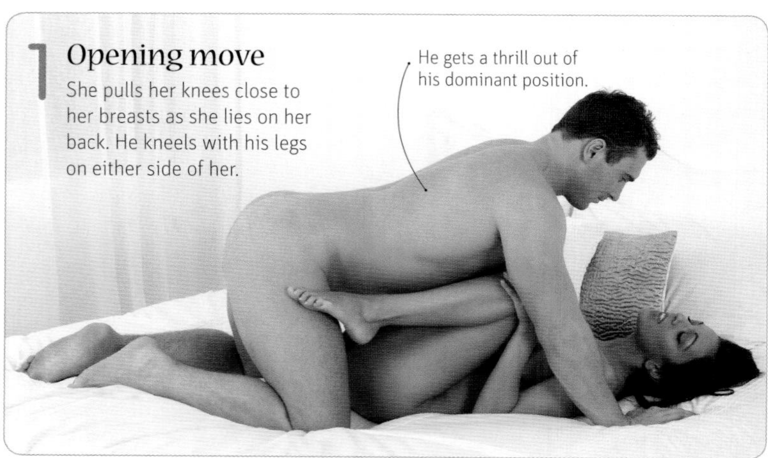

He gets a thrill out of his dominant position.

1 Opening move

She pulls her knees close to her breasts as she lies on her back. He kneels with his legs on either side of her.

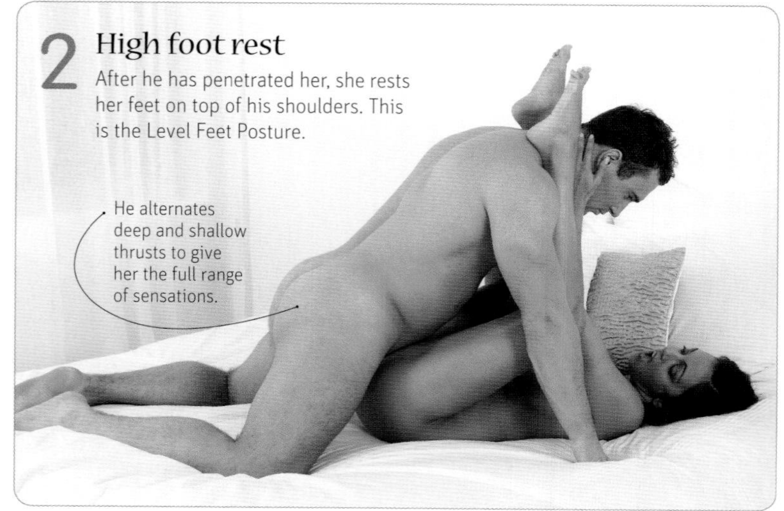

He alternates deep and shallow thrusts to give her the full range of sensations.

2 High foot rest

After he has penetrated her, she rests her feet on top of his shoulders. This is the Level Feet Posture.

"Uttana-bandha is the style of position named by men well versed in the art of love when a woman lies on her back." THE PERFUMED GARDEN

Taking it further

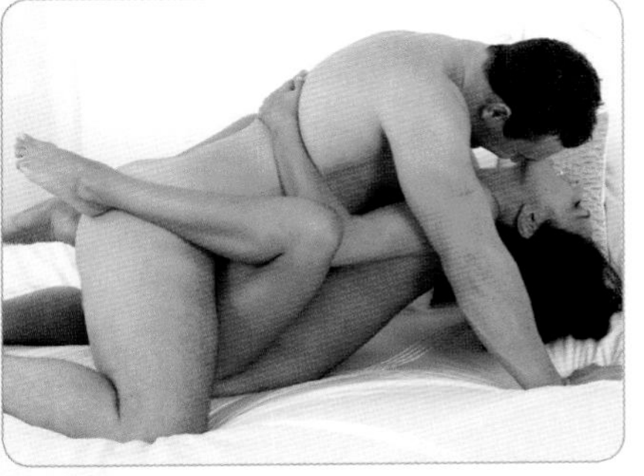

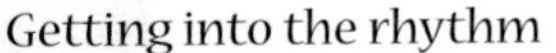

Getting into the rhythm

She takes a more active role, sitting up slightly, reaching through her thighs, and grabbing him around the waist to grind against him.

3 Low foot rest

She slides her feet down to his waist in a slow, teasing movement. He bends forward over her body. This is the Raised Feet Posture.

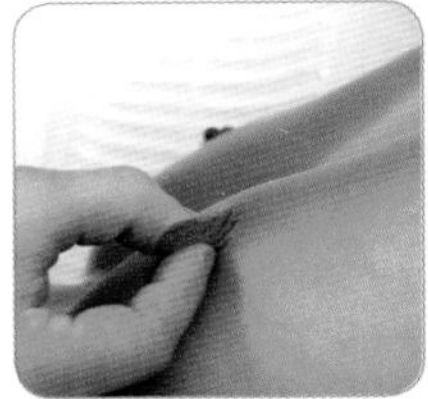

He can make her melt by rolling her nipple between his thumb and forefinger.

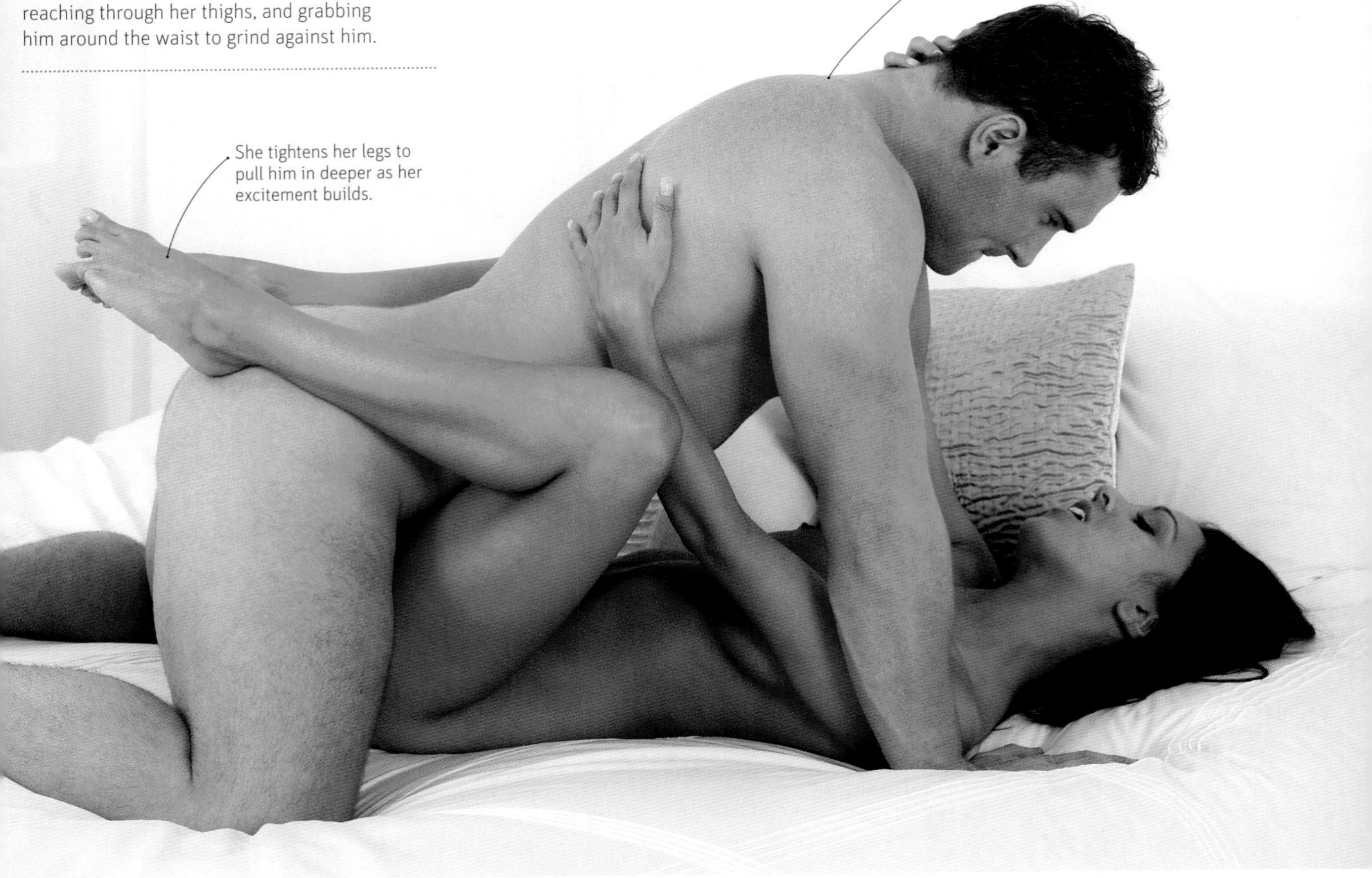

She tightens her legs to pull him in deeper as her excitement builds.

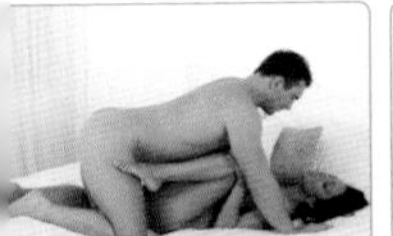
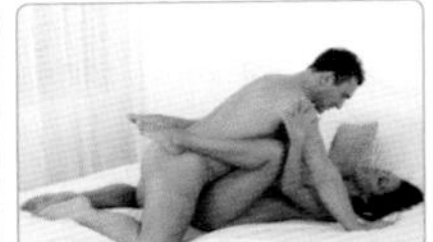
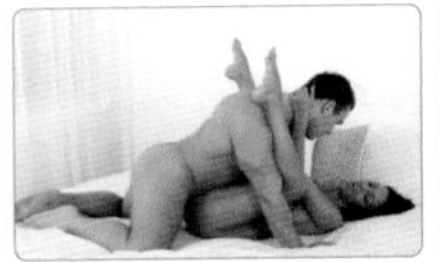
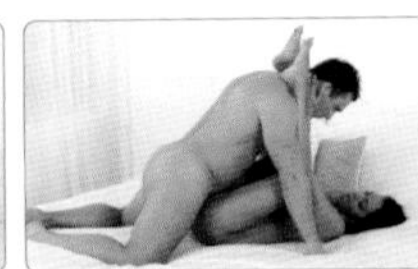
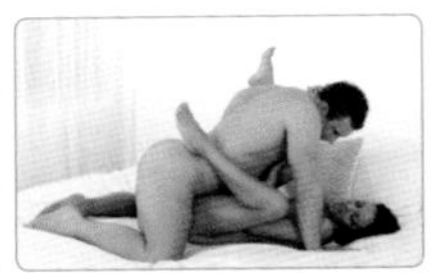
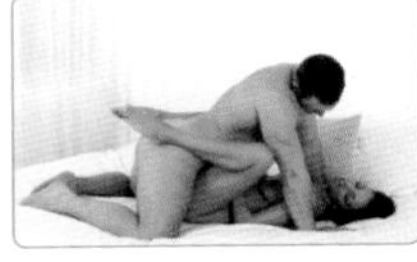

Interchange of coition

☆☆☆☆ Kama sensation rating

Tired of him being on top in the missionary position? She can forcefully overthrow him so that he's lying flat on his back with his legs spread, while she climbs on top in the traditionally masculine half push-up. Think of it as a sexual coup.

Why it works

– Her legs are together, which produces a satisfyingly snug fit between the two of you.

– She makes sparks fly for both of you by jerking her pelvis rapidly back and forth. This mimics the pumping action of his penis.

– She can pull things back from the brink with seductive feminine movements such as slow hip circles.

– There's little pressure on him to perform; he just has to lie back.

– He loves the sight of her on top of him and the sensation of her breasts caressing his chest as she moves.

Turn on…

… Concentrate on movements that take you to orgasm. If you find the right angle and motion, you'll feel lots of clitoral friction from his pubic bone and the base of his penis. The fact that your legs are together may also help you to climax.

Turn off…

… Don't stay in a half push-up if you're getting tired. Lean forward and cuddle him for a moment of deep and soulful union.

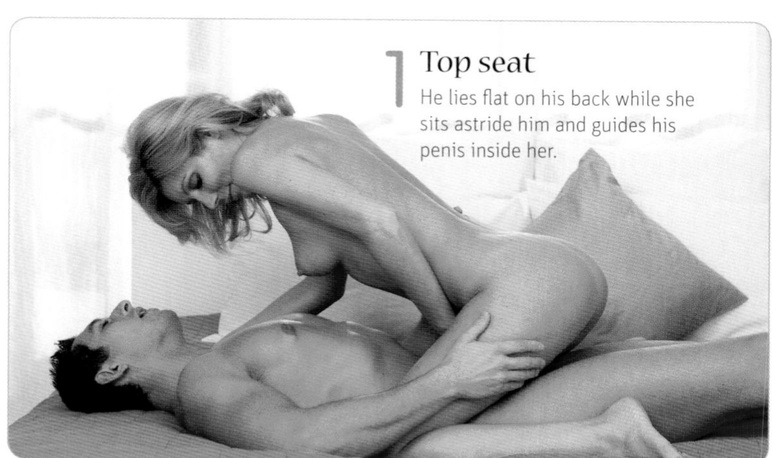

1 Top seat
He lies flat on his back while she sits astride him and guides his penis inside her.

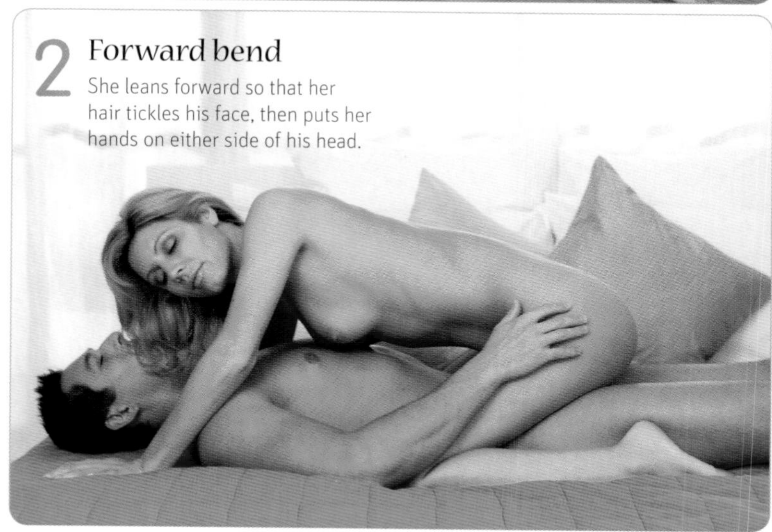

2 Forward bend
She leans forward so that her hair tickles his face, then puts her hands on either side of his head.

"She moves on him with exactly the sexual strokes that he would use on her." KAMA SUTRA

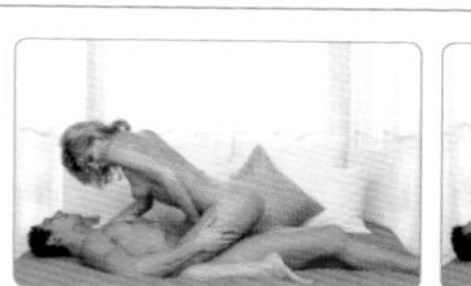

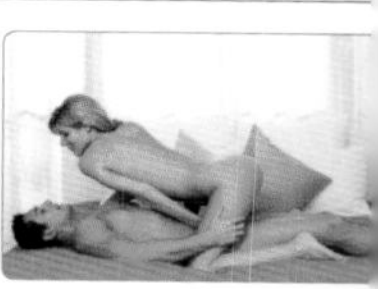

Taking it further

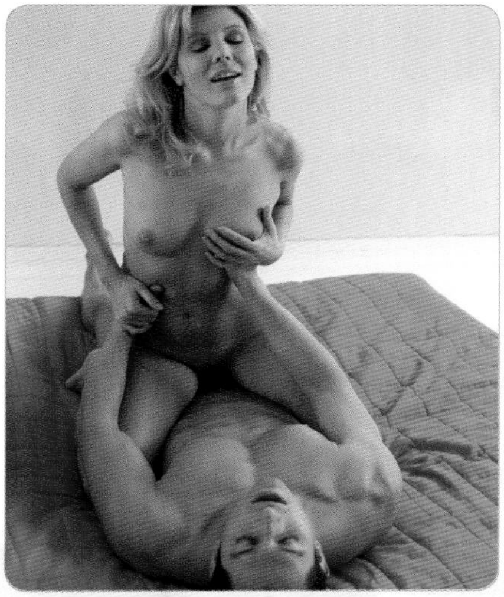

Cowgirl-style

She brings her knees up to straddle him as in a cowgirl-style position, opening her legs up and allowing him to thrust too.

3 Half push-up

She straightens her legs so that she's in a half push-up position. He bends his knees and encloses her between his legs.

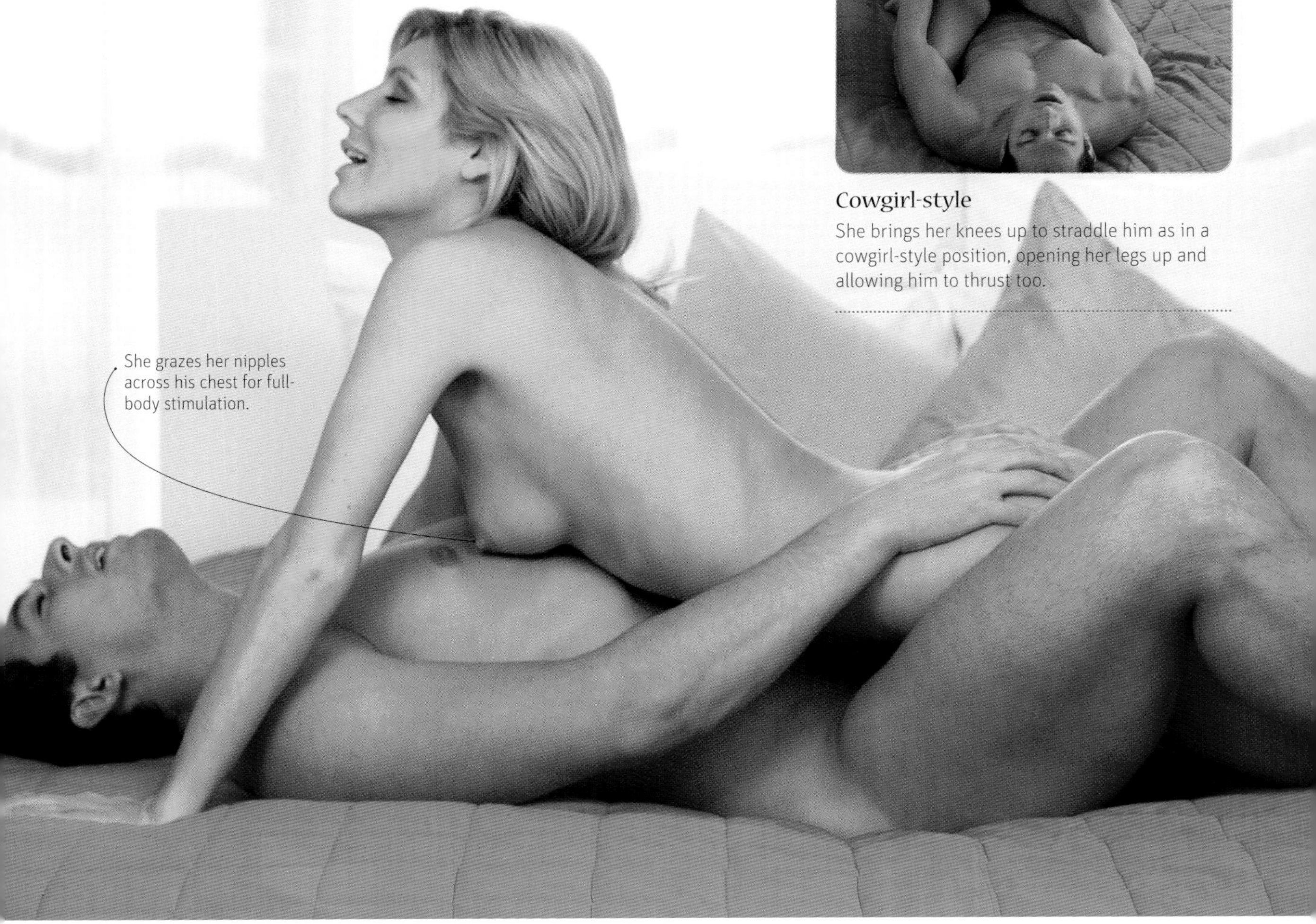

She grazes her nipples across his chest for full-body stimulation.

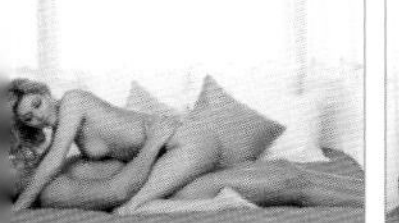
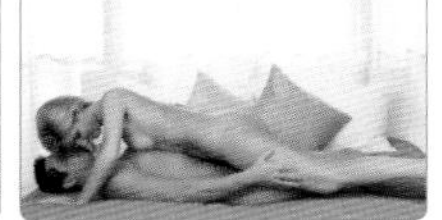
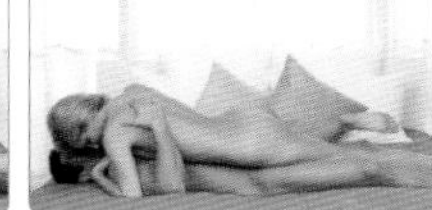
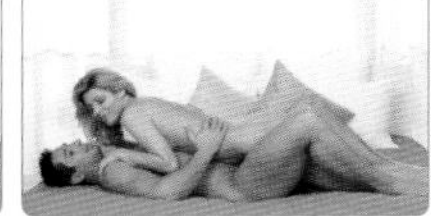
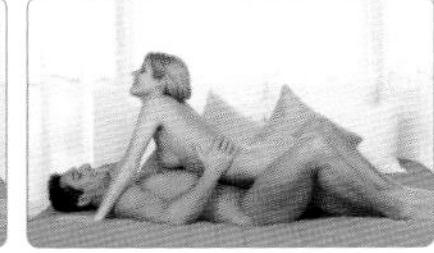

Driving the peg home

Reserve this position for moments of grand passion. It's exciting, rampant, and immediate. For the ultimate in spontaneous kicks, do it anywhere that's not at home. Suitable venues include the spare room at a party, a deserted corridor, an office (after-hours), a quiet backstreet, or a patch of secluded woodland (pick a tree that won't graze her back).

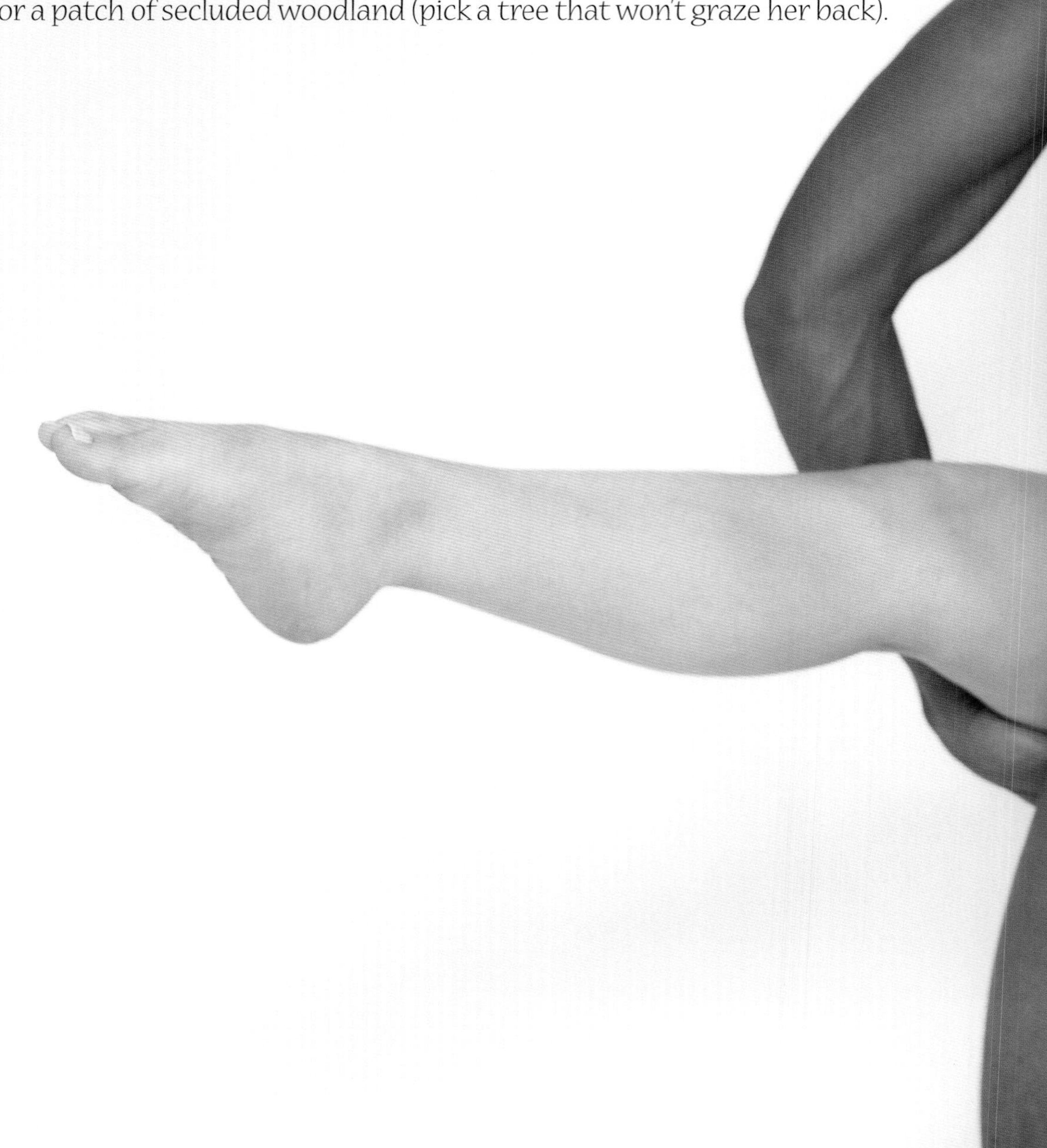

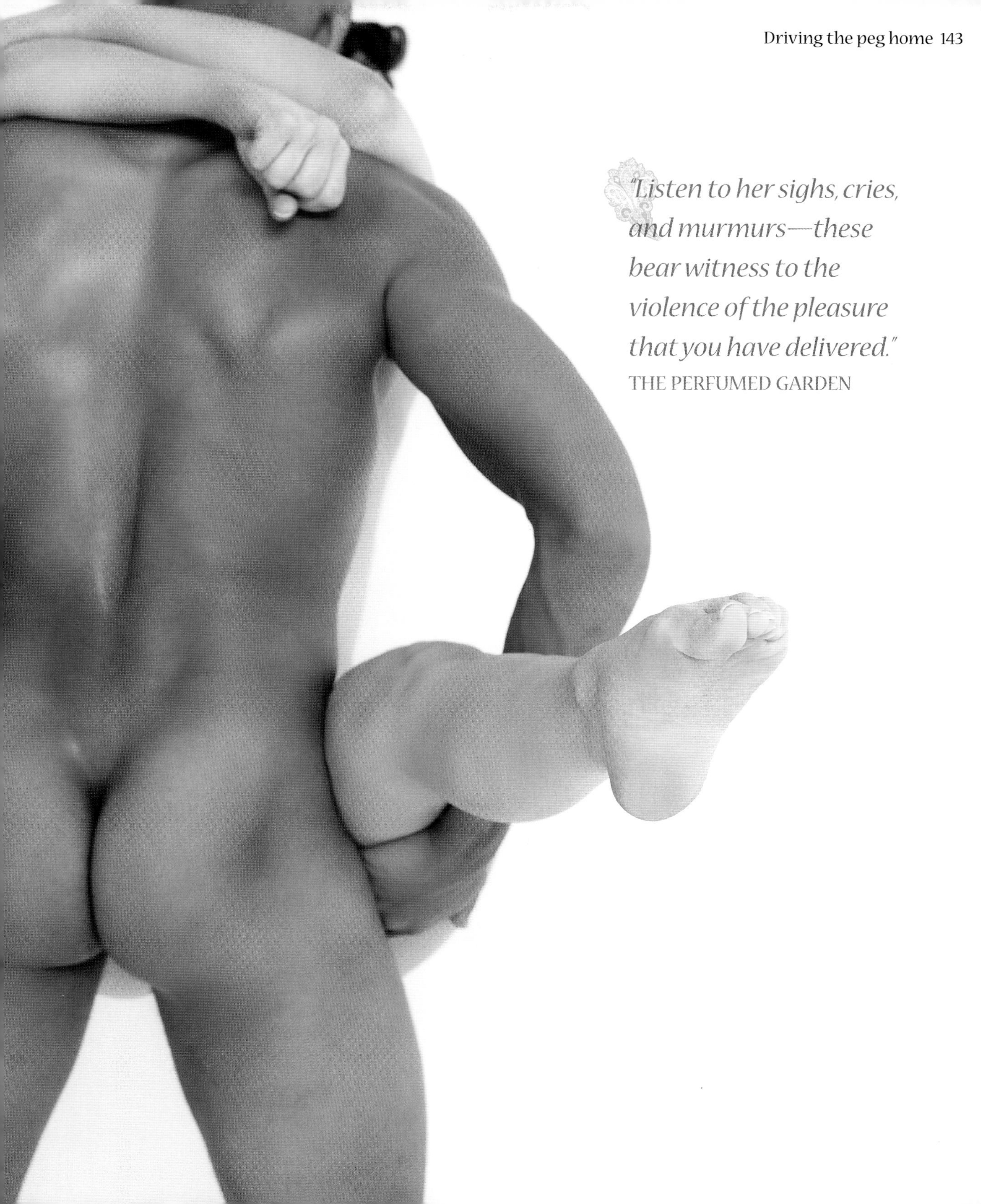

"Listen to her sighs, cries, and murmurs—these bear witness to the violence of the pleasure that you have delivered."
THE PERFUMED GARDEN

Driving the peg home

☆☆☆☆
Kama sensation rating

Why it works

– She feels thoroughly penetrated as he drives his peg home.

– The wall behind her back supports and stabilizes the position as he thrusts.

– If you're near a bed, you can use this position as a sexy mode of transport. When you arrive at the bed, he can lower her on to the mattress, then pounce on top.

– She loves feeling swept away by the force and strength of his passion.

– He loves feeling powerful and in control.

– It gives you the thrill of just-can't-wait-another-second passion.

– If there's even a small possibility of being caught, this adds to the sense of lustful and naughty urgency.

Turn on...

... Try it the other way around as well; he has his back to the wall, and she presses against the wall with her feet. If she's light and he's strong, she may be able to push on and off him while he stands still.

Turn off...

... Doing your back in. Do cheat if she's heavy or he's struggling. She can sit on a high counter so that he doesn't have to support her weight.

1 Wall press

He presses her up against a wall and kisses her passionately, his hands roaming over her body.

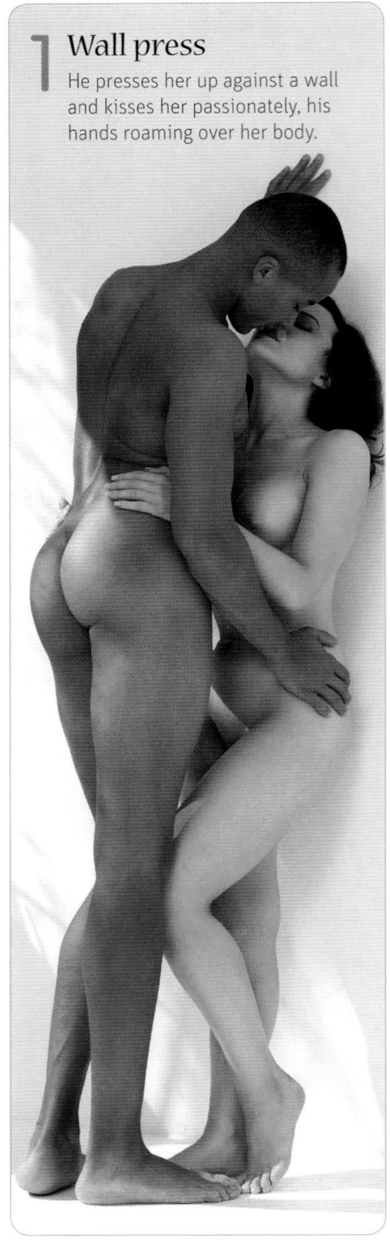

2 The descent

He slides slowly down her body, pausing on the way down to kiss, lick, and fondle all her most sensitive and intimate areas.

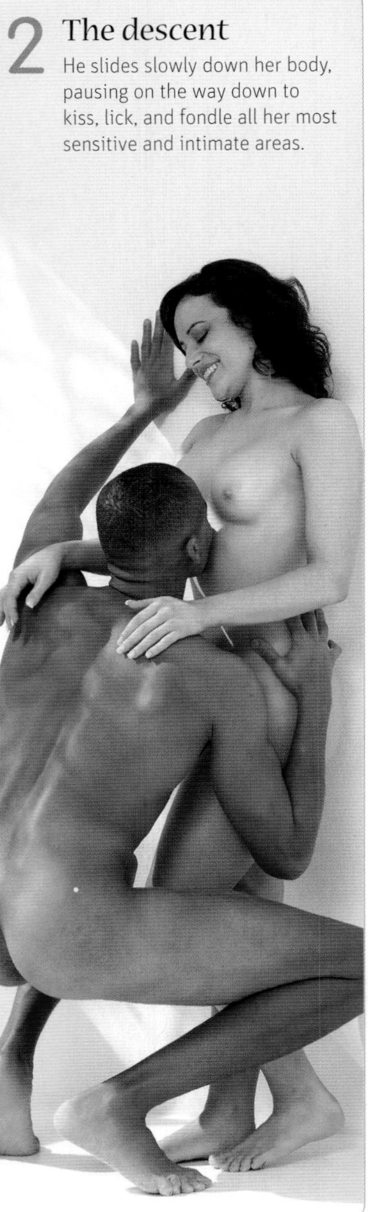

"When the man introduces his member, it is as if the woman is sitting on a peg." THE PERFUMED GARDEN

Taking it further

Leaning back

She changes the angle of penetration by leaning back and bracing her shoulders against the wall, giving him more freedom to thrust.

3 Mounting

He crouches, and she mounts him, crossing her ankles behind his back for support.

4 Tight clasp

He straightens up as she clasps him tightly with her arms and legs. He presses her against the wall as he moves inside her.

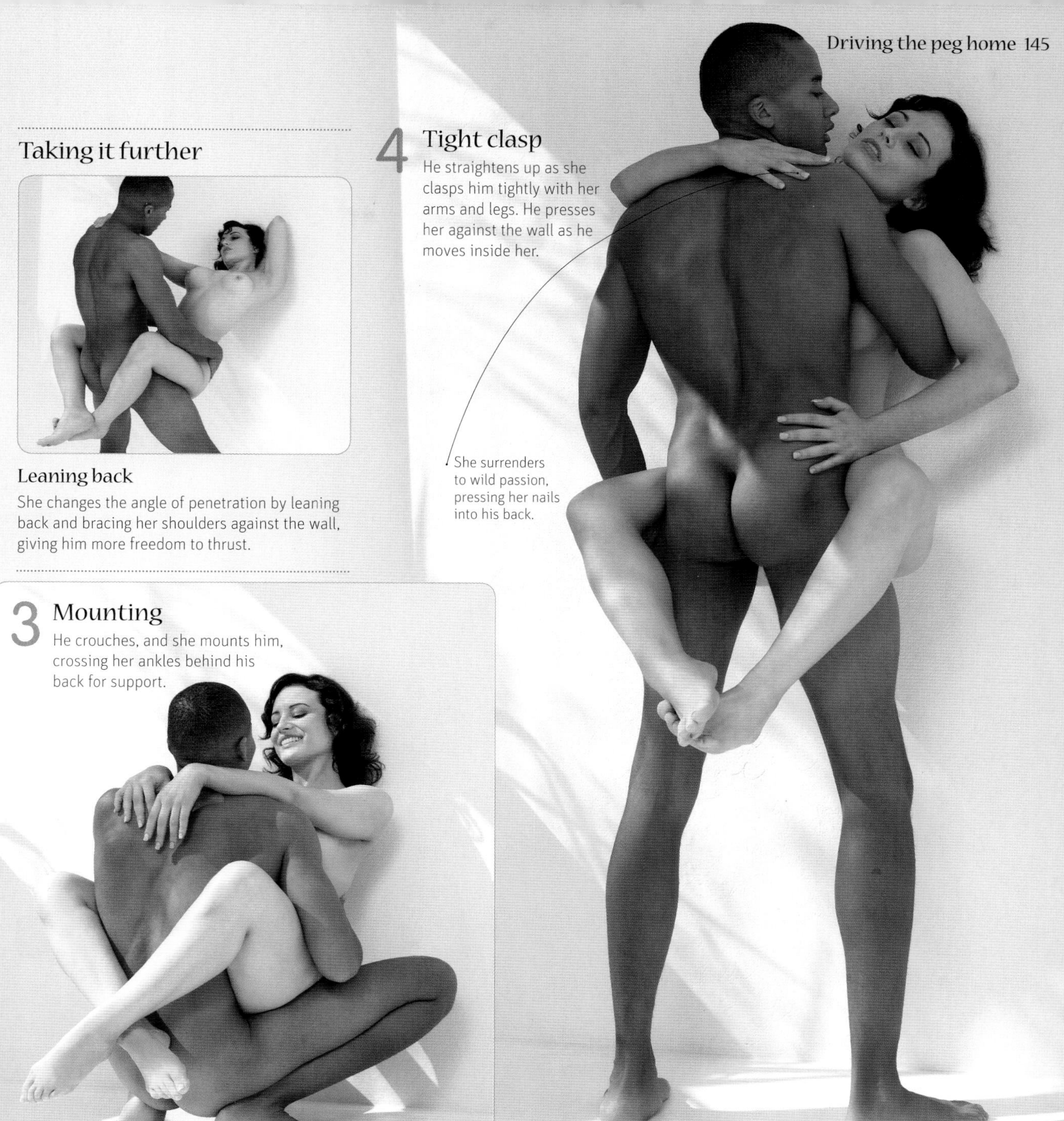

She surrenders to wild passion, pressing her nails into his back.

If you liked this, try…

– Turning around so his back is against the wall in Suspended Congress (see page 186).

– The weight-free Supported Congress, if you're flagging (see page 90).

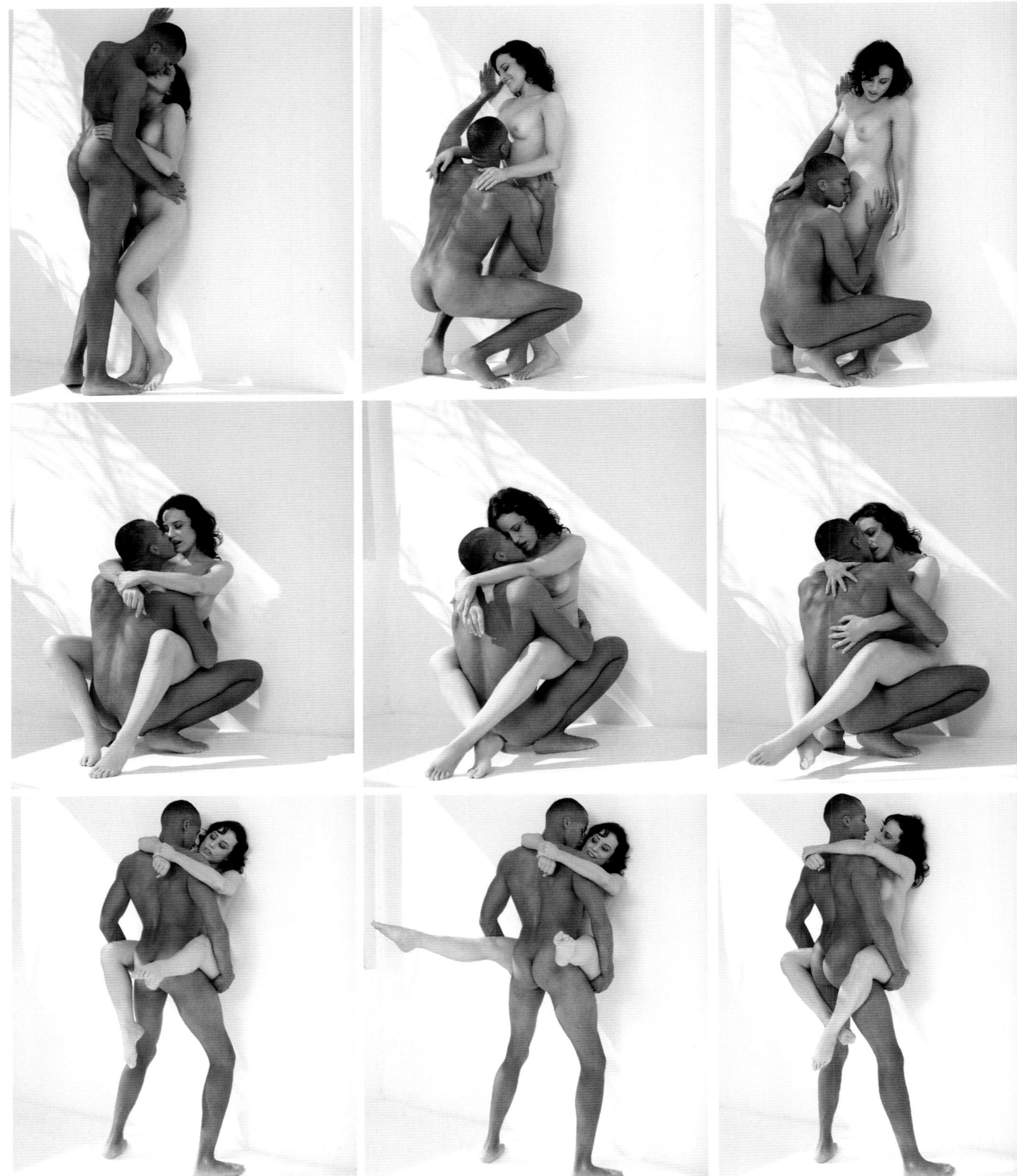

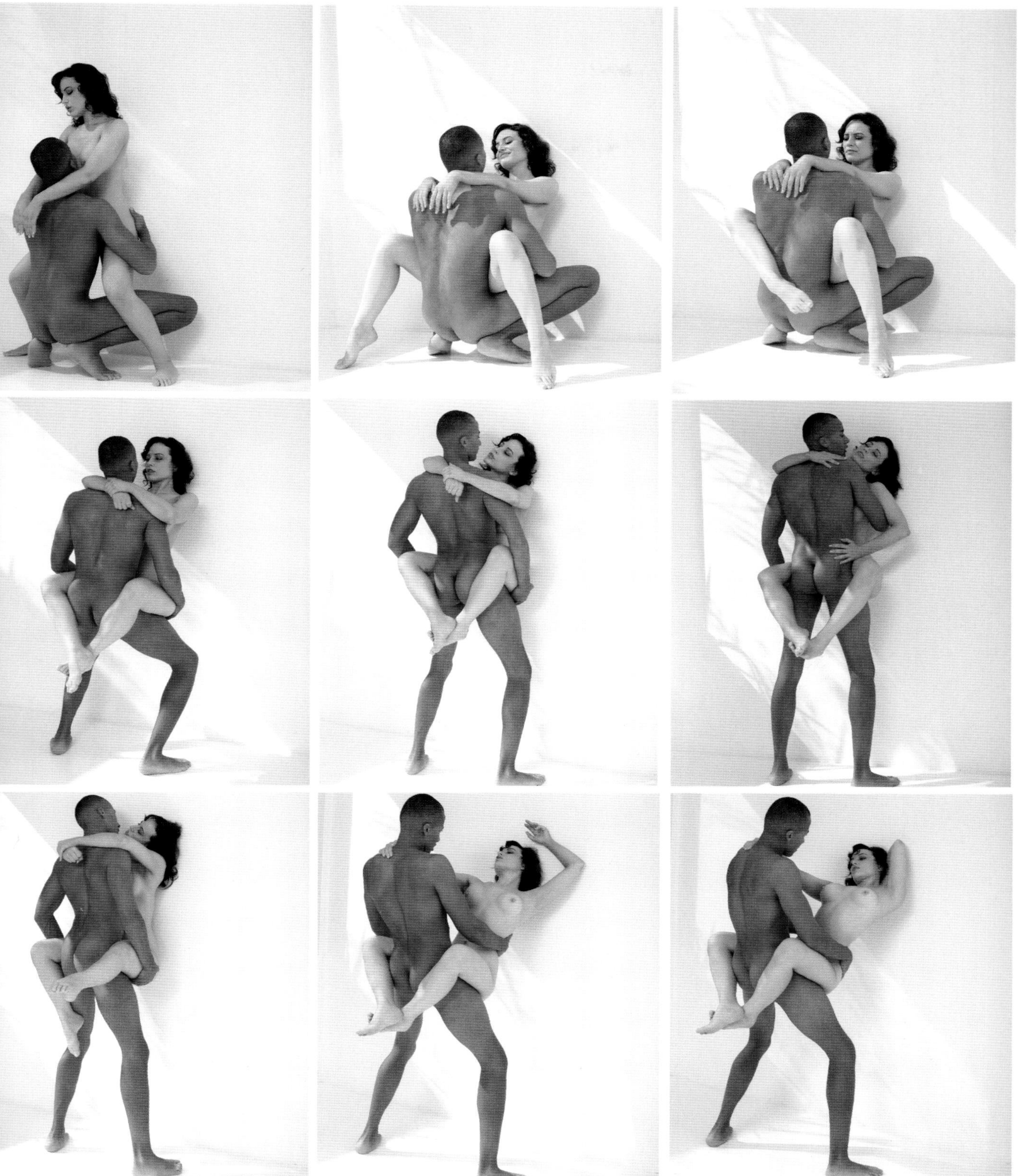

Phoenix playing in a red cave

☆☆☆☆☆ Kama sensation rating

This position sounds deliciously Eastern, erotic, and exotic. Happily, it lives up to its name in terms of sensation by allowing deep, intense penetration. He feels sucked in (in more ways than one) as she draws her knees to her chest in the ultimate "come-on-in" gesture.

Why it works

– Her vagina is contracted, so she feels every sensation exquisitely. This position is good for couples with low union (see page 128).

– Her clitoris is exposed, so it's an ideal position for top-up clitoral stimulation with his fingers or a sex toy.

– He enjoys physical barrier-free penetration and can plunge deeply.

– Apparent vulnerability meets sexual power as she raises her legs for him in an intimate sexual invitation.

– He can give her melting sensations by stroking the backs of her thighs.

Turn on...

... Talk dirty. Use whatever language comes naturally to you. If it turns you on to talk about "his phoenix" or "her red cave," go ahead.

Turn off...

... Don't neglect foreplay; she'll need to be as wet as possible because penetration is deep in this position. If she's not ready, penetration may be uncomfortable, and her cervix may take a pounding.

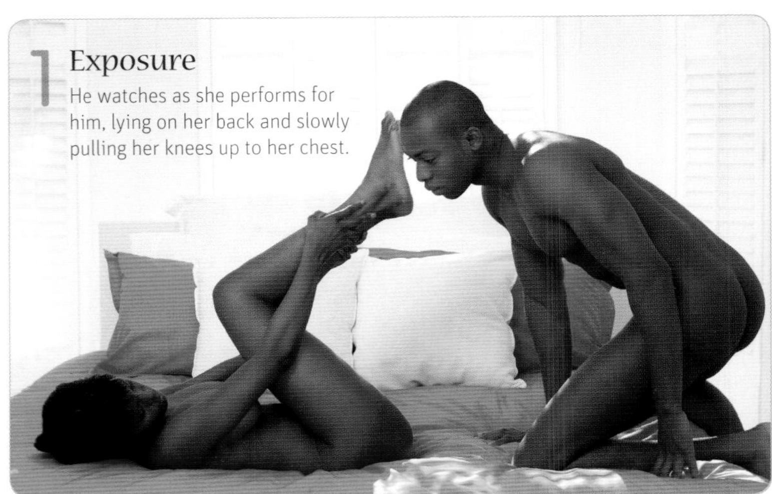

1 Exposure
He watches as she performs for him, lying on her back and slowly pulling her knees up to her chest.

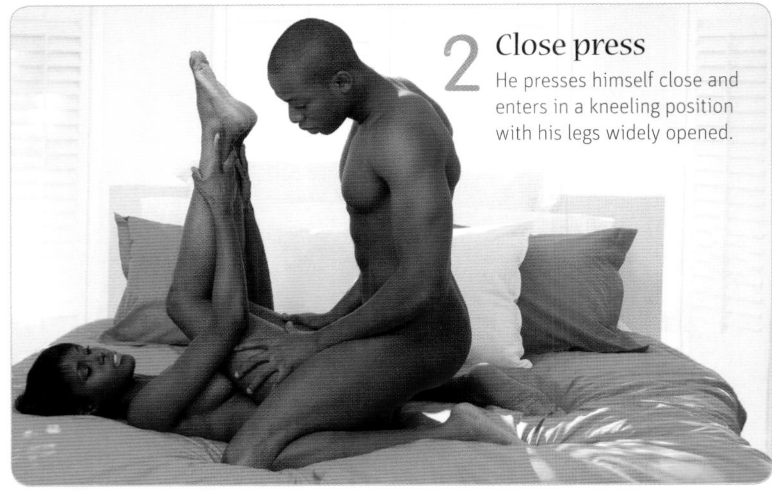

2 Close press
He presses himself close and enters in a kneeling position with his legs widely opened.

"Seek ardently to arouse her sucker, so will your work be worthily crowned." THE PERFUMED GARDEN

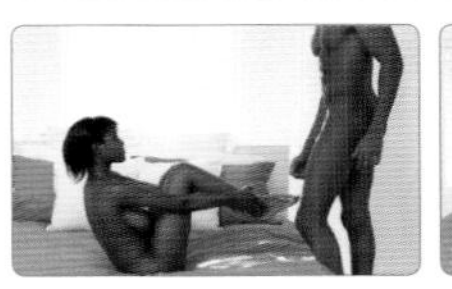

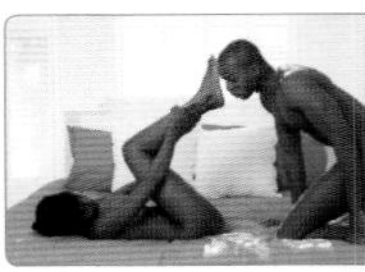

Taking it further

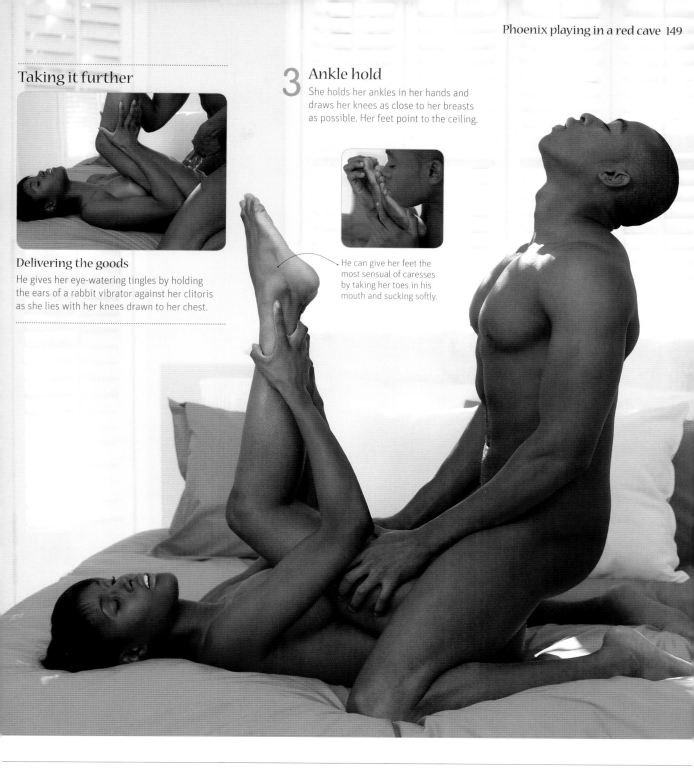

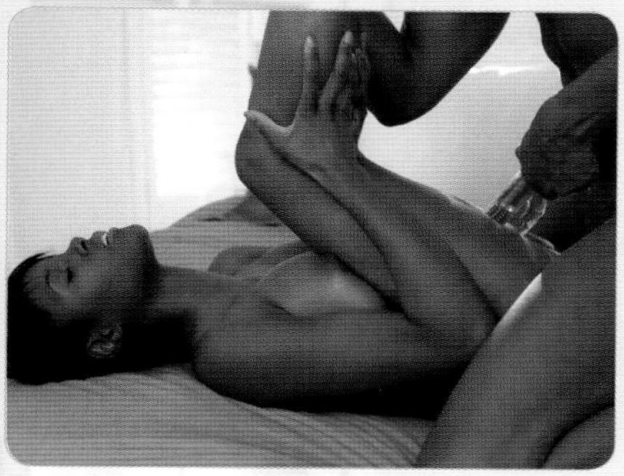

Delivering the goods

He gives her eye-watering tingles by holding the ears of a rabbit vibrator against her clitoris as she lies with her knees drawn to her chest.

3 Ankle hold

She holds her ankles in her hands and draws her knees as close to her breasts as possible. Her feet point to the ceiling.

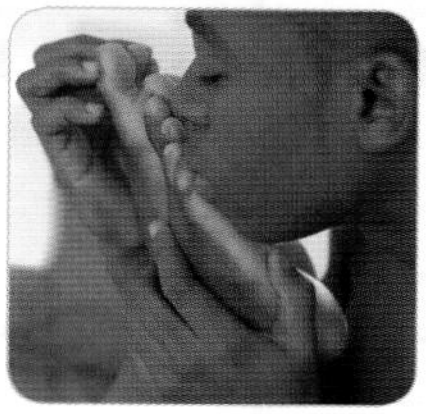

He can give her feet the most sensual of caresses by taking her toes in his mouth and sucking softly.

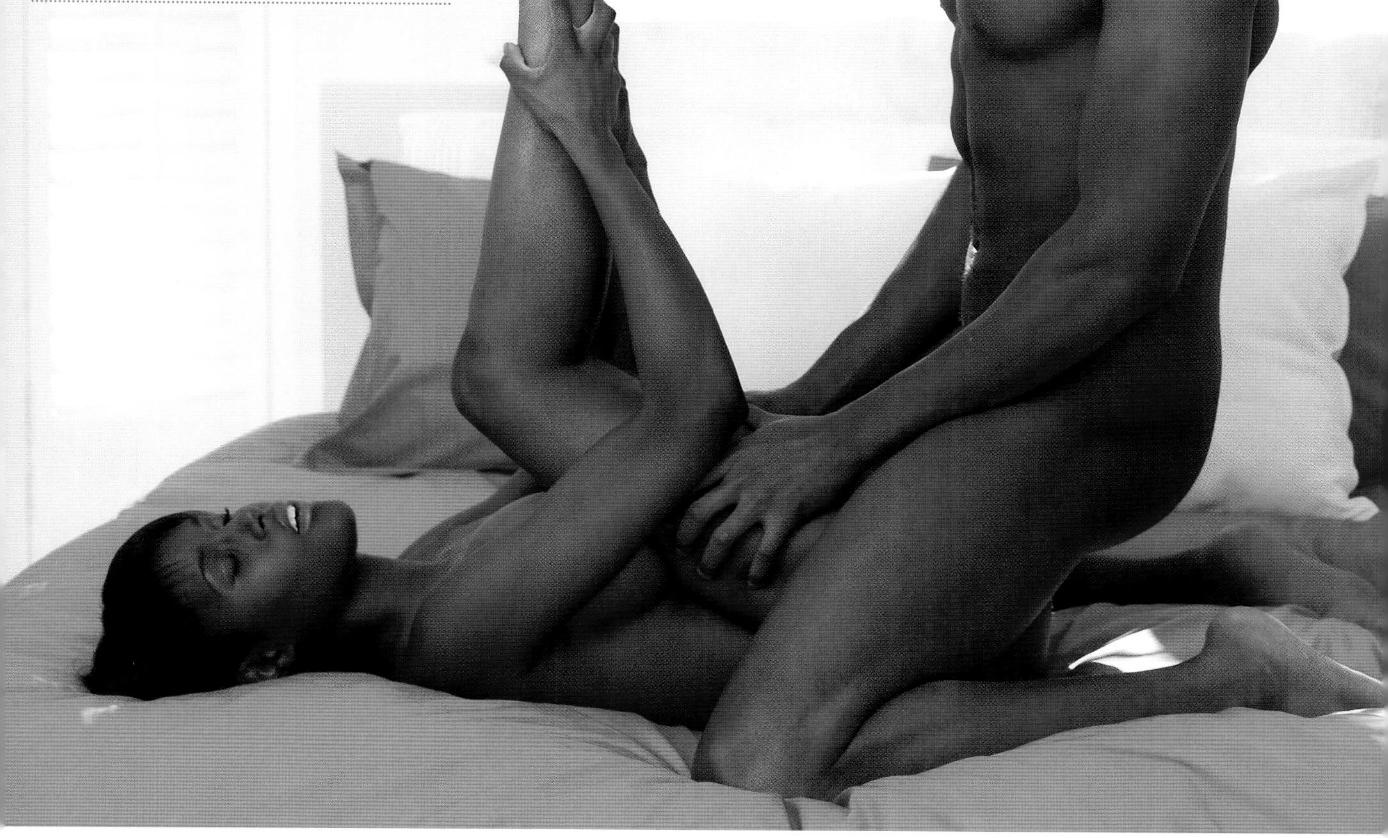

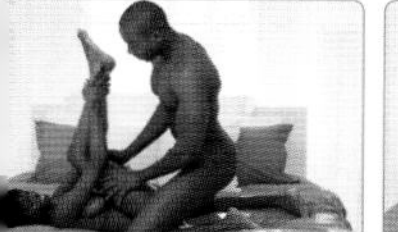
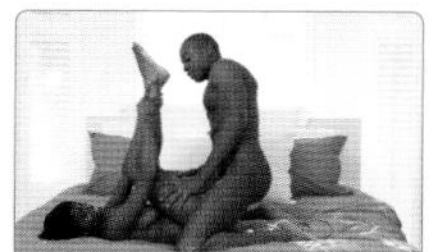
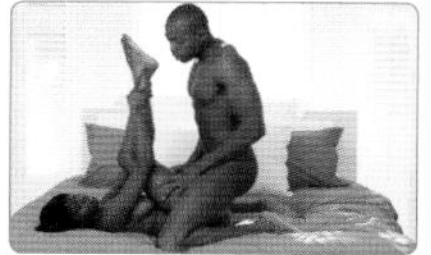
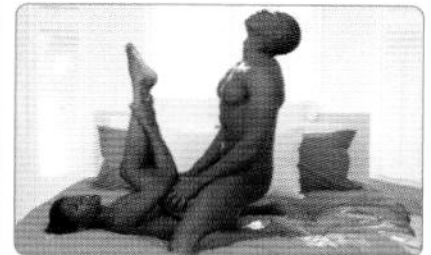
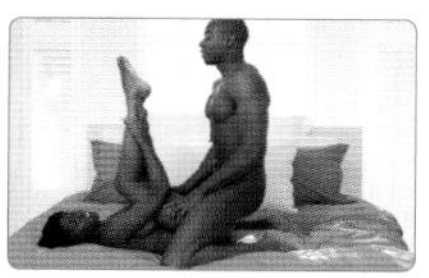

Pressed and Half-pressed positions

☆☆☆☆ Kama sensation rating

The eroticism of these two positions comes from the mix of resistance and compliance; the fact that you're pushing against one another creates an enticingly erotic struggle. And, despite the fact that he's in a dominant position, she can use her legs to push him away in a second.

Why they work

– Pressed Position feels tight and compact; she pushes against him with her feet, and he pushes back with his thrusts.

– Her knees are packed tightly against her breasts, which shortens her vagina.

– You can both use your hands to massage each other's thighs (or, if you're having sex that's too wild and uncontained for massage, you can pinch, grab, and slap instead).

– Switching from Pressed to Half-Pressed Position changes the tension with which her vagina grips his penis; if this feels good, you can keep doing it with alternate legs.

Turn on...

... Make the most of the proximity of her foot to his mouth. You don't have to be a foot fetishist to enjoy some mid-sex toe-sucking; the sensations of her toes enclosed in his warm mouth can be sublime.

Turn off...

... Don't make these positions the exclusive focus of a sex session if your legs can't go the distance. Mix them up with other sex positions that are easier on the thigh muscles.

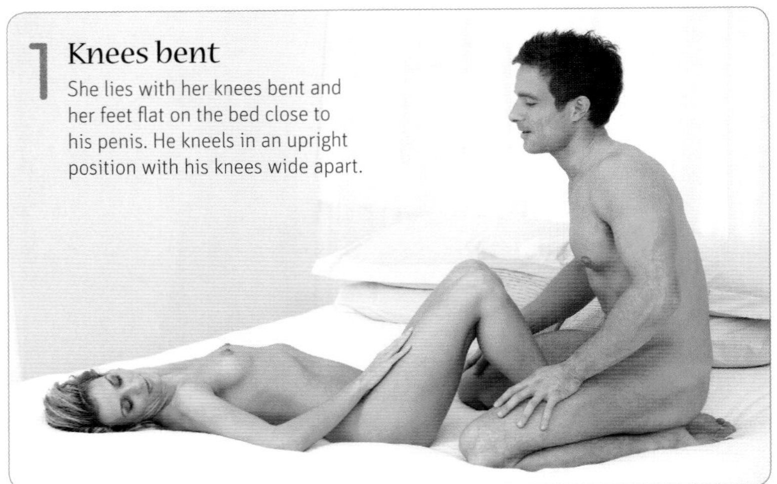

1 Knees bent

She lies with her knees bent and her feet flat on the bed close to his penis. He kneels in an upright position with his knees wide apart.

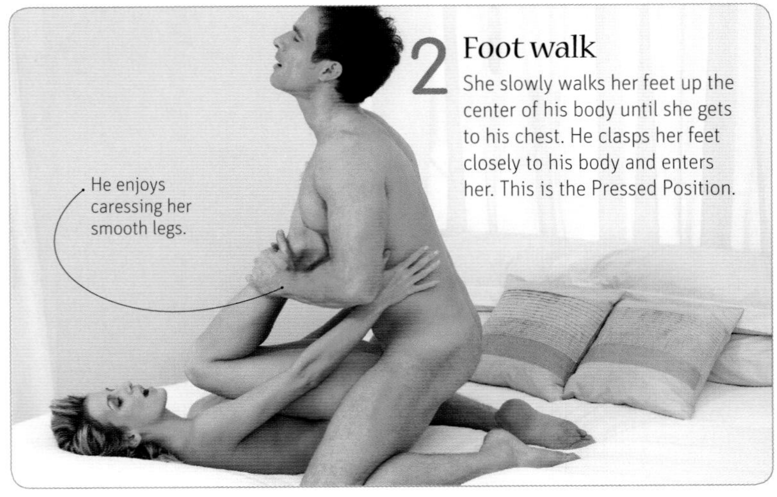

2 Foot walk

She slowly walks her feet up the center of his body until she gets to his chest. He clasps her feet closely to his body and enters her. This is the Pressed Position.

He enjoys caressing her smooth legs.

"When the woman presses her lover with her legs, it is called the Pressing Position." KAMA SUTRA

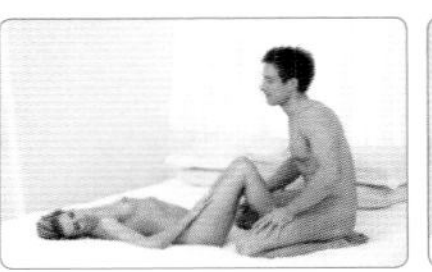

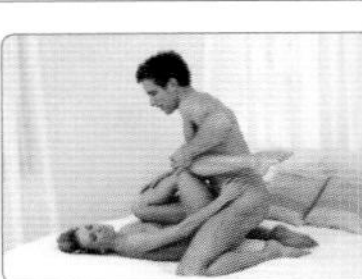

Taking it further

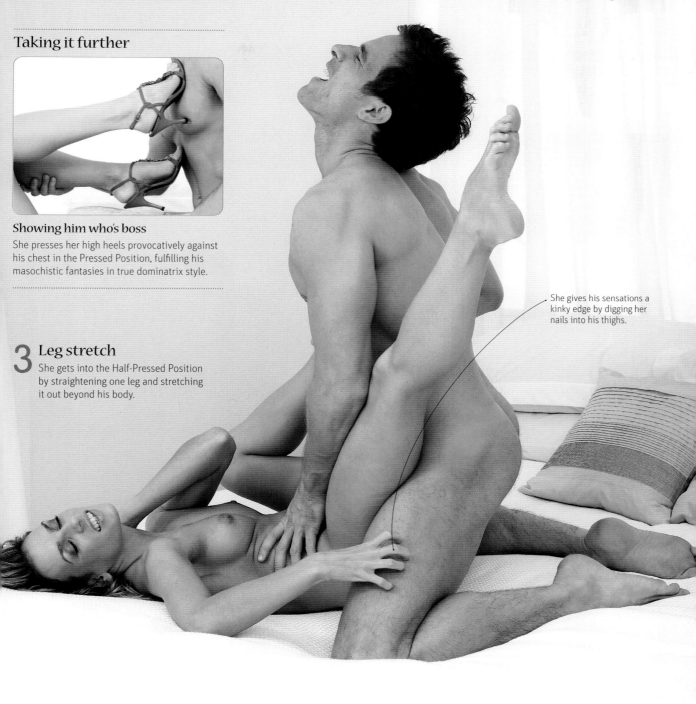

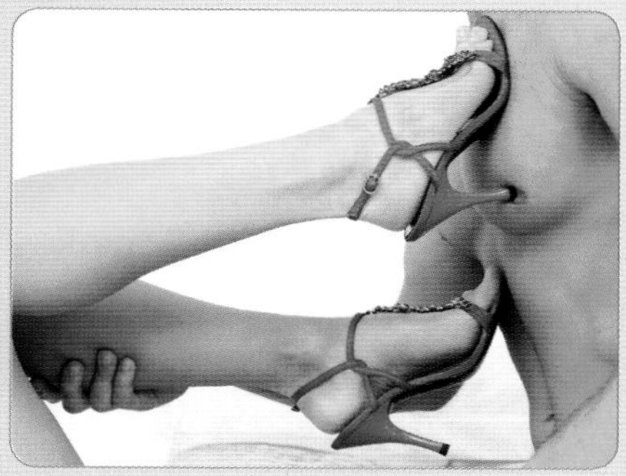

Showing him who's boss

She presses her high heels provocatively against his chest in the Pressed Position, fulfilling his masochistic fantasies in true dominatrix style.

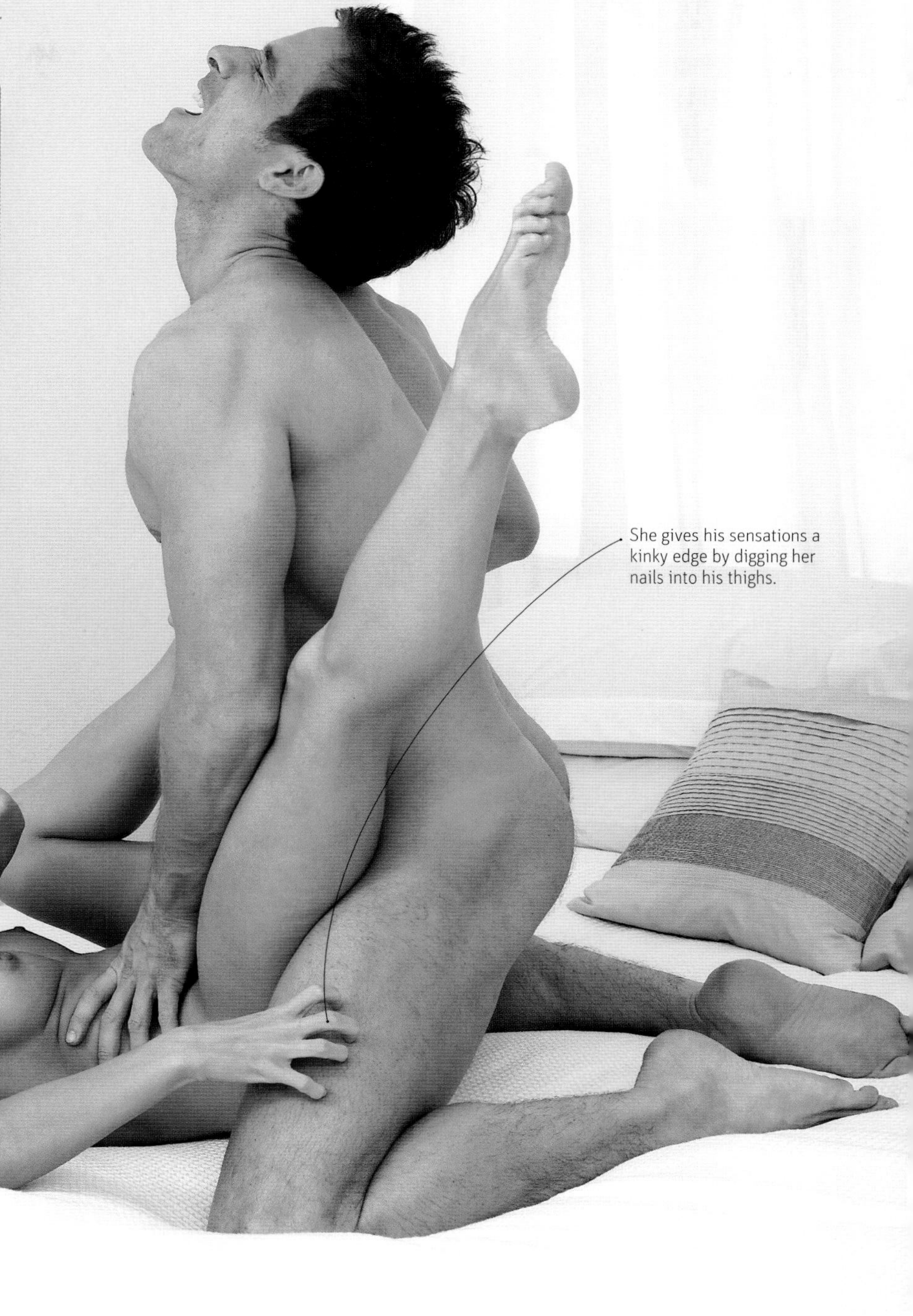

She gives his sensations a kinky edge by digging her nails into his thighs.

3 Leg stretch

She gets into the Half-Pressed Position by straightening one leg and stretching it out beyond his body.

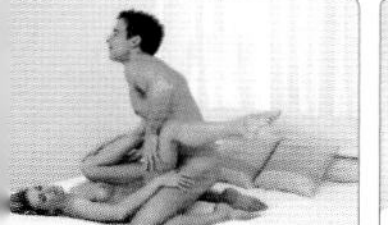
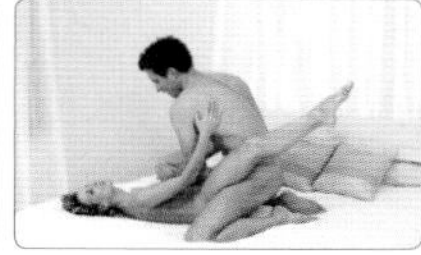
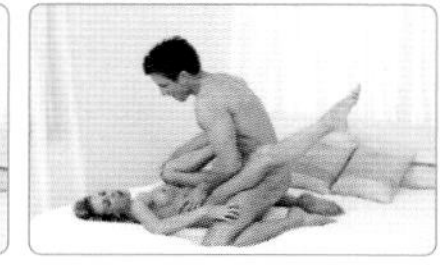
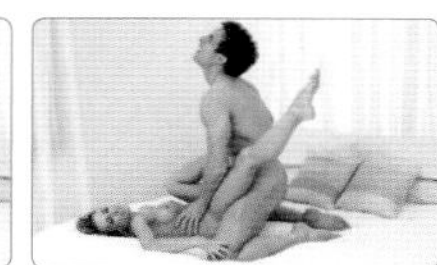
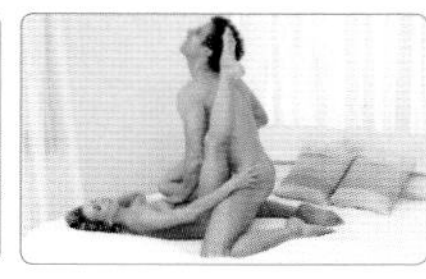

Refined position

☆☆☆☆☆ Kama sensation rating

This is precision sex: her vagina is exactly opposite his penis as he kneels upright. As a result he can glide in and out like a piece of well-oiled machinery, and the smooth, regular, rhythmic repetition should take both of you straight to sex heaven.

Why it works

- Sex feels effortlessly pleasurable because her pelvis is raised to the perfect height.
- His entry is slick and smooth.
- He can thrust with wild abandon or gentle restraint, depending on her mood.
- She feels comfortably supported in a wide-open, ready-to-receive-him position.
- He can support each swing of his pelvis by gripping her waist or hips.
- Four hands make light work of stimulating her breasts and clitoris to bring her to a fantastically speedy climax.

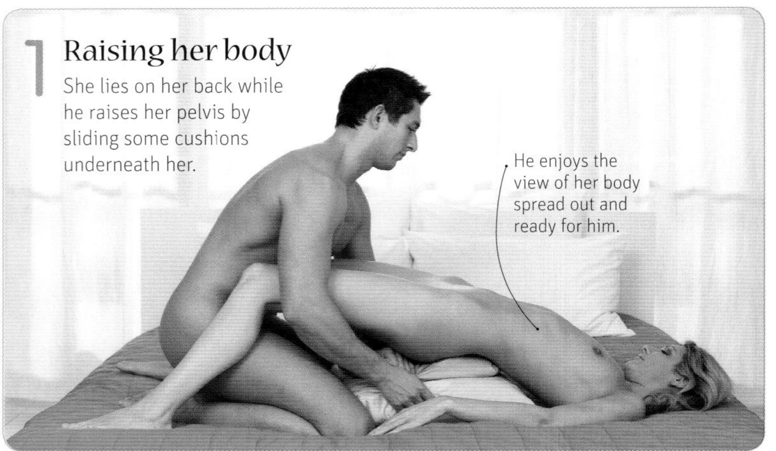

He enjoys the view of her body spread out and ready for him.

1 Raising her body

She lies on her back while he raises her pelvis by sliding some cushions underneath her.

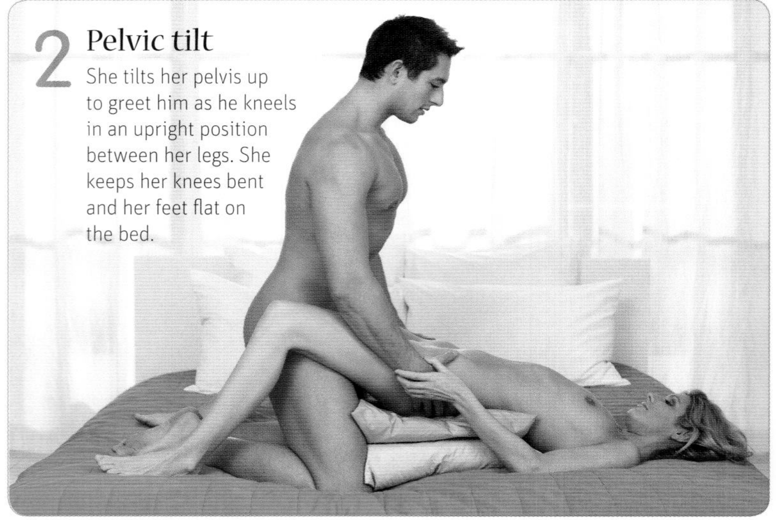

2 Pelvic tilt

She tilts her pelvis up to greet him as he kneels in an upright position between her legs. She keeps her knees bent and her feet flat on the bed.

Turn on...

... Make sure you're both lying/kneeling comfortably. Comfort may not sound sexy, but if you don't have to worry about carpet burns/wobbly cushions/ back strain, you can surrender to the moment.

Turn off...

... Don't attempt this position on a soft mattress; you need firm support underneath you to support those piston-like thrusts. If your bed doesn't do the job, transfer to the floor.

"The husband raises the seat of pleasure by placing pillows or pads under her head and hips this is an admirable form of congress and is greatly enjoyed by both." ANANGA RANGA

Taking it further

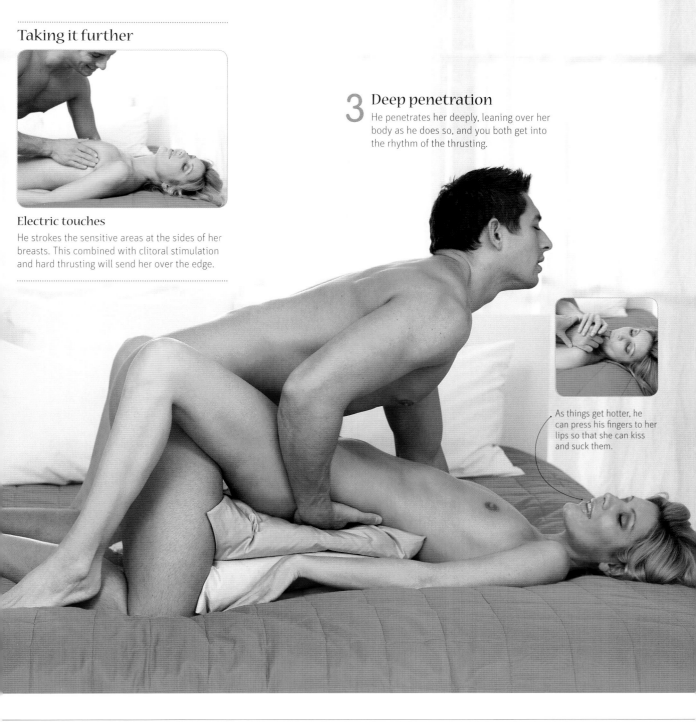

Electric touches

He strokes the sensitive areas at the sides of her breasts. This combined with clitoral stimulation and hard thrusting will send her over the edge.

3 Deep penetration

He penetrates her deeply, leaning over her body as he does so, and you both get into the rhythm of the thrusting.

As things get hotter, he can press his fingers to her lips so that she can kiss and suck them.

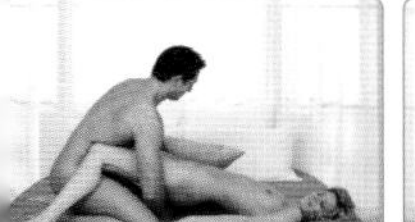
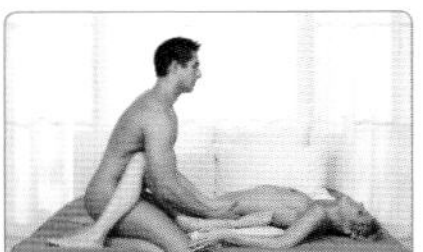
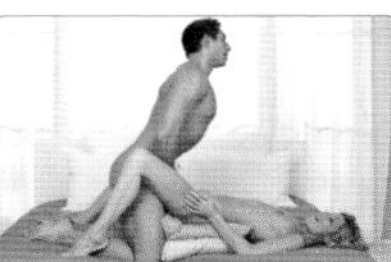
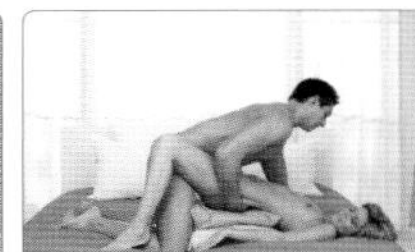
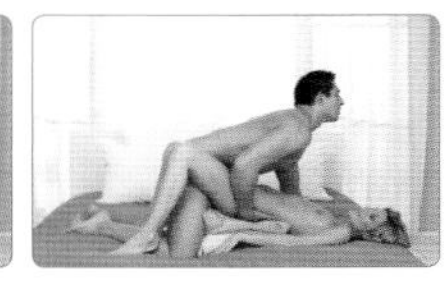

The tenth posture

☆☆☆☆☆ Kama sensation rating

Try this position when you want thunderous sex that threatens to overcome you or when there's enormous sexual tension simmering below the surface. It's great for unleashing your emotions, throwing each other on the bed, and slamming your bodies into each other.

Why it works

- No-holds-barred, mattress-pounding sex is powerful and liberating for both of you.
- It's a great tension diffuser; if you're feeling frustrated or irritable, wild sex acts as a fabulous stress-buster.
- The headboard acts as a brace and a shock absorber, which allows you to move as freely as you want.
- You have to creatively devise a way of pushing and pulling against each other.
- Afterward he can fall beside her, and you can cuddle each other knowing that all your passion and energy has been spent.

Turn on...

... Use sex to express dark and powerful emotions. This doesn't mean shouting angry criticisms at your partner; it means allowing wild movements to possess your body and making lots of noise.

Turn off...

... Don't try The Tenth Posture when you're feeling vulnerable or tender. Turn to Chapter 2 for loving and intimate sex positions (see pages 26–103).

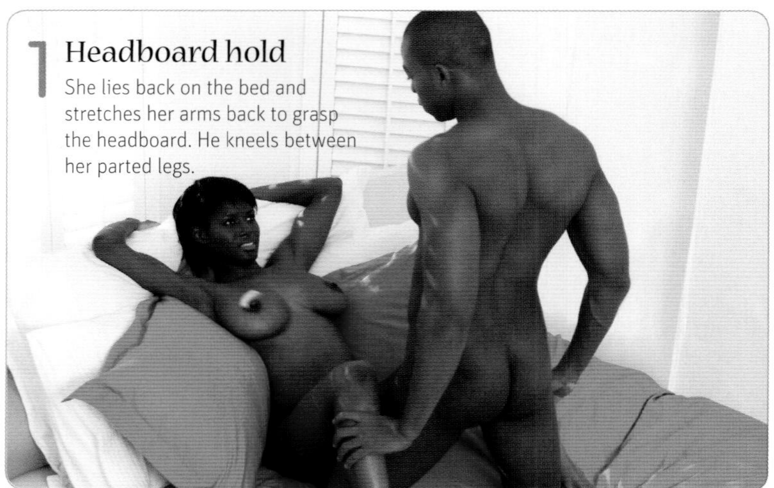

1 Headboard hold
She lies back on the bed and stretches her arms back to grasp the headboard. He kneels between her parted legs.

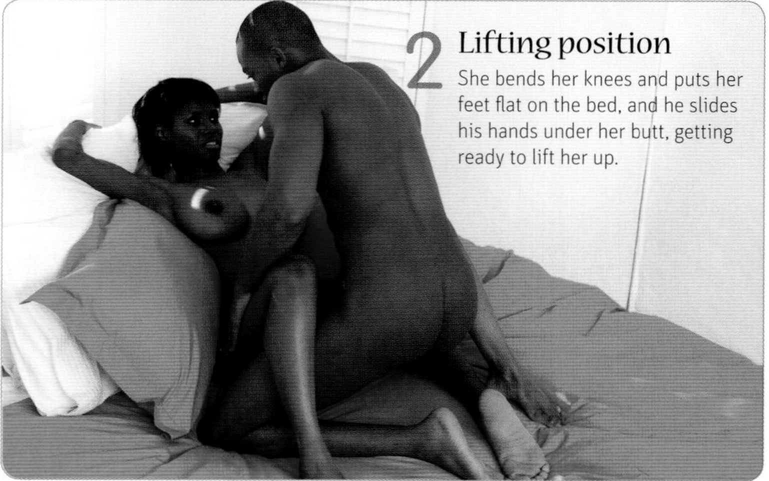

2 Lifting position
She bends her knees and puts her feet flat on the bed, and he slides his hands under her butt, getting ready to lift her up.

"Several agents may achieve their goals at the same time as we see when two rams batter one another… or two wrestlers are locked together in a fight." KAMA SUTRA

3 Hand on hand

He lifts her and slides his penis into her as he kneels upright. Then he leans over her body and puts his hands on top of hers.

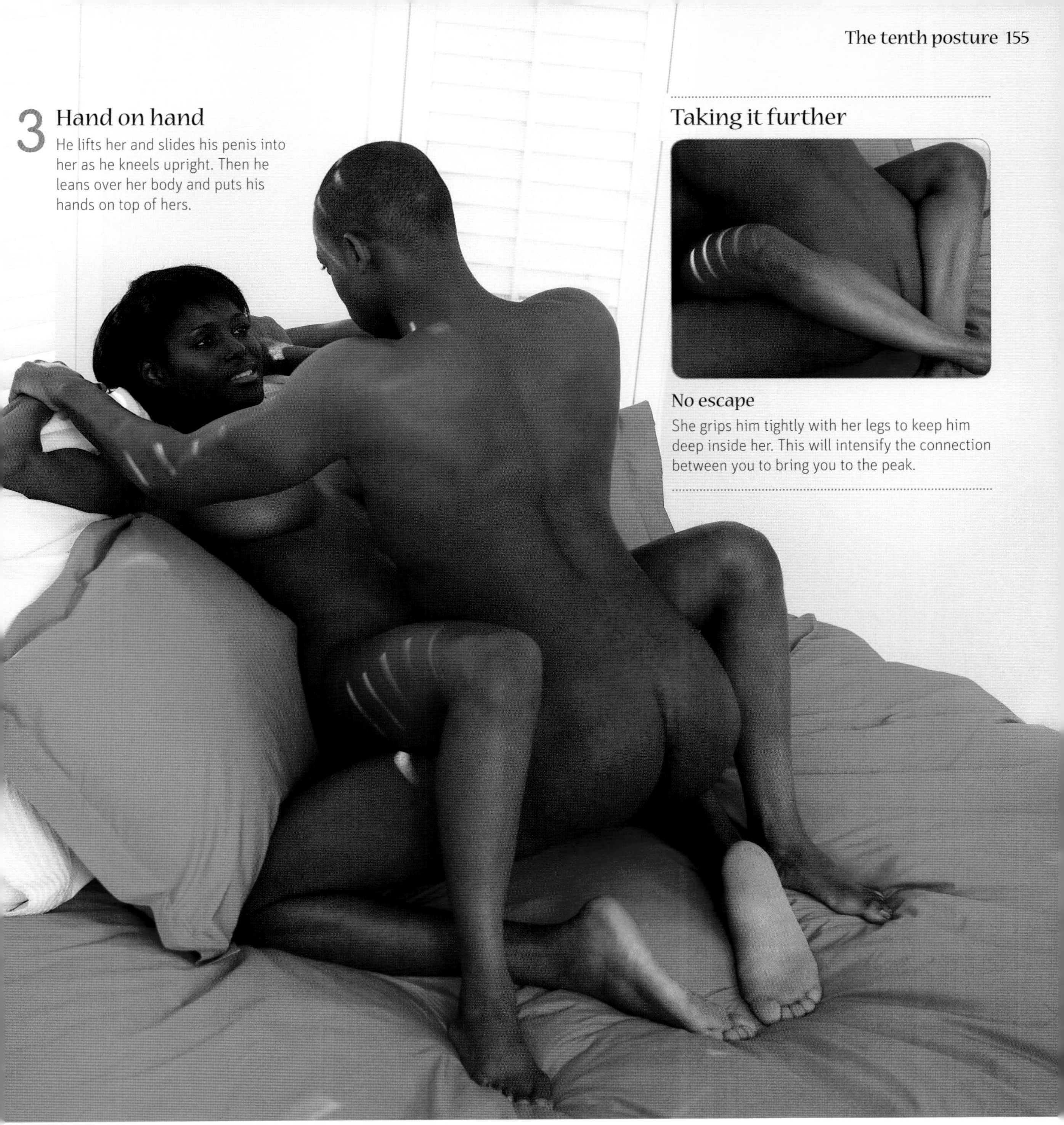

Taking it further

No escape

She grips him tightly with her legs to keep him deep inside her. This will intensify the connection between you to bring you to the peak.

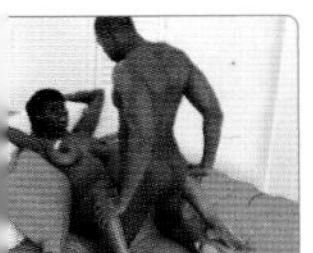
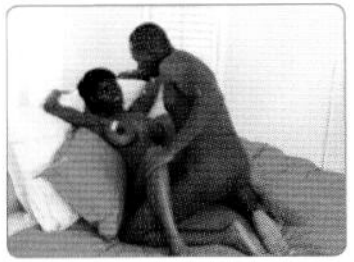
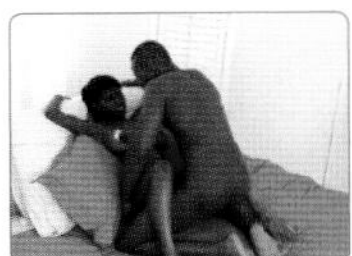
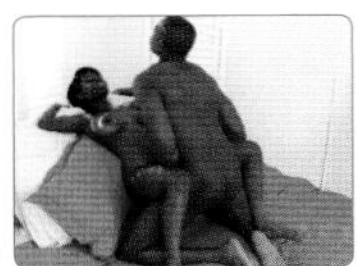
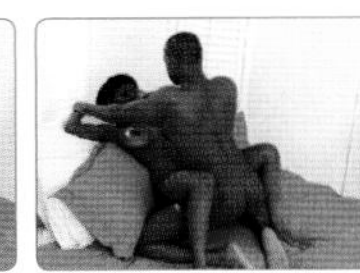

The gaping position

☆☆☆☆ Kama sensation rating

Although the word "gaping" might not fire your erotic imagination, the woman's wide-open legs and invitingly raised hips make sex in this position deeply penetrating and fulfilling. She feels taut and sexy, and he feels manly and in control.

Why it works

- He can hold her around the waist and pull her firmly on to him.
- He feels tightly gripped by her thighs.
- She can reach up to stroke his face or grab his hair in the throes of passion.
- She can take a turn at moving by pressing down through her feet and moving her hips.
- He can plunge in all the way for that pleasurable engulfed feeling.
- She can arch her back to push her breasts out; she feels sexy and gorgeous, and he enjoys taking in the view.

Turn on...

... Change the mood and tempo by sitting up on his lap for a mid-sex cuddle. You could kiss him hard on the lips and bounce or wiggle to keep him hard.

Turn off...

... Don't worry if this position doesn't notch up five stars on your personal sensation rating. Having her legs wide apart may weaken vaginal sensation for her and penile sensation for him because the vagina is widened rather than narrowed.

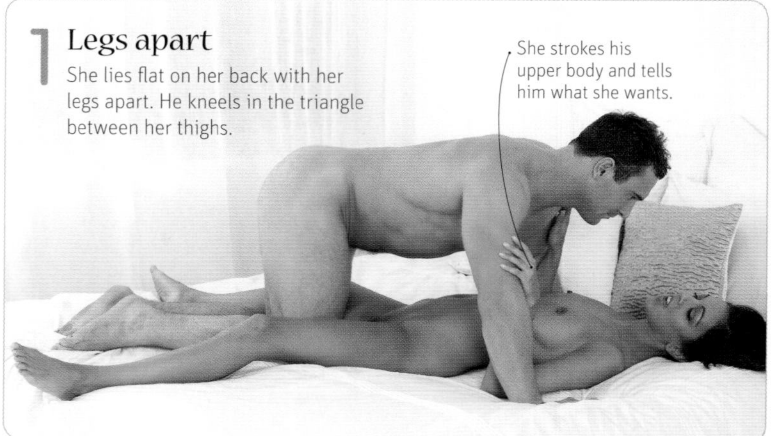

She strokes his upper body and tells him what she wants.

1 Legs apart
She lies flat on her back with her legs apart. He kneels in the triangle between her thighs.

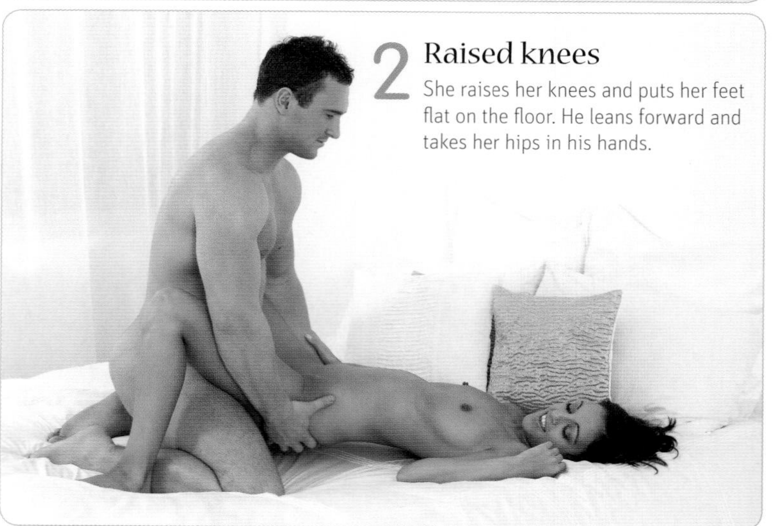

2 Raised knees
She raises her knees and puts her feet flat on the floor. He leans forward and takes her hips in his hands.

"Women differ greatly in the seasons which they prefer enjoyment, according to their class and temperament." ANANGA RANGA

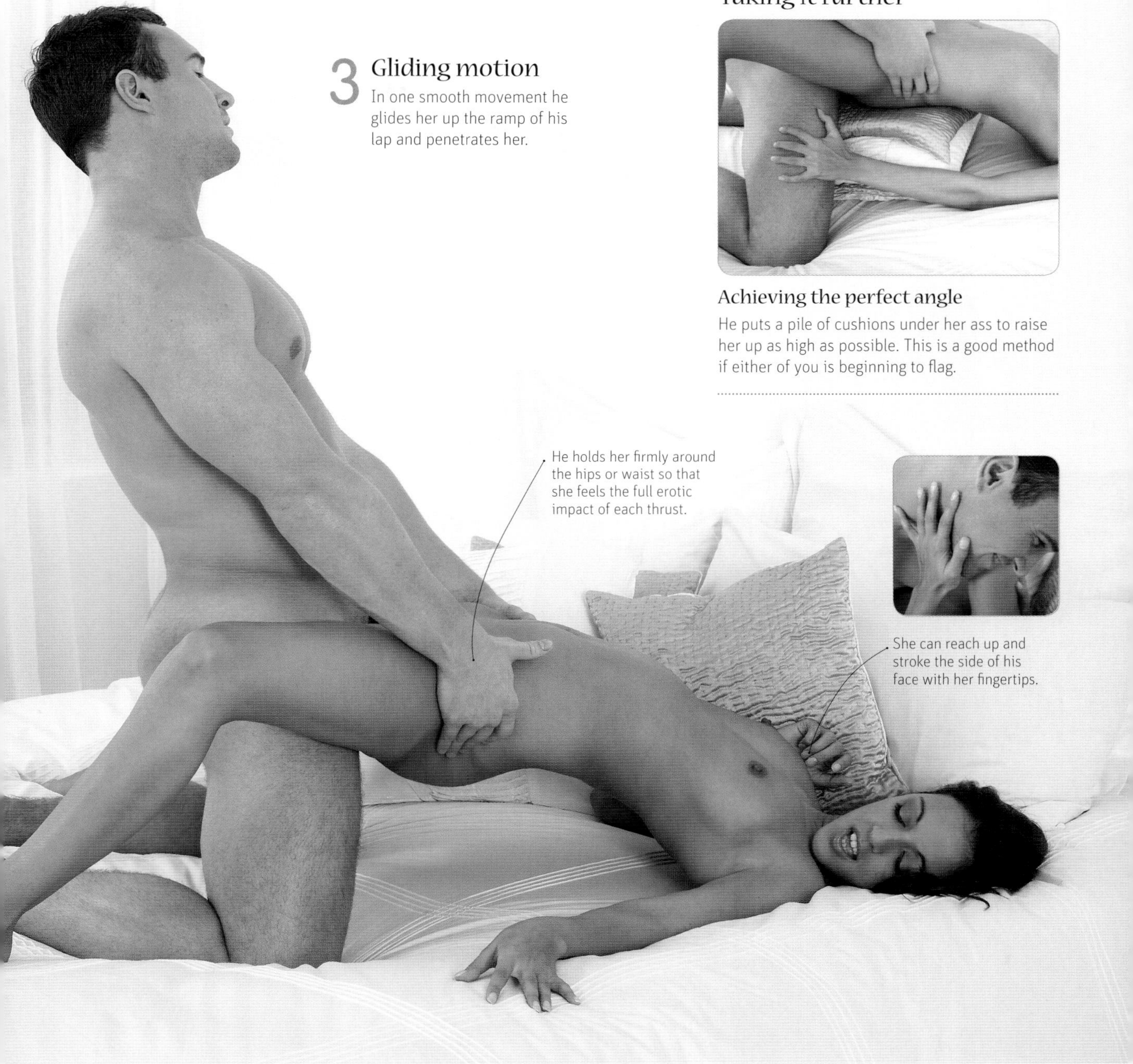

3 Gliding motion

In one smooth movement he glides her up the ramp of his lap and penetrates her.

He holds her firmly around the hips or waist so that she feels the full erotic impact of each thrust.

She can reach up and stroke the side of his face with her fingertips.

Taking it further

Achieving the perfect angle

He puts a pile of cushions under her ass to raise her up as high as possible. This is a good method if either of you is beginning to flag.

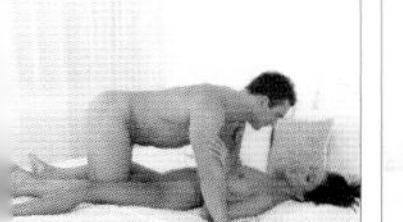
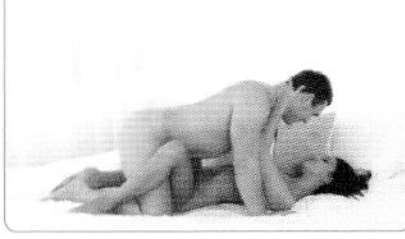
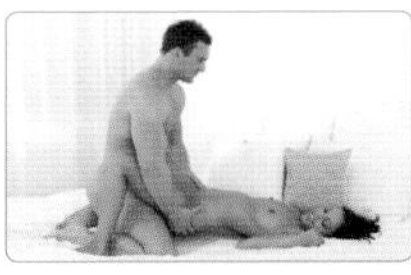
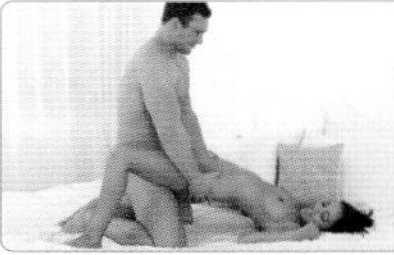
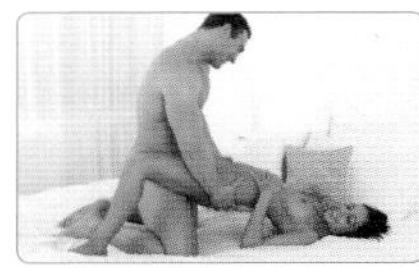

Orgasmic role reversal

☆☆☆☆☆ Kama sensation rating

"Allowing" the woman a turn on top was recommended for occasions when a man was "no longer capable of muscular exertion." Fortunately a woman no longer needs to wait until her lover is limp and inert to try this position—she can hop on top whenever she fancies.

Why it works

– She's in charge of her own pleasure; she can masturbate with him inside her, she can squat and thrust, she can circle her hips, or she can sit still and relish the connection.

– He can lie there and experience the sexy gratification of being used and abused.

– If she has strong thighs, she can bob up and down on the tip of his penis for a few strokes, then lower herself to enclose the whole of his shaft. Frequent repetition of this technique should take him to boiling point.

– He gets a great view of her writhing and churning on top of him.

Turn on…

… Lie back and relax while she does the work. If she's reproducing your thrusting movements, enjoy your passive role to the full.

Turn off…

… Bobbing up and down for any length of time is the equivalent of a thigh workout. Don't forget to lend her a hand if she needs it; you can give her some sexy support by cupping her buttocks.

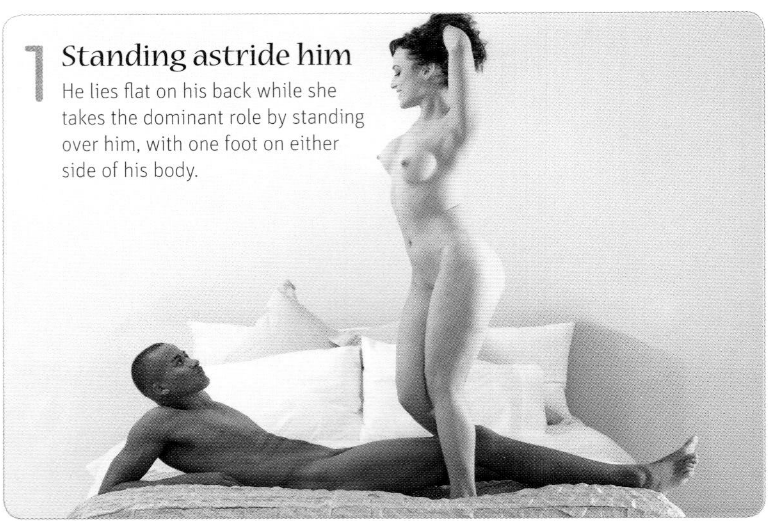

1 Standing astride him

He lies flat on his back while she takes the dominant role by standing over him, with one foot on either side of his body.

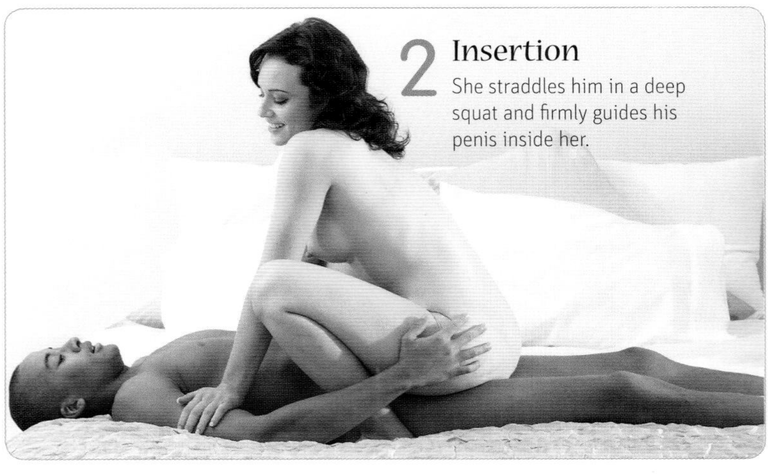

2 Insertion

She straddles him in a deep squat and firmly guides his penis inside her.

"Moving her waist in a circular form she enjoys her husband and thoroughly satisfies herself." ANANGA RANGA

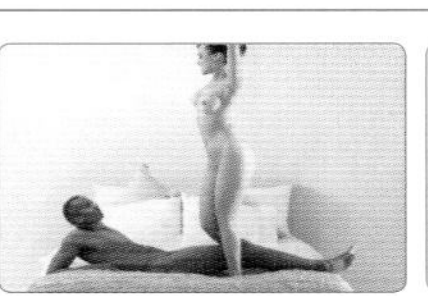

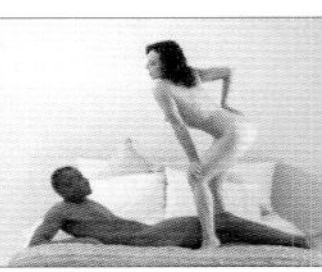

Taking it further

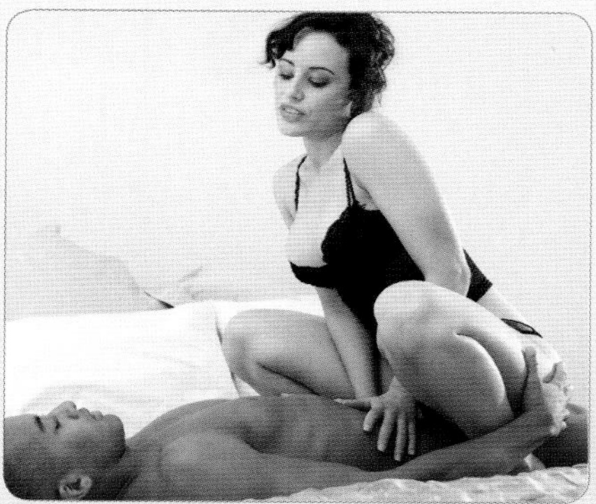

Tantalizing textures

She casts off her work clothes and slips into something super-sexy to mark the start of the evening's erogenous zone.

3 Knees together

She brings her knees together and leans backward or forward to support herself on his body as she moves.

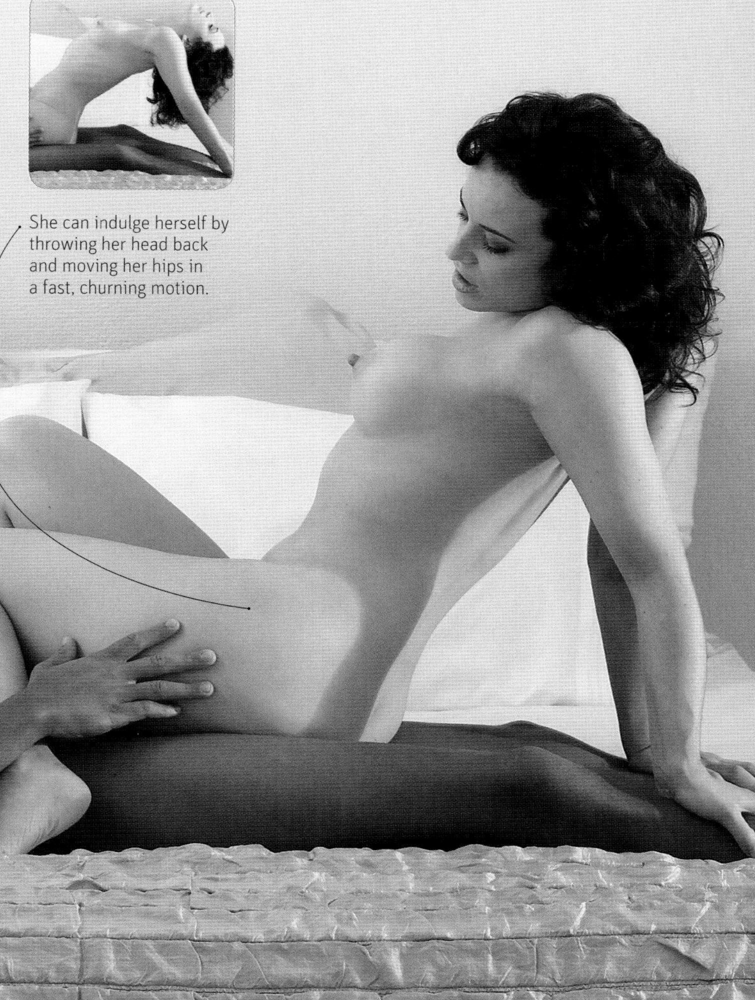

She can indulge herself by throwing her head back and moving her hips in a fast, churning motion.

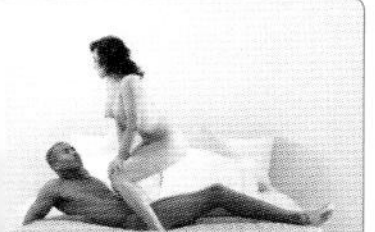
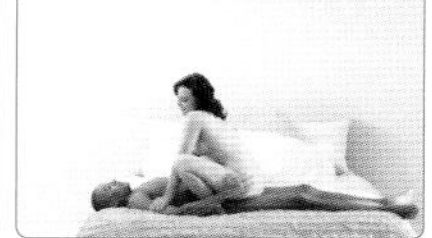
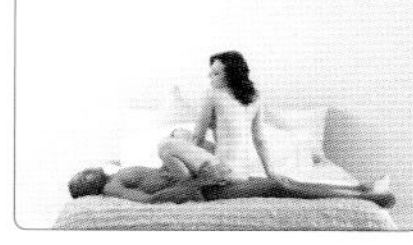
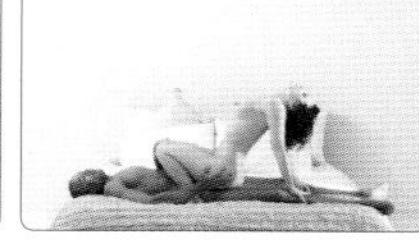
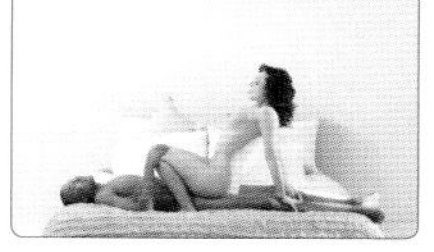
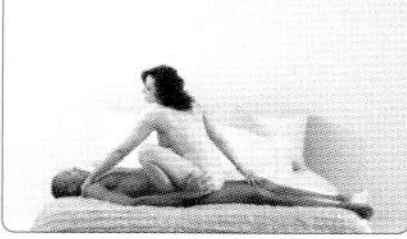

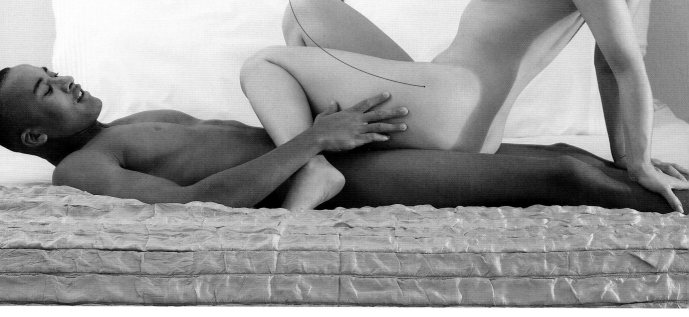

Turning

This is a classic from the *Kama Sutra* hall of fame; you can't claim *Kama Sutra* sexpert status unless you've done it (or attempted it) at least once. It starts off in a standard man-on-top position—so far so good—but then he completes a 180-degree turn so he ends up nuzzling her toes. And if that isn't tricky enough, he must stay inside her for the duration of the turn.

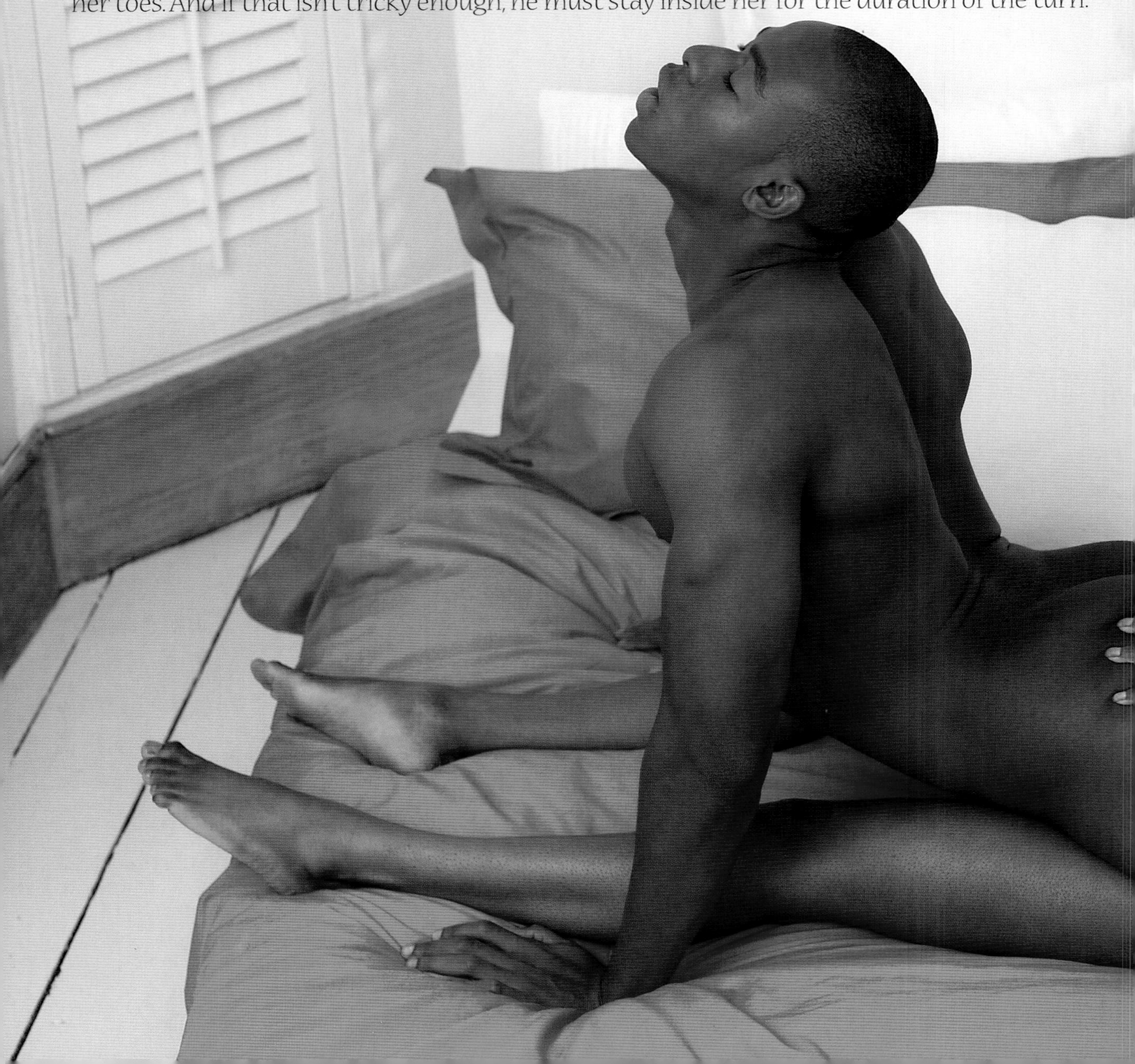

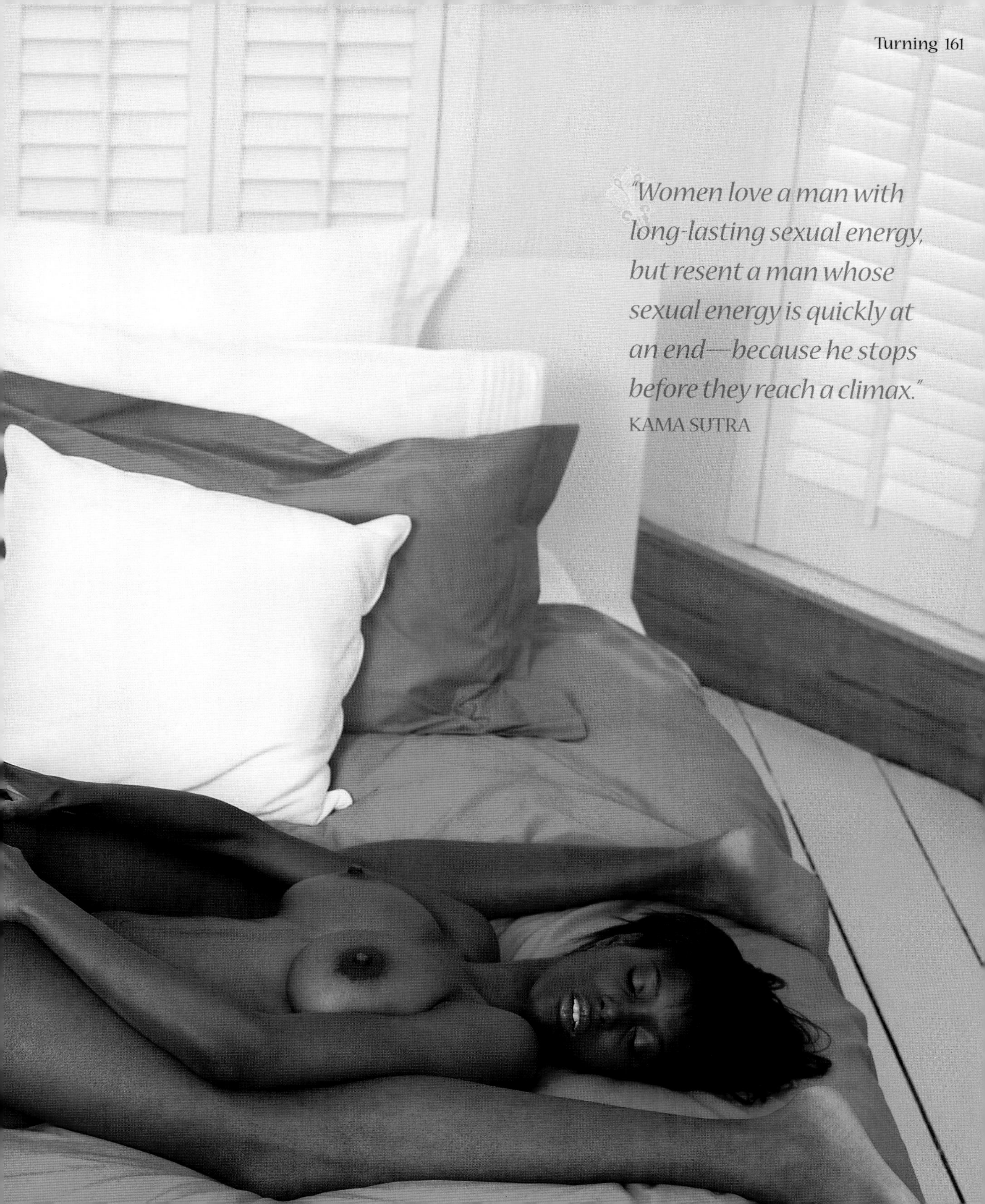

"Women love a man with long-lasting sexual energy, but resent a man whose sexual energy is quickly at an end—because he stops before they reach a climax."
KAMA SUTRA

Turning

☆☆☆☆

Kama sensation rating

Why it works

– It's one of those novelty positions you can boast about afterward.

– She meets the challenge of keeping him erect not by external movements, but by being lewd and suggestive.

– You both discover exciting new sensations and angles of penetration.

– His glans and shaft press against the sides of her vagina (conventional sex usually involves penile pressure on just the front and back vaginal walls).

– If he successfully completes the turn, he's entitled to challenge her to do the equivalent (see The Top on page 226).

Turn on…

… Make sure that he's equipped for the journey before he sets off. Two essential tools are a vat of lube to smooth his turn and a sturdy erection (plenty of pre-coital oral sex can help). She can cheer him on from underneath by squeezing him with her vaginal muscles and talking dirty.

Turn off…

… Falling off the bed. Unless you own a king-size bed, the best bet is to decamp to the floor. Throw some soft blankets and cushions on the ground, and spend some time canoodling in the missionary position before you start your spin cycle.

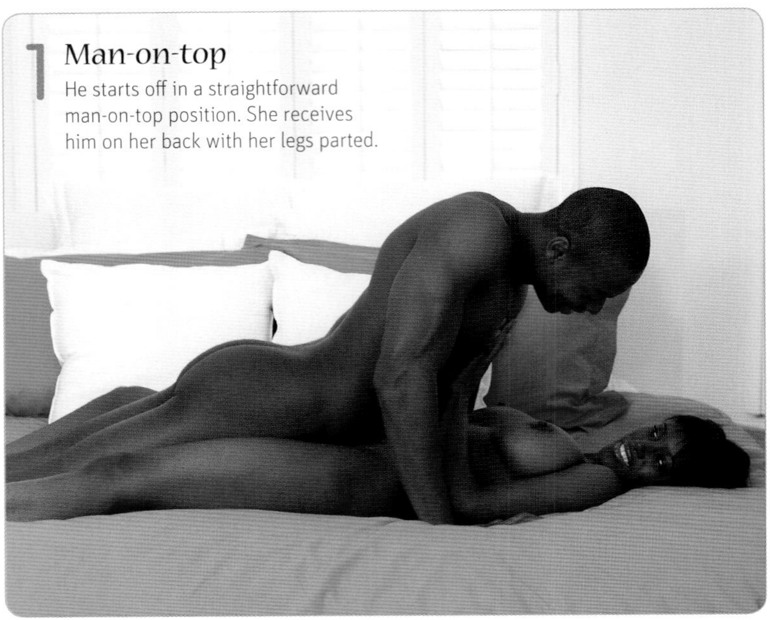

1 Man-on-top
He starts off in a straightforward man-on-top position. She receives him on her back with her legs parted.

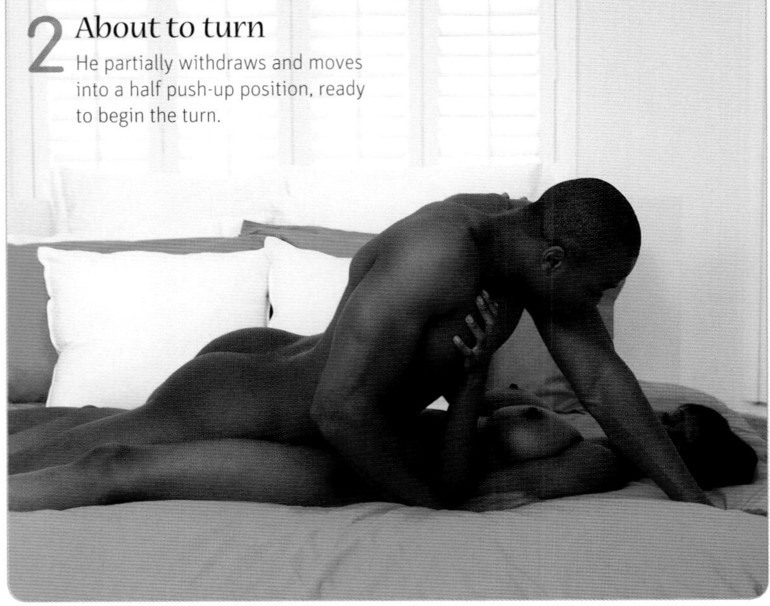

2 About to turn
He partially withdraws and moves into a half push-up position, ready to begin the turn.

"When he turns around with his back to her and she caresses his back, this is called 'turning'. It can be done only with practice." KAMA SUTRA

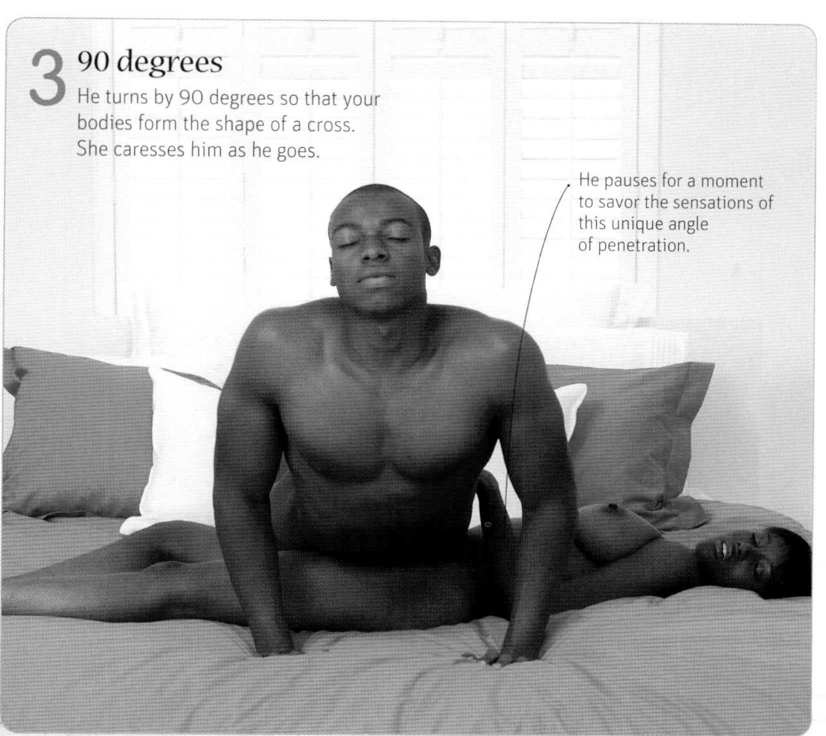

3 90 degrees

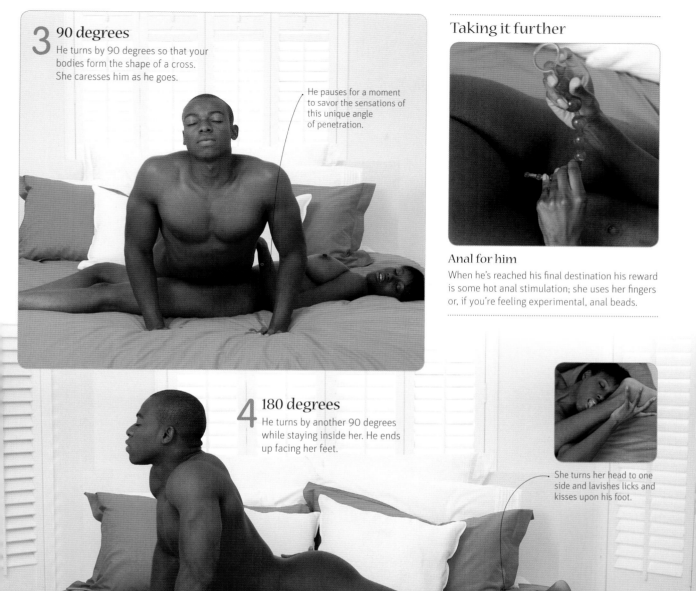

He turns by 90 degrees so that your bodies form the shape of a cross. She caresses him as he goes.

He pauses for a moment to savor the sensations of this unique angle of penetration.

Taking it further

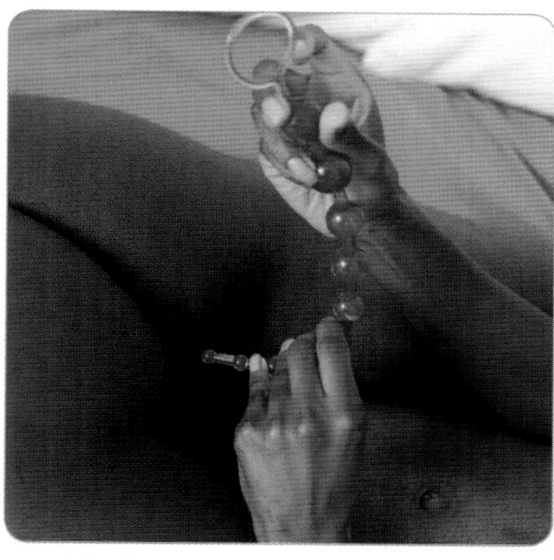

Anal for him

When he's reached his final destination his reward is some hot anal stimulation; she uses her fingers or, if you're feeling experimental, anal beads.

4 180 degrees

He turns by another 90 degrees while staying inside her. He ends up facing her feet.

She turns her head to one side and lavishes licks and kisses upon his foot.

If you liked this, try…

- Letting her take the lead in The Top (see page 226).
- Lotus-like position (see page 192) for another *Kama Sutra* sex challenge.

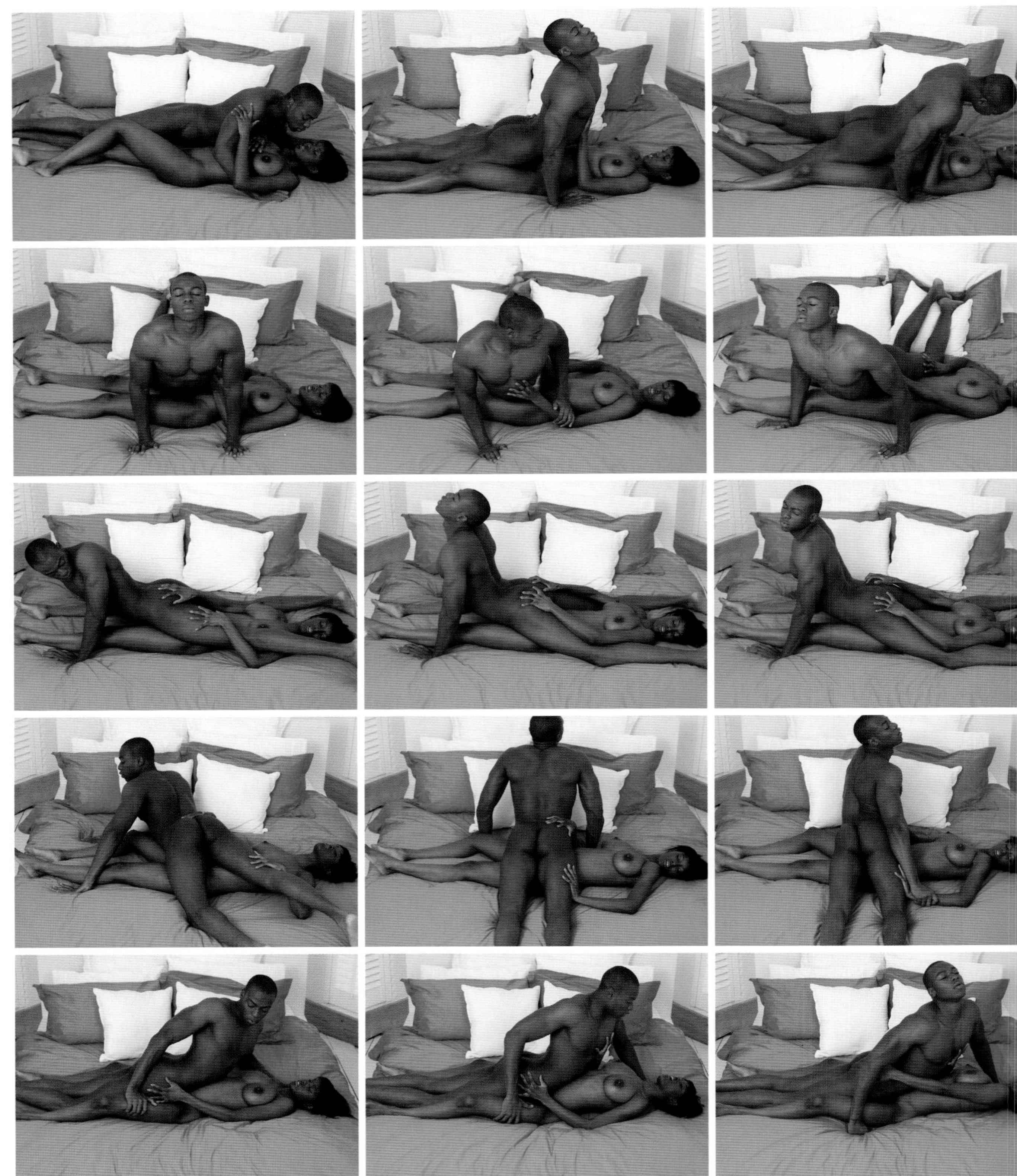

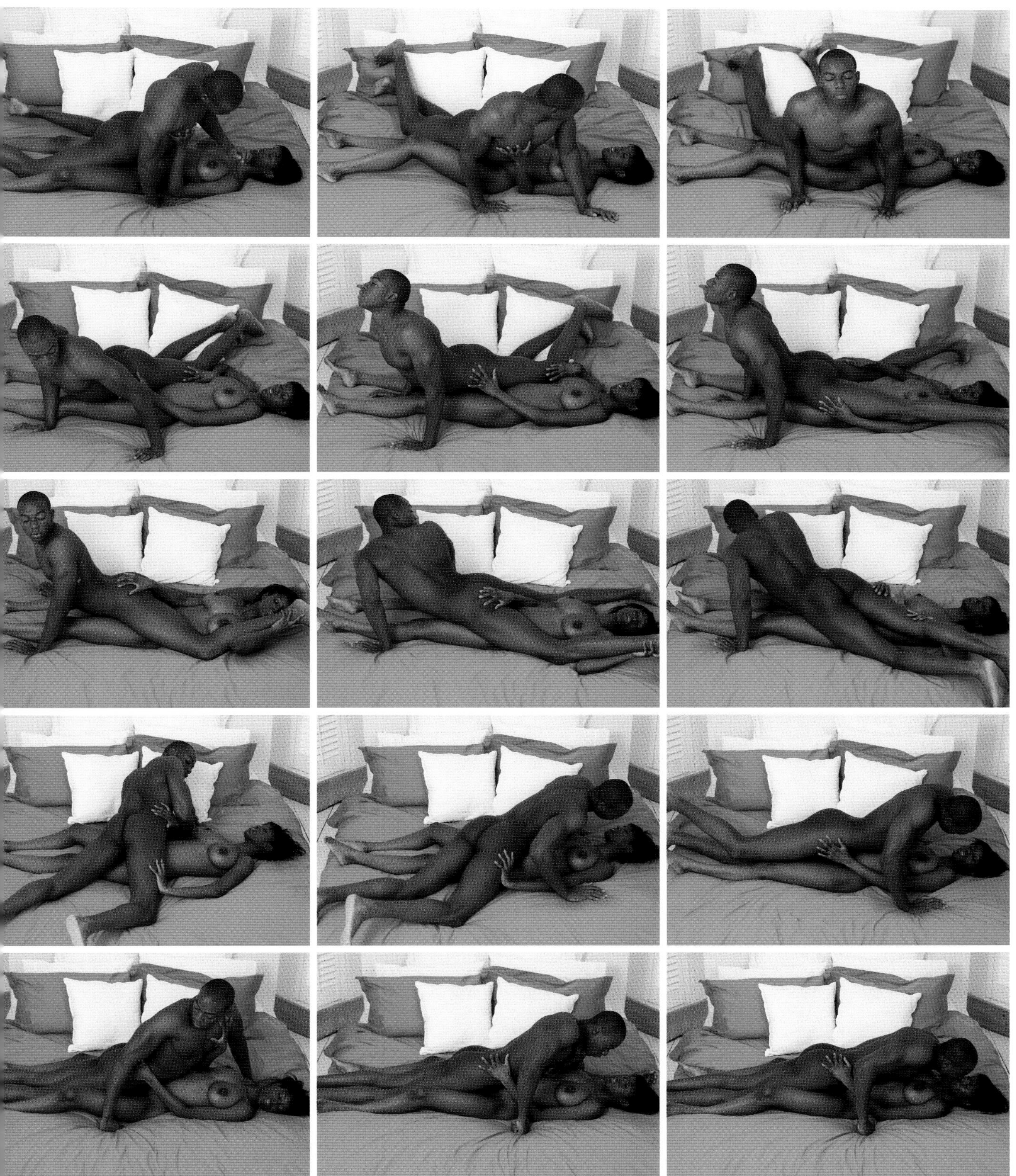

The splitting position

☆☆☆ Kama sensation rating

This position is perfect when she wants to put her feet up. As long as she's supple, she can make it look effortlessly casual and laid-back. On the other hand, if you want to try some mild BDSM, just a couple of kinky accessories can change the mood from decent to depraved.

Why it works

- He fully penetrates her, then moves in small in-out movements that bump you both to extreme arousal.
- If she's been "bad," he can restrain her legs.
- He can turn to kiss and bite her calf.
- He can peer around her legs for some face-to-face smoochiness.
- Her legs are together, which creates a nice tight fit between the two of you. This means that she feels sensations more acutely, and he feels pleasantly gripped; a feeling she can enhance by giving him rhythmic squeezes with her vaginal muscles.

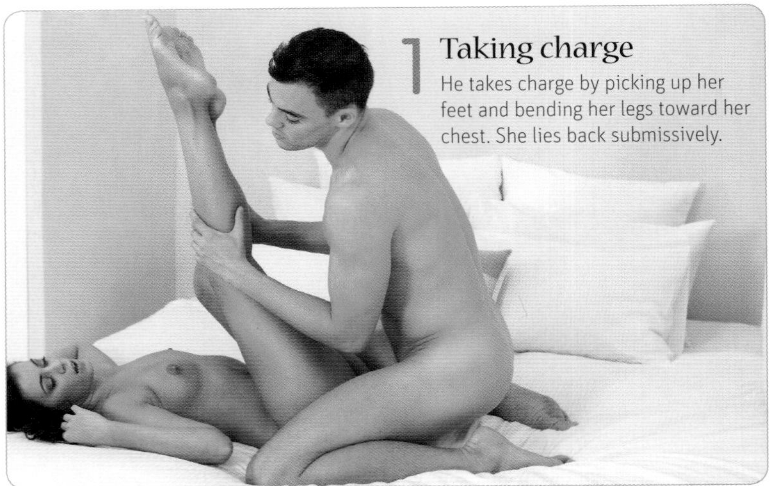

1 Taking charge
He takes charge by picking up her feet and bending her legs toward her chest. She lies back submissively.

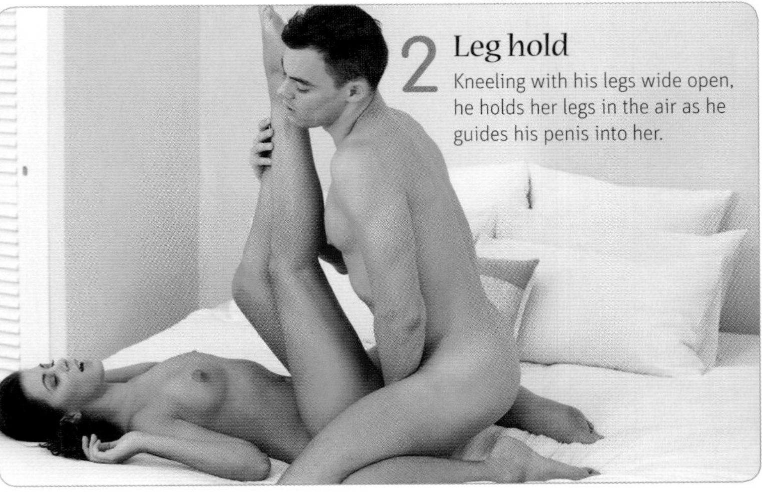

2 Leg hold
Kneeling with his legs wide open, he holds her legs in the air as he guides his penis into her.

Turn on...

... Slide your hands slowly up and down her thighs and breasts to enjoy their smooth silkiness. Add some massage oil to make things even silkier.

Turn off...

... Don't neglect her clitoris. It's tucked away in this position and receives only indirect stimulation. A solution is for her to put a leg on each shoulder to create some hand room for either of you.

"Woman resembles a fruit that yields its fragrance only when rubbed by the hands." THE PERFUMED GARDEN

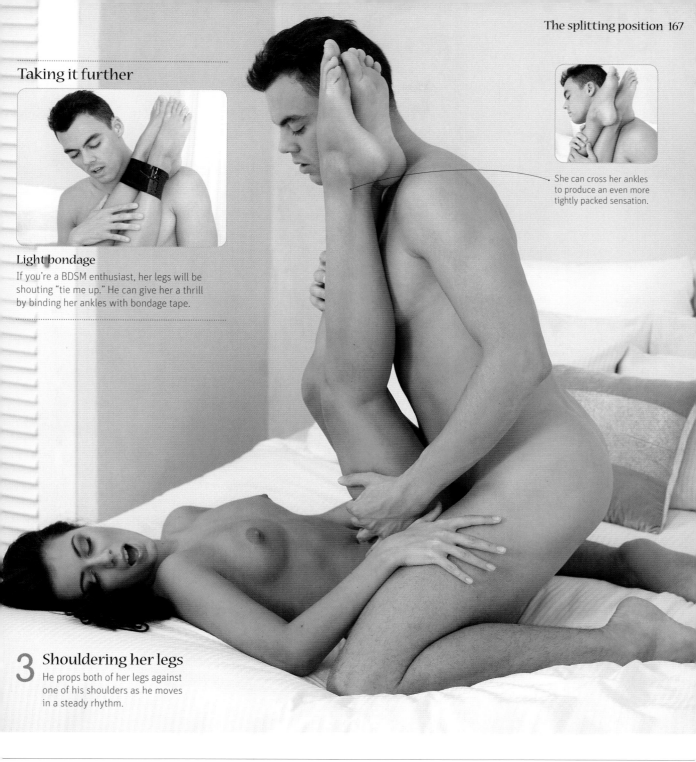

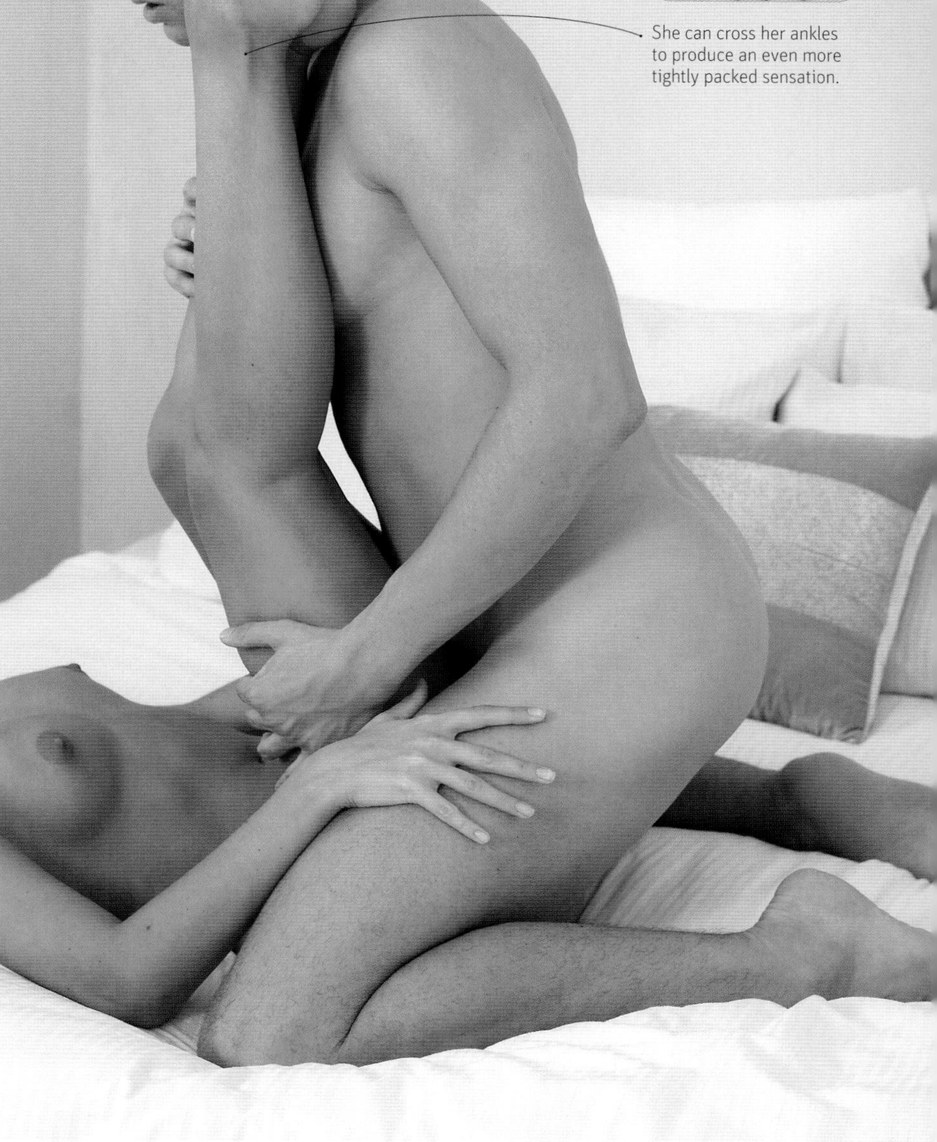

Taking it further

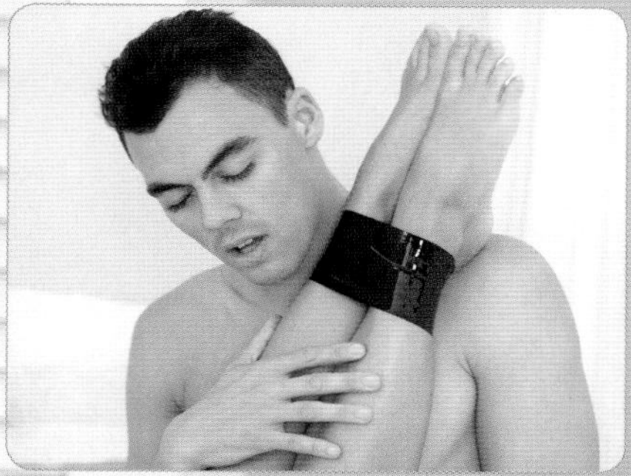

Light bondage

If you're a BDSM enthusiast, her legs will be shouting "tie me up." He can give her a thrill by binding her ankles with bondage tape.

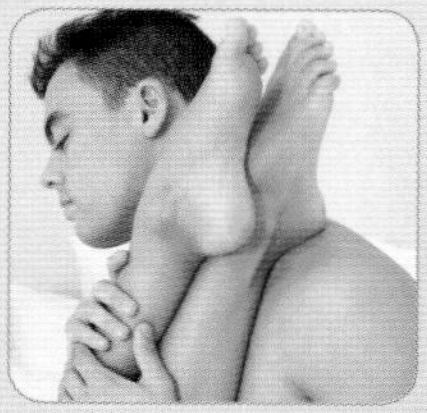

She can cross her ankles to produce an even more tightly packed sensation.

3 Shouldering her legs

He props both of her legs against one of his shoulders as he moves in a steady rhythm.

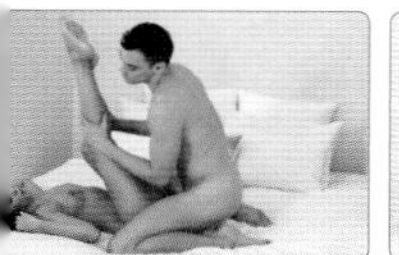
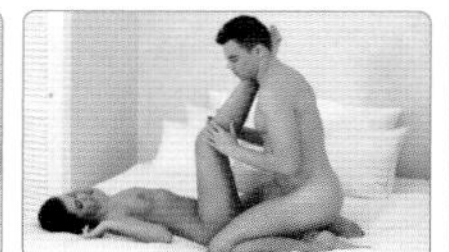
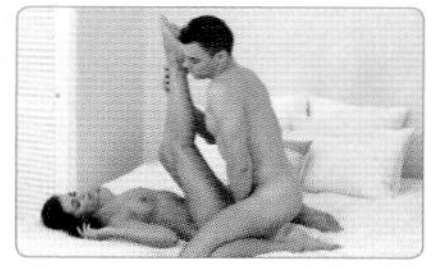
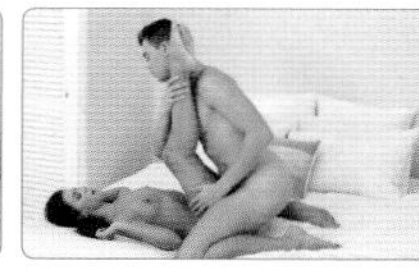
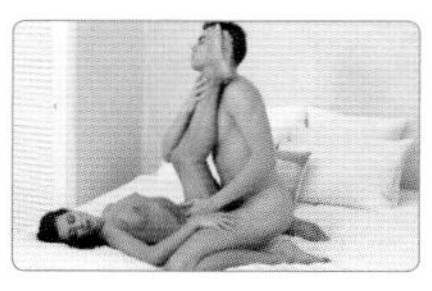

The seducer

☆☆☆ Kama sensation rating

The man takes on the role of the passionate Lothario to his partner's naïve virgin in this steamy position. Play your roles to the hilt: she feigns innocence, while he seduces her with wine and chocolates before luring her to the bedroom for a good ravishing.

Why it works

– He can rock her to orgasm using his hands or penis, with maximum face-to-face intensity and sizzling eye contact.

– She can slip her fingers into his mouth to increase the heat levels.

– If he wants to really go deep, it's easy for him to move her legs up to shoulder level.

– He can stay still and slide her on and off him with his hands, pausing to stroke her clitoris if he needs to slow down.

– He can move fast, but not too fast, enabling him to stay on the edge of ecstasy without tipping over before he wants to.

Turn on...

... Clasp your legs tightly around his body so he feels like he's penetrating you to the maximum. And if you can manage some wiggling, jiggling hip moves, this will add to his joy.

Turn off...

... Using this when you've got a deadline or you're desperate for a quickie. It's hot and sexy, but it's not the fastest way to raise the roof.

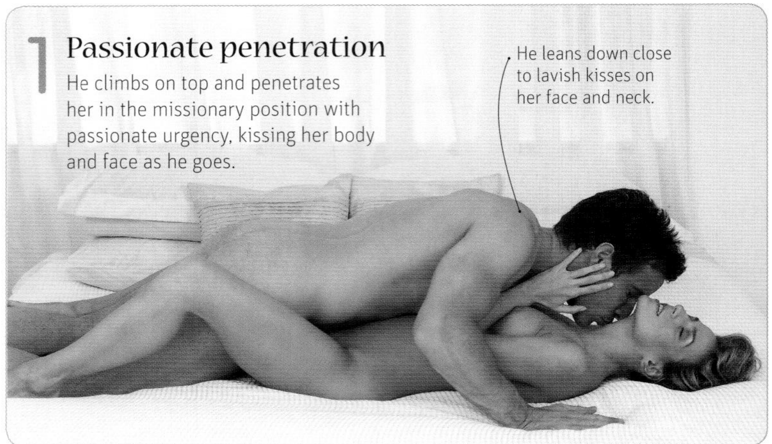

1 Passionate penetration He climbs on top and penetrates her in the missionary position with passionate urgency, kissing her body and face as he goes.

He leans down close to lavish kisses on her face and neck.

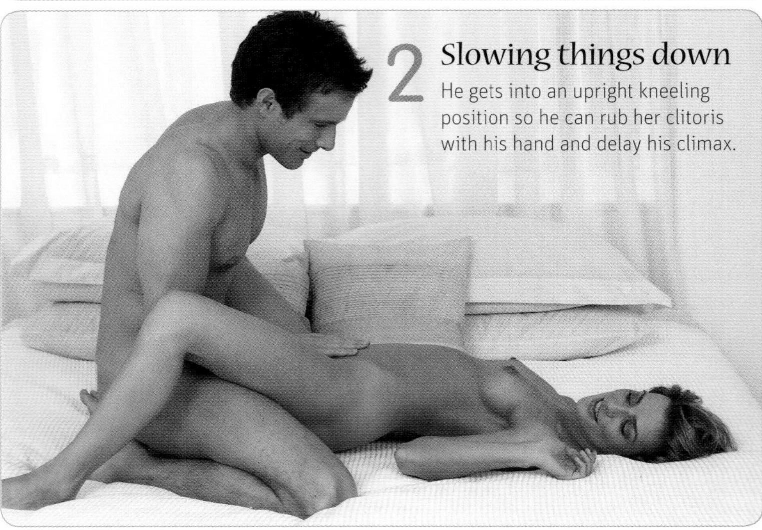

2 Slowing things down He gets into an upright kneeling position so he can rub her clitoris with his hand and delay his climax.

"The woman lying on her back, the man sits between her legs; he raises and separates her thighs, then takes her around the waist." THE PERFUMED GARDEN

Taking it further

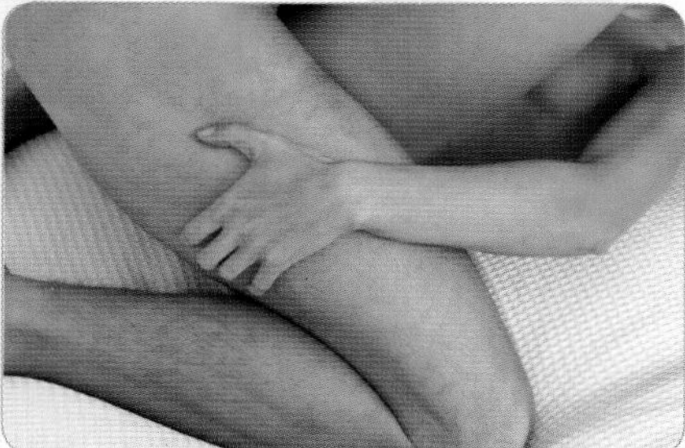

The thigh grip

She grips his thighs tightly with her hands to help communicate her urgency, and so that her whole body moves in time with his thrusts.

3 The final act

She encloses him between her thighs and crosses her ankles behind his back as he moves in close for the final act.

As well as thrusting in and out, he moves his hips from side to side to stimulate all of her vaginal hot spots.

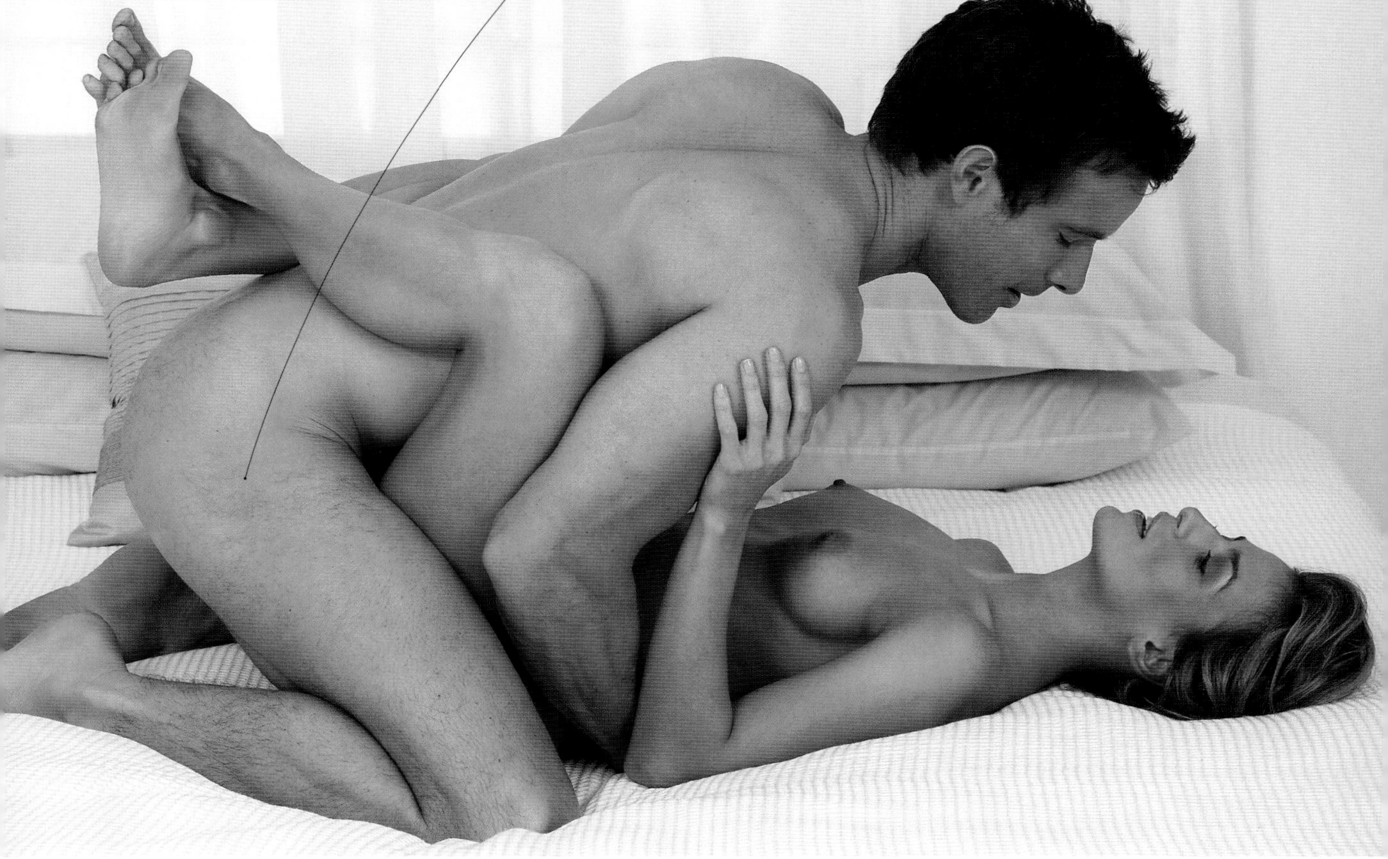

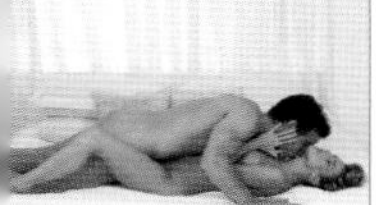
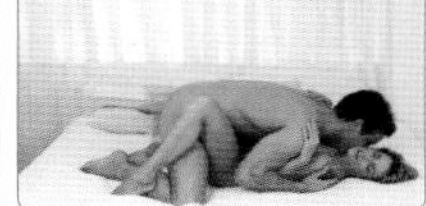
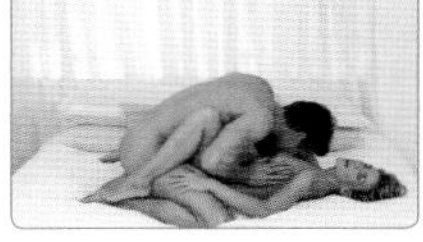
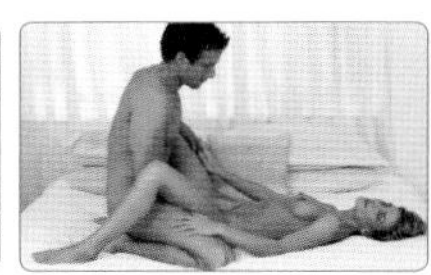
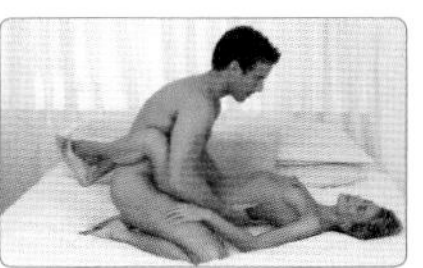
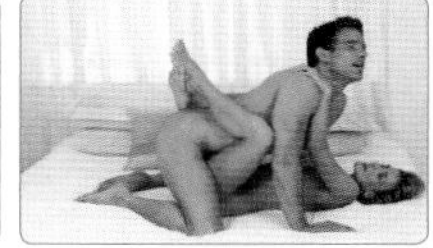

Keeping it varied

As the ancient texts say, it is the "want of varied pleasures" that drives lovers to the embraces of strangers. So don't wait until familiarity and monotony set in, keep the sexual tension crackling between you on a daily basis by taking every possible opportunity to be naughty.

It's possible for lovers to see each other every day and sleep together every night without actually looking at each other. Keeping it varied will force you to sit up and not just notice your partner, but fancy, fetishize, and salivate over them.

Showing off Exhibitionism can mean casually bending over with no panties on, or serving dinner wearing nothing but a dog collar. If you don't count yourself as a natural exhibitionist, follow these tips:

- Maximize your positive points. If you have great legs, highlight them with stockings.
- Do a striptease, with your favorite music as backing to give you a confidence boost.
- Treat your lover to a tantalizing lap dance.
- Radiate sexual confidence and give your lover a wicked smile. This beats a perfect body every time.

Accessorize If you're sex toy-shy, it's worth reviewing your attitude. Sometimes anus-friendly beads or G-spot dildos are exactly what you need to land yourself a monumentally mind-bending orgasm. (Although do note that anything that goes up anyone's butt *must* have a flared base.) Even the *Kama Sutra* recommends accessorizing sex, after a fashion; men can either wear penis rings or insert objects into holes pierced in the penis.

The secret of enjoying sex toys is to use them on each other (rather than in solitude) and to add them to your sex life as you'd add condiments to a fantastic meal. Choose them carefully, and use them sparingly. They're there to enhance rather than to dominate your menu (and they're certainly not there to disguise the fact that something's not working).

Battery-powered sex It may be the fact that a toy targets your clitoral head/G spot/P-spot with scientific accuracy, or that a sex toy doesn't get tired like your lover's hand, or it may simply be that frisson of naughtiness that turns you on like nothing else. Whatever the reason, vibrators can put the oh-my-God back into sex. Sex-toy novices: start with a simple, no-frills vibrator, and use it on his hot spots as well as hers.

Anywhere but the bedroom If you revisit your juiciest memories, chances are they are of sex that took place outside the bedroom: that time you did it on a swing, a park bench, a moonlit beach, in the break room at work, or up a mountain. Your lifestyle (not to mention the law) may not permit you to shag in weird or exotic locations, but you can mix up your sex life simply by trying a no-sex-in-the-bedroom policy. Be creative.

Out of your mind Sometimes it's good to change personality during sex. This is where role play comes in: you can give up your mild manners and become a dominatrix, or stop being the pants-wearing boss and obey like a frightened puppy. Because you're suddenly free from your normal script, you can relate to your partner in a different way and, best of all, have a different kind of sex. You don't need to set up complicated scenarios for role play; you can simply wear a costume that you wouldn't usually wear.

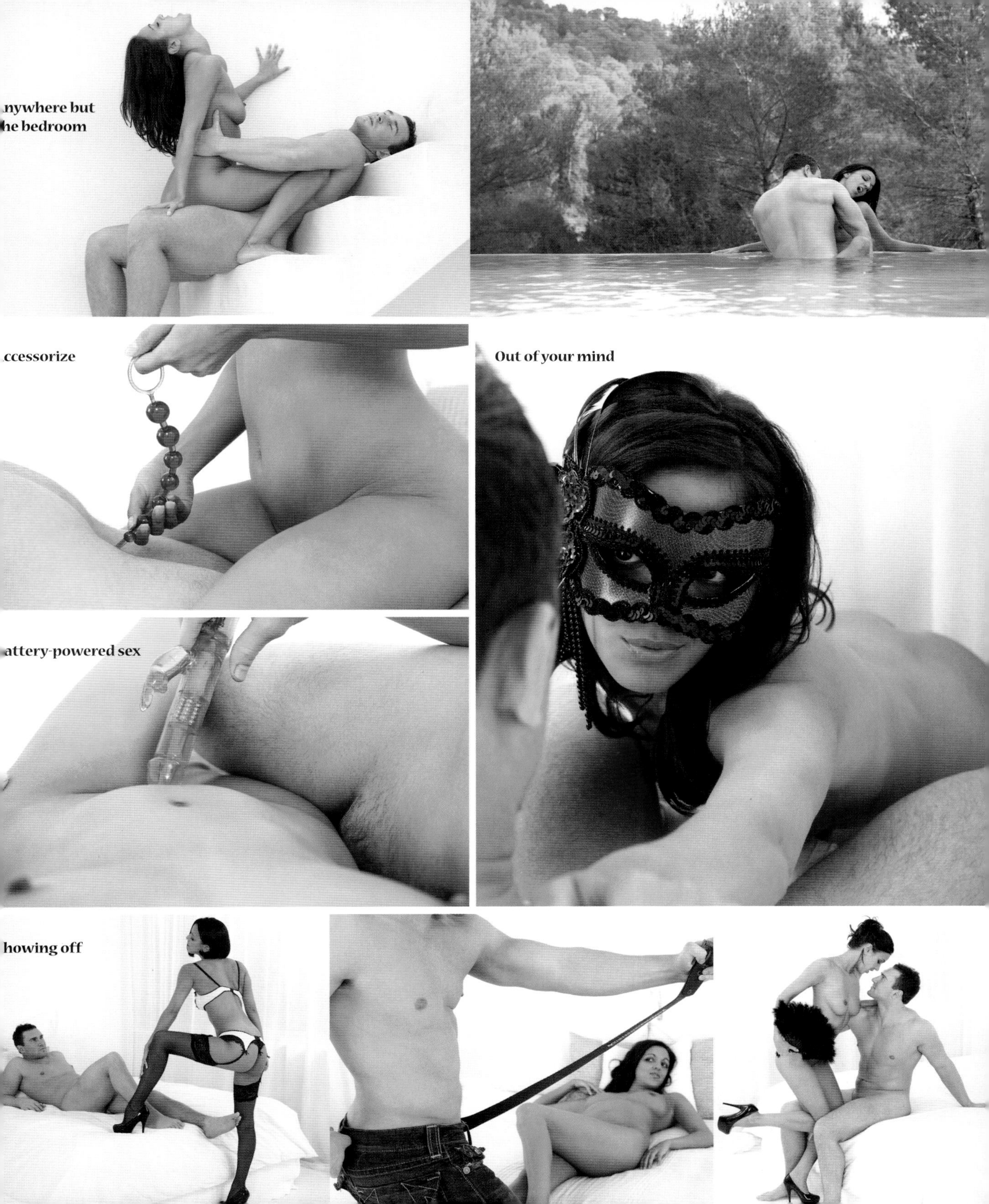

nywhere but
he bedroom

ccessorize

Out of your mind

attery-powered sex

howing off

The fitting on of the sock

☆☆☆☆ Kama sensation rating

Her clitoris is firmly center stage in this woman-on-top position. Before he penetrates he takes his penis firmly in his hand and uses it like a vibrator around her clitoral hood. Then when she's wet and writhing, he plunges in to do some interior work.

Why it works

– If she doesn't come from intercourse alone, this position is ideal for top-up stimulation. He holds his shaft in his hand and flicks his glans to and fro across her clitoris (he can do this both before and during sex).

– He becomes an elite member of the cliterati; by using his penis as a sex toy, he learns exactly what kind of pace, pressure, and rhythm she needs to reach orgasm.

– He gets to enjoy sex with her when she's at boiling point; her extreme arousal will be super-infectious, especially if she lets him know how turned on she is.

Turn on...

... Take your cues from her. Watch her body language, and listen to her moans to gauge how close she is to coming. If you're in doubt about what she wants, ask. Keep questions to one-worders: "Harder?", "More?"

Turn off...

... Don't conduct a NASA-level exploration in which she feels under pressure to come. Too much attention can give her stage fright; keep things light and interactive.

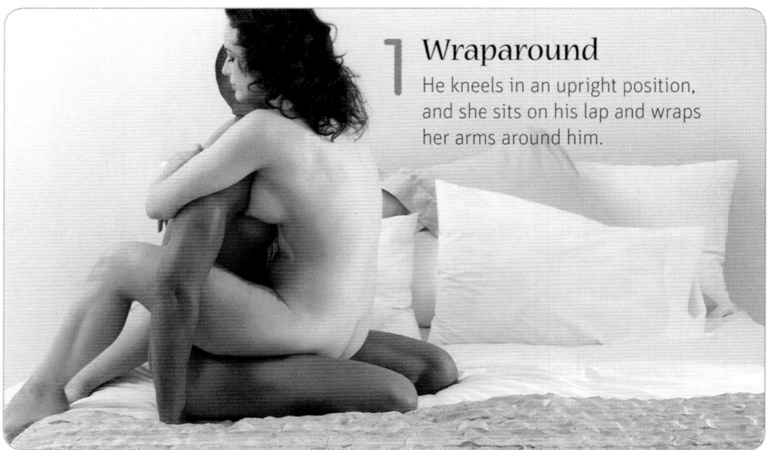

1 Wraparound
He kneels in an upright position, and she sits on his lap and wraps her arms around him.

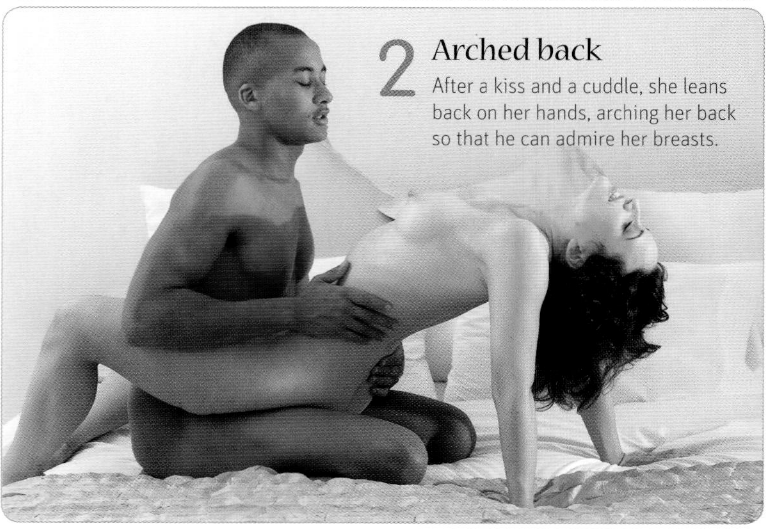

2 Arched back
After a kiss and a cuddle, she leans back on her hands, arching her back so that he can admire her breasts.

"Place your member between her lips... use it to rub her vulva... Having given her a foretaste of pleasure, you may penetrate her completely." THE PERFUMED GARDEN

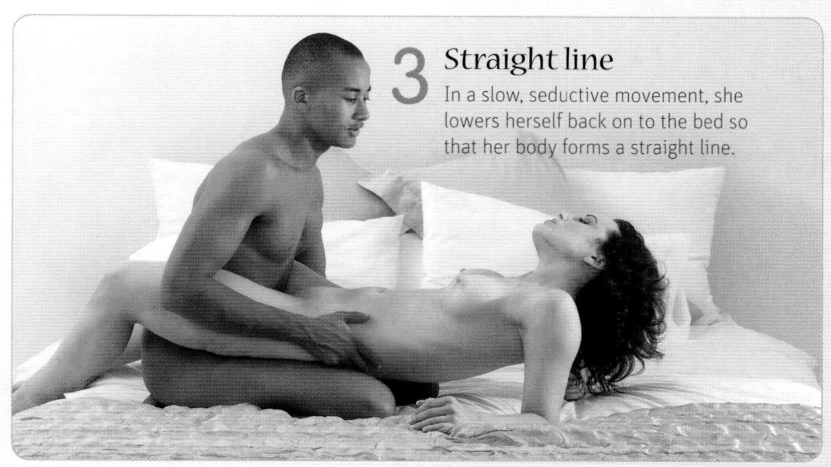

3 Straight line

In a slow, seductive movement, she lowers herself back on to the bed so that her body forms a straight line.

Taking it further

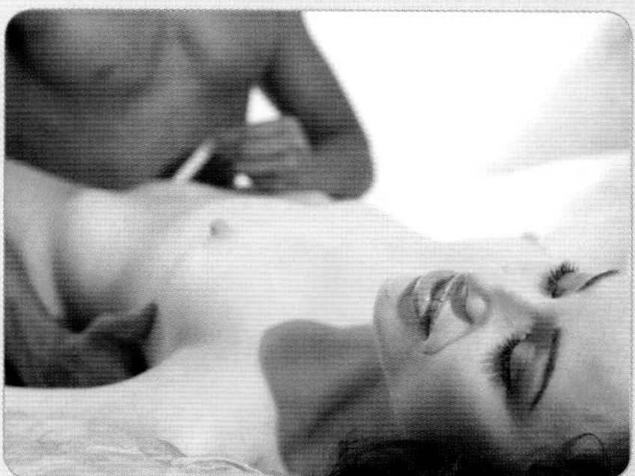

Good vibrations

If she gets off on fast, powerful vibrations, a vibrator is a vital addition to this position. Either of you can hold it against her clitoris as he thrusts.

4 Long and taut

She makes her body long and taut by raising her arms above her head. He uses the head of his penis to stroke, rub, and flick her clitoris before he enters.

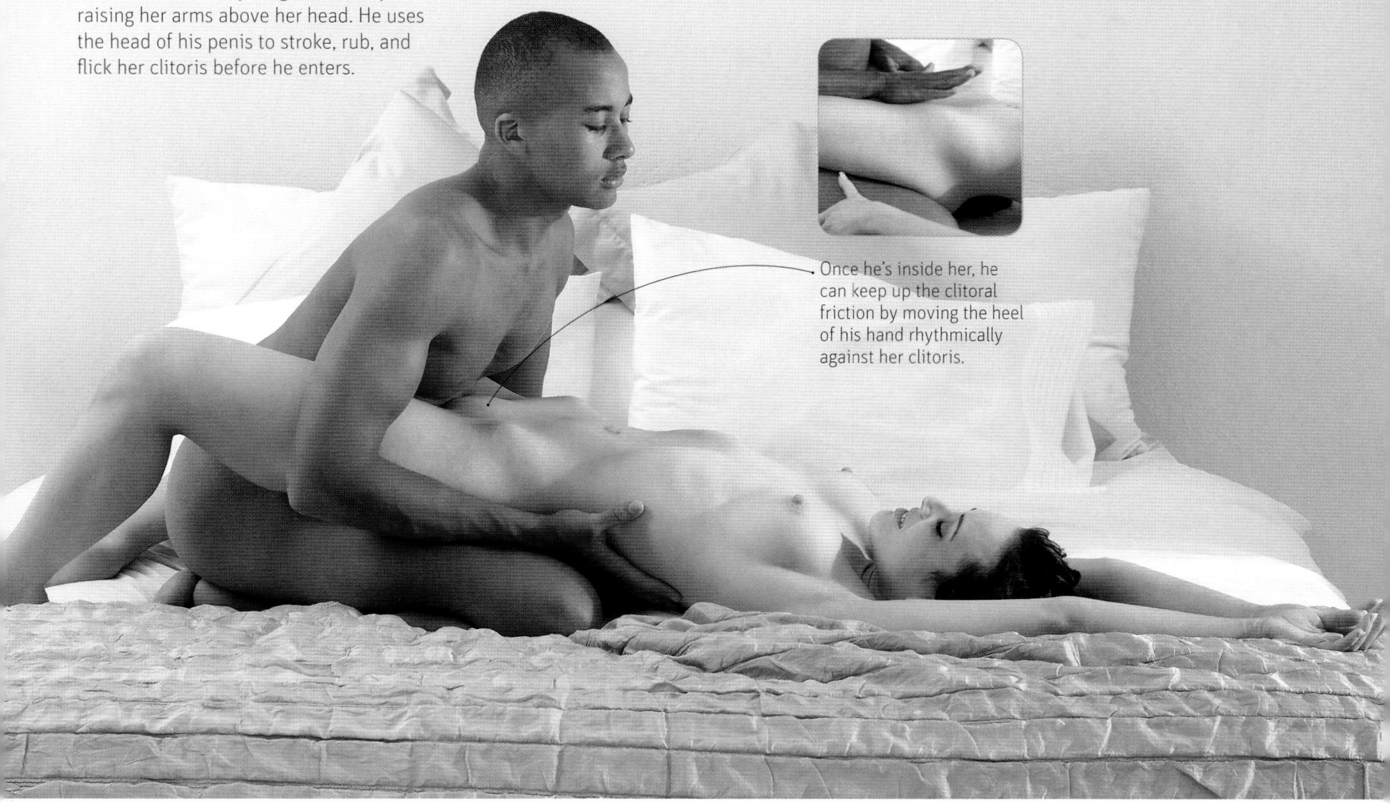

Once he's inside her, he can keep up the clitoral friction by moving the heel of his hand rhythmically against her clitoris.

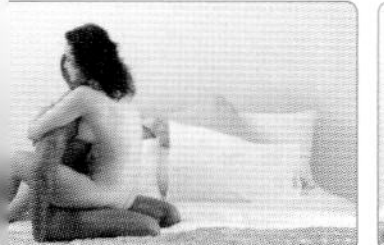
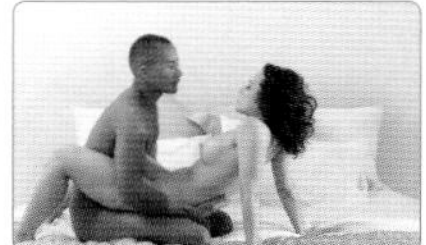
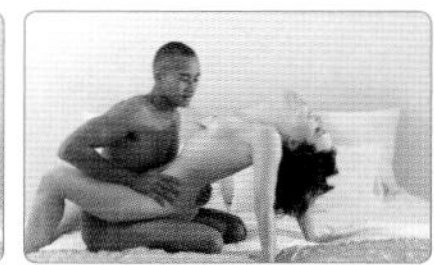
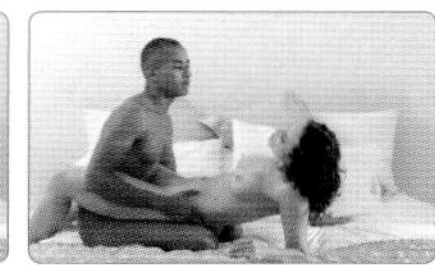
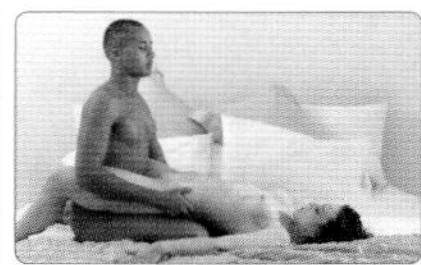
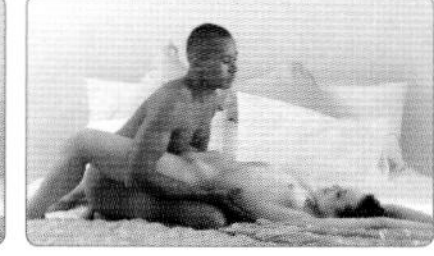

Late spring donkey

☆☆☆☆ Kama sensation rating

If you think your sex life is too squeaky clean, you can use the raunchy Late Spring Donkey to sex things up. It's primal, animalistic, and naughty, and there's no room for manners, romance, or politeness... which can sometimes be exactly what you need.

Why it works

– It's raw and ready no-frills sex; you'll both love its bend-over and slip-it-in immediacy.

– She gets a rush from being pounded from behind while the blood rushes to her head.

– If she's G-spot-sensitive, the drumming on the front wall of her vagina can lead to a body-quaking G-spot orgasm.

– A well-timed spank on her buttocks will give her a jolt of sudden pleasure.

– She can try a new move: rapidly shaking her legs while he stays still. The vibes will reverberate throughout your bodies.

Turn on...

... Take a breather midway through. It's easy to become desensitized to rhythmic pounding, so take the occasional pause in which you simply stay still and steady your breathing.

Turn off...

... Saying please and thank you. The whole point of this position is to hump like animals, so save any tender asides, sweet nothings, or sensitive whispers for another, more intimate time.

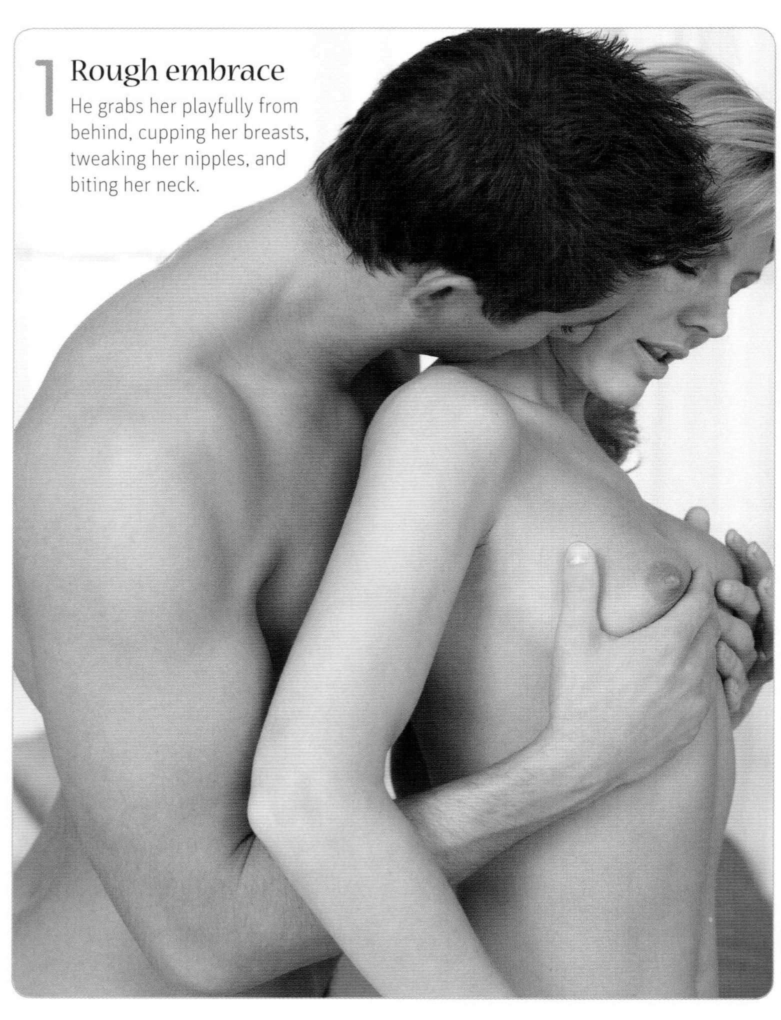

1 Rough embrace
He grabs her playfully from behind, cupping her breasts, tweaking her nipples, and biting her neck.

"When the woman's sucker is in action, she will be possessed of the most violent love for her partner..." THE PERFUMED GARDEN

2 Half bend

She puts her hands on her knees and bends over with her spine straight. He holds on to her hips.

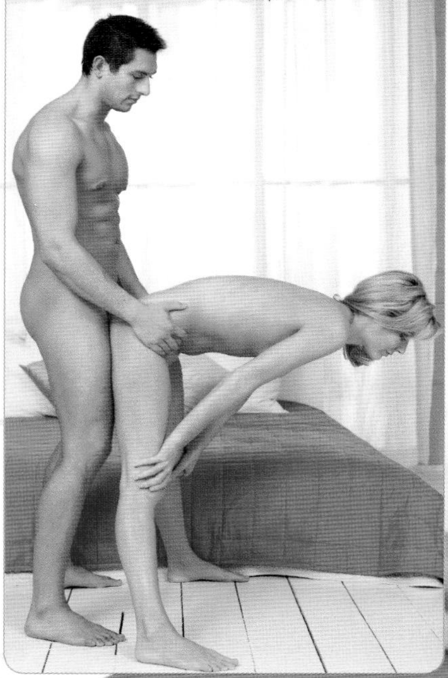

3 Full bend

She bends over completely and puts her hands on the floor. He steadies her with a hand on her ass, then enters her.

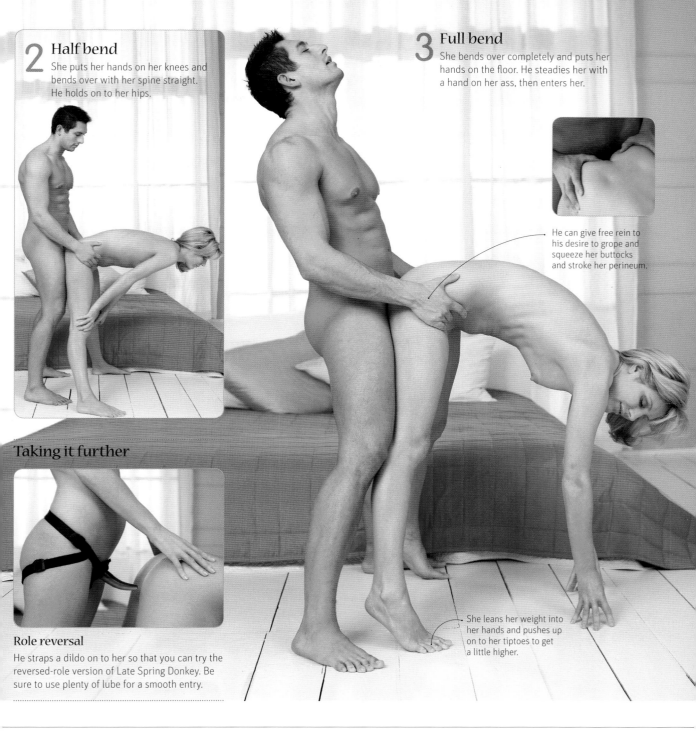

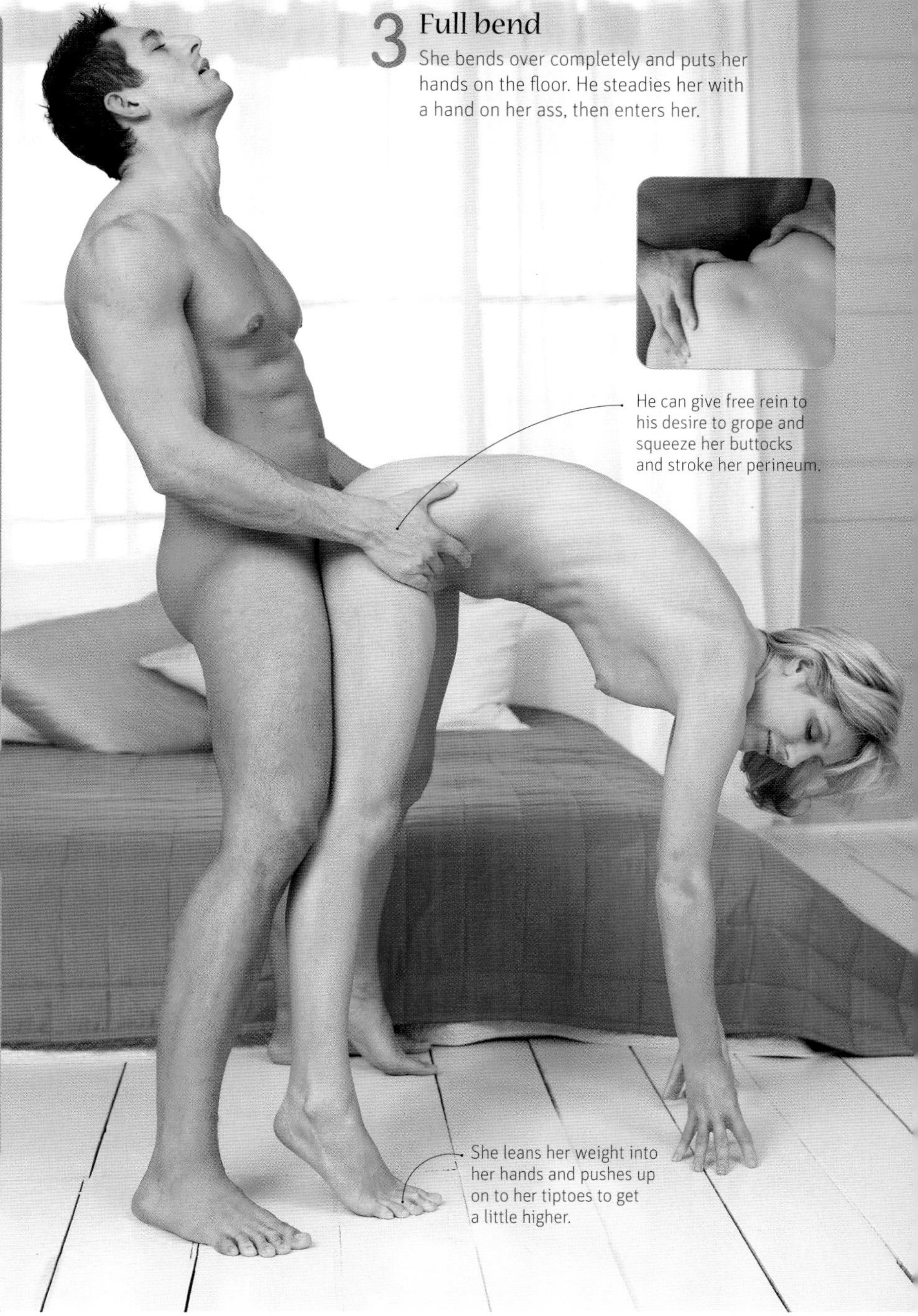

He can give free rein to his desire to grope and squeeze her buttocks and stroke her perineum.

She leans her weight into her hands and pushes up on to her tiptoes to get a little higher.

Taking it further

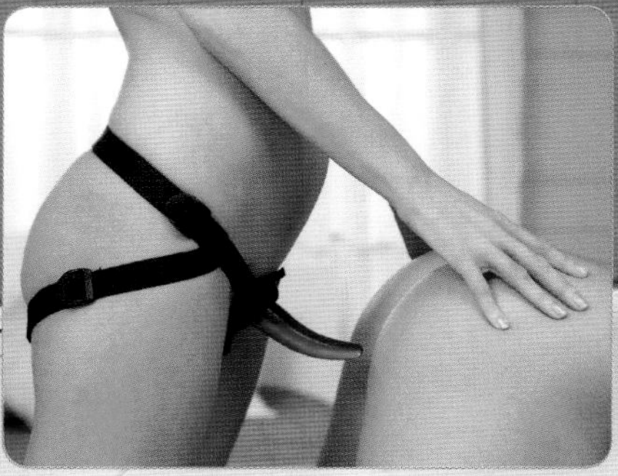

Role reversal

He straps a dildo on to her so that you can try the reversed-role version of Late Spring Donkey. Be sure to use plenty of lube for a smooth entry.

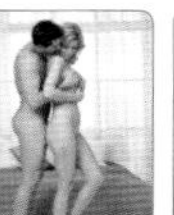
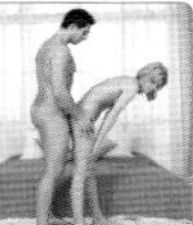
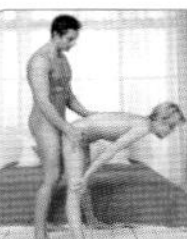
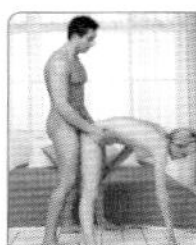
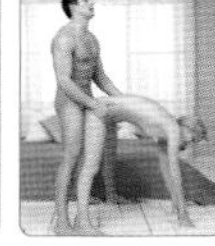

Reciprocal sights of the posterior

Also known in the trade as "I'll show you my mine if you'll show me yours," this is a novel way of ogling each other's nether regions. He lifts his head to see the cleft of her buttocks provocatively perched on top of him. She, meanwhile, leans forward to see not just his ass and his balls, but the sexy spectacle of his penis plunging into her.

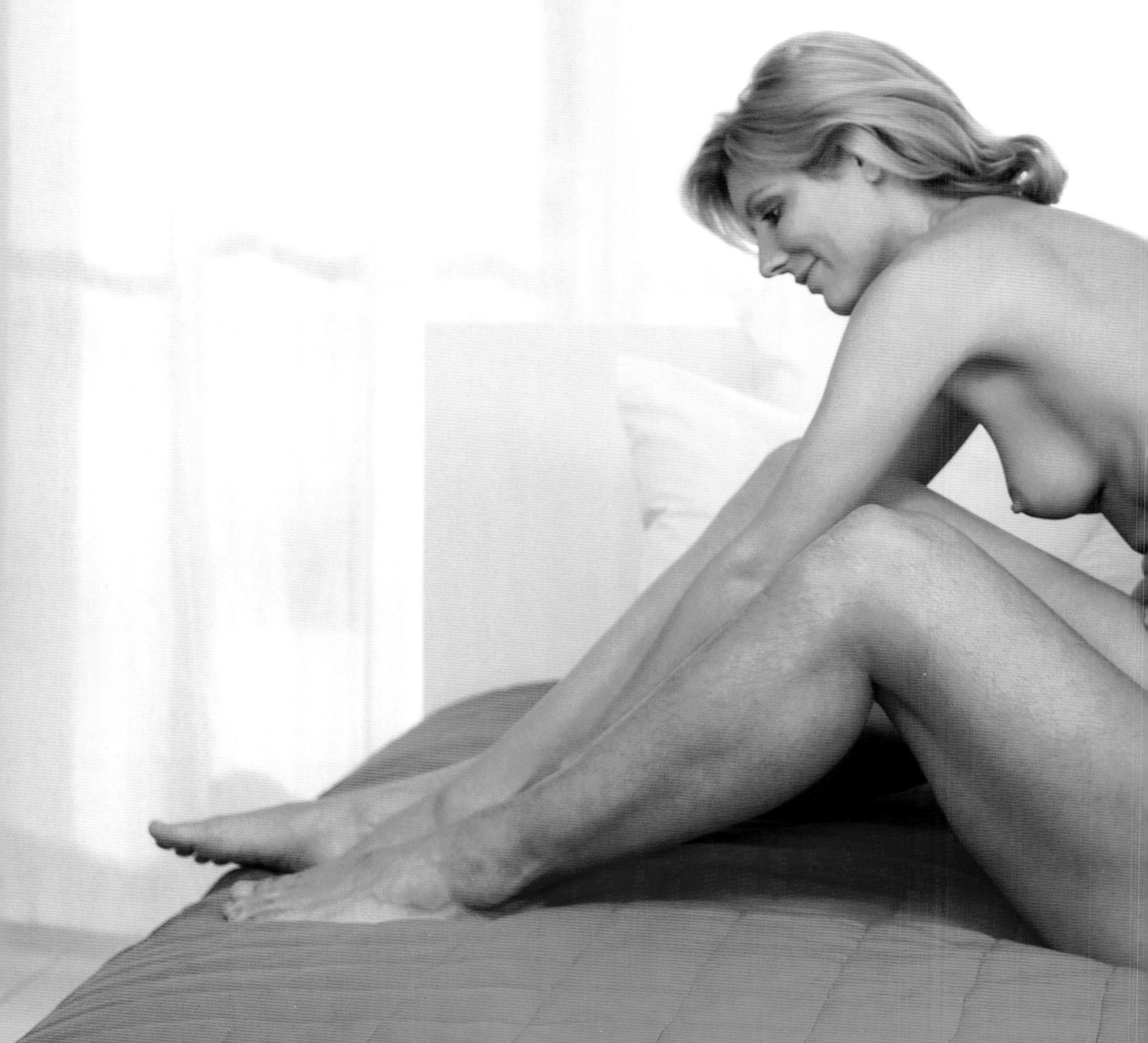

"The man clasps her body between his legs and she leans over until she can touch the floor. Supported in this way, she is able to see his buttocks and he can see hers. She can move conveniently in this position."

THE PERFUMED GARDEN

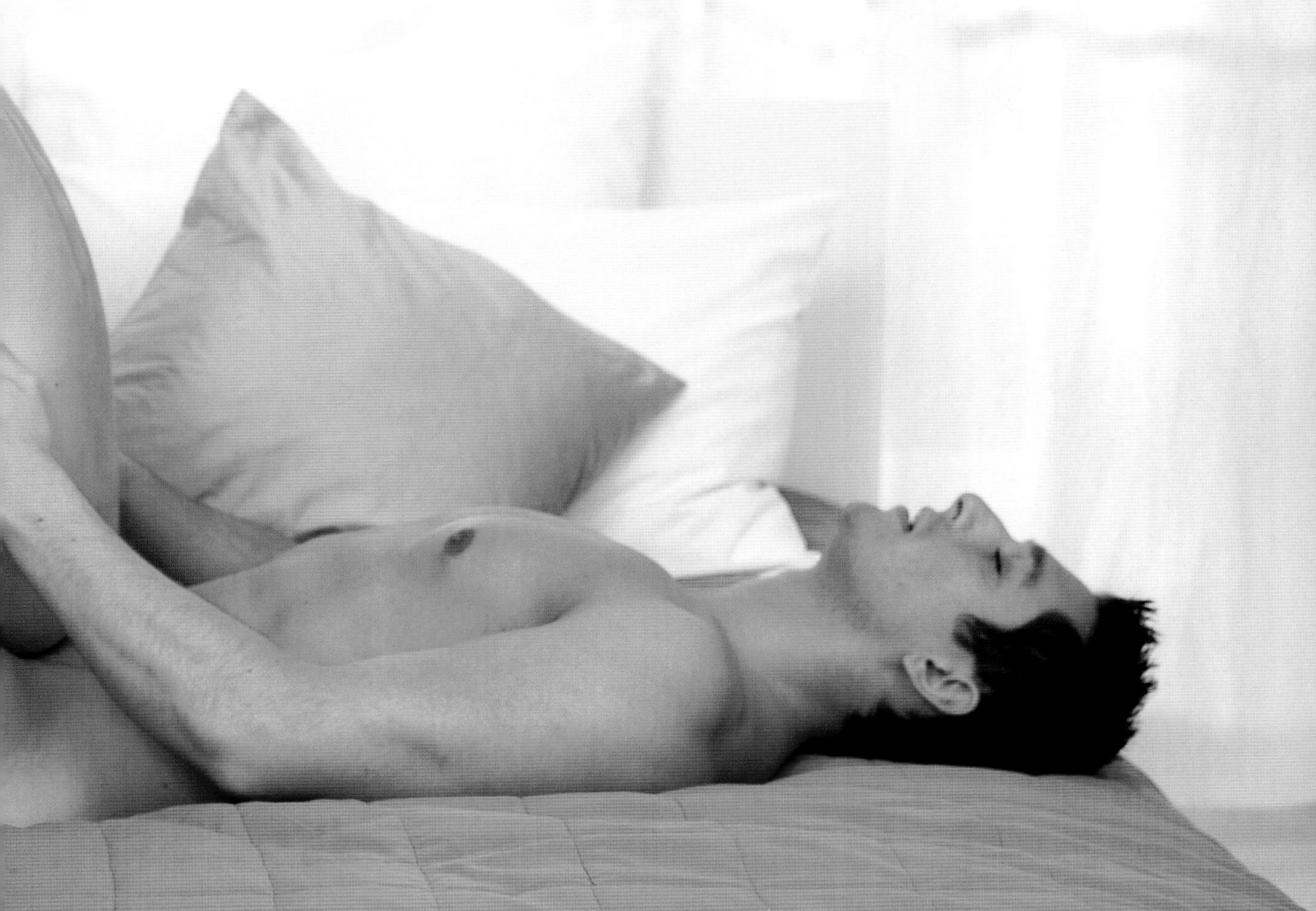

Reciprocal sights of the posterior

☆☆☆☆

Kama sensation rating

Why it works

– If she likes porn-style close-ups, she's scored the best seat in the house.

– If both of you like porn-style close ups, she can video the action from where she's sitting. Watch the footage back afterward, and find yourselves getting horny all over again.

– He can get all hot and bothered by the sight of her ass rising and falling on his belly.

– Her buttocks spread out as she nestles tightly against him; the result is hot friction between her perineum and his abdomen.

– She gets to make the moves: long, slick up-and-down strokes, internal contractions, or wiggles that bring his penile head into perfect alignment with her G-spot.

– You're in your own separate worlds, so you can make your thoughts as bargain-basement dirty as you like.

Turn on...

... Go easy on his shaft. The further forward you lean, the more his erect penis bends toward his feet, which goes against the normal order of things.

Turn off...

... Don't drift too far off into your separate worlds. You can keep in touch with moans and compliments.

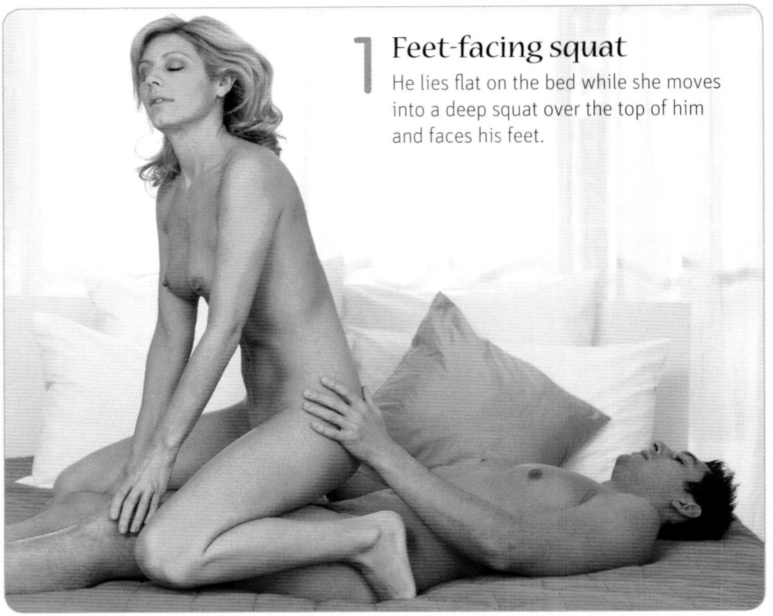

1 Feet-facing squat
He lies flat on the bed while she moves into a deep squat over the top of him and faces his feet.

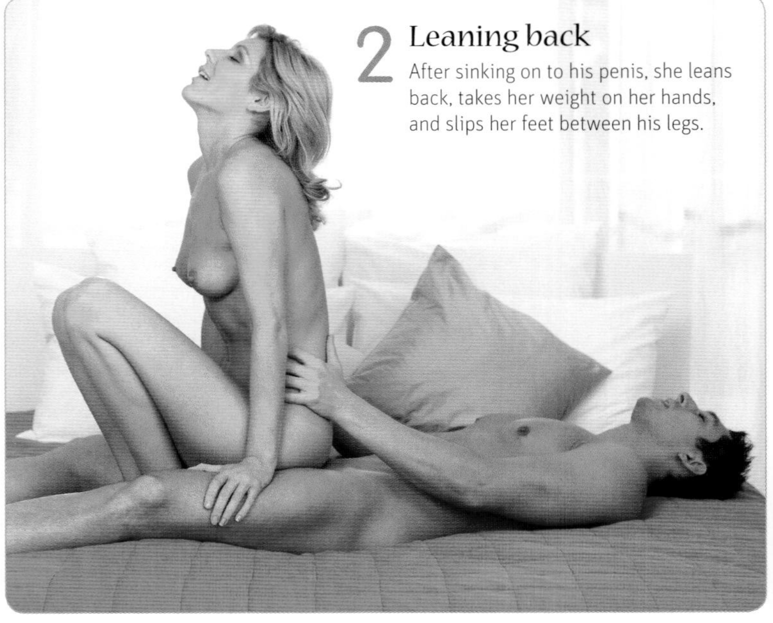

2 Leaning back
After sinking on to his penis, she leans back, takes her weight on her hands, and slips her feet between his legs.

"Explore her with all possible enjoyment, and let your mind be empty of all other thoughts." THE PERFUMED GARDEN

Taking it further

Taking in the view

She leans further forward and looks down to catch more of the action. The increased tension of this angle of penetration can work wonders.

3 Leaning forward

She leans forward and rests her hands on the bed between his legs. He encloses her in the position with his bent knees.

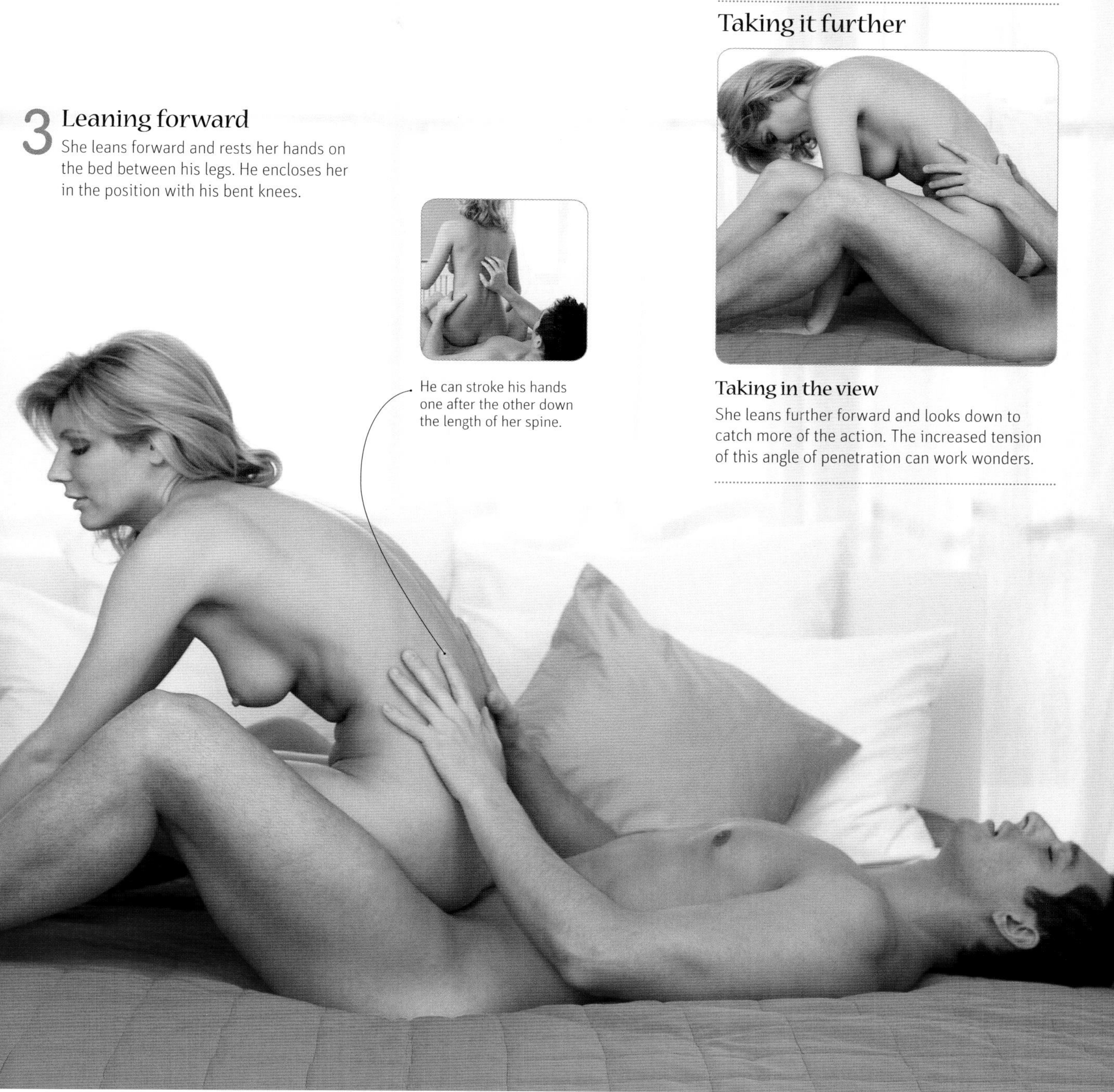

He can stroke his hands one after the other down the length of her spine.

If you liked this, try…

– Getting a bit closer in The Mare (see page 126).
– Making it part of a sequence in The Top (see page 226).

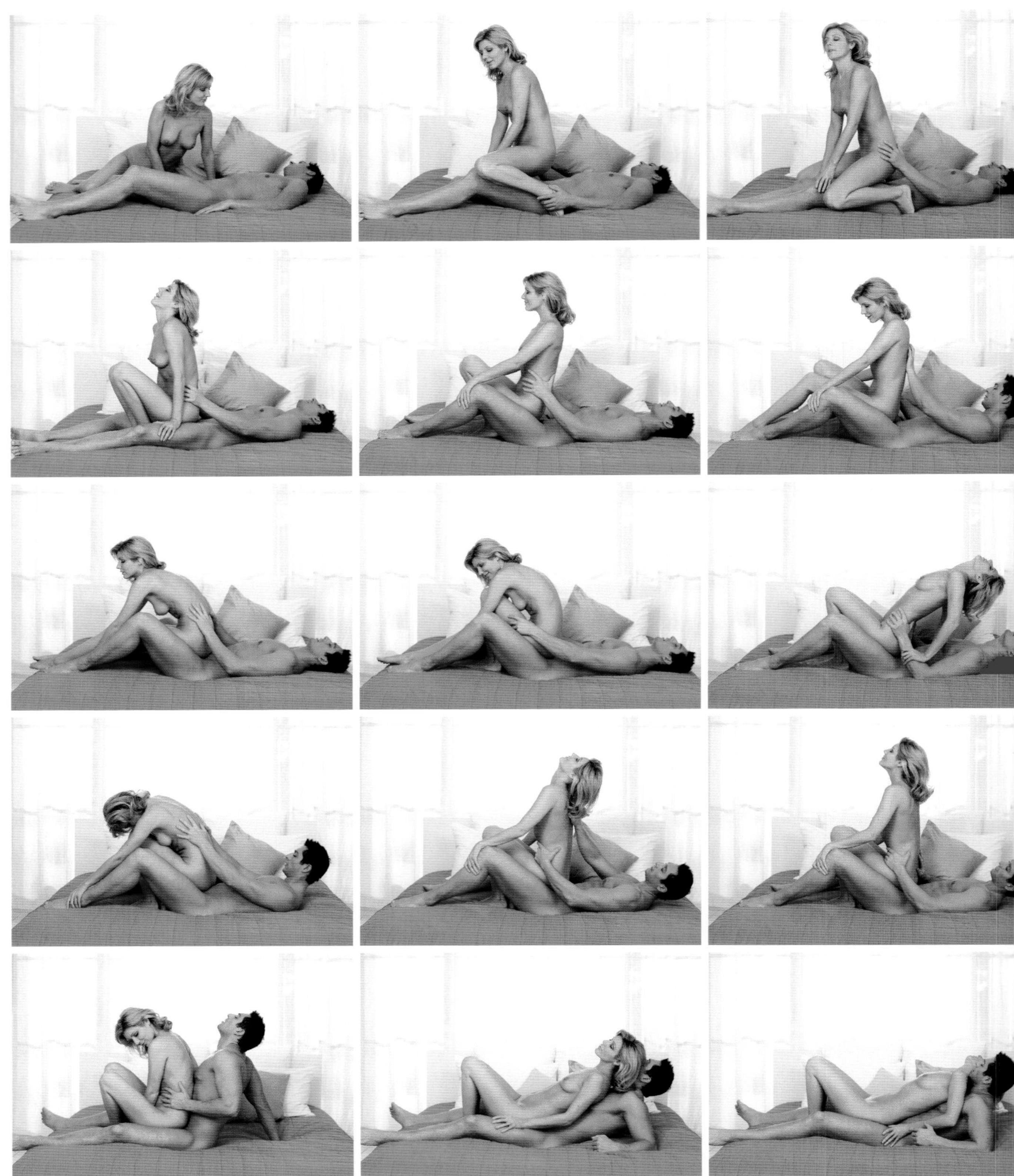

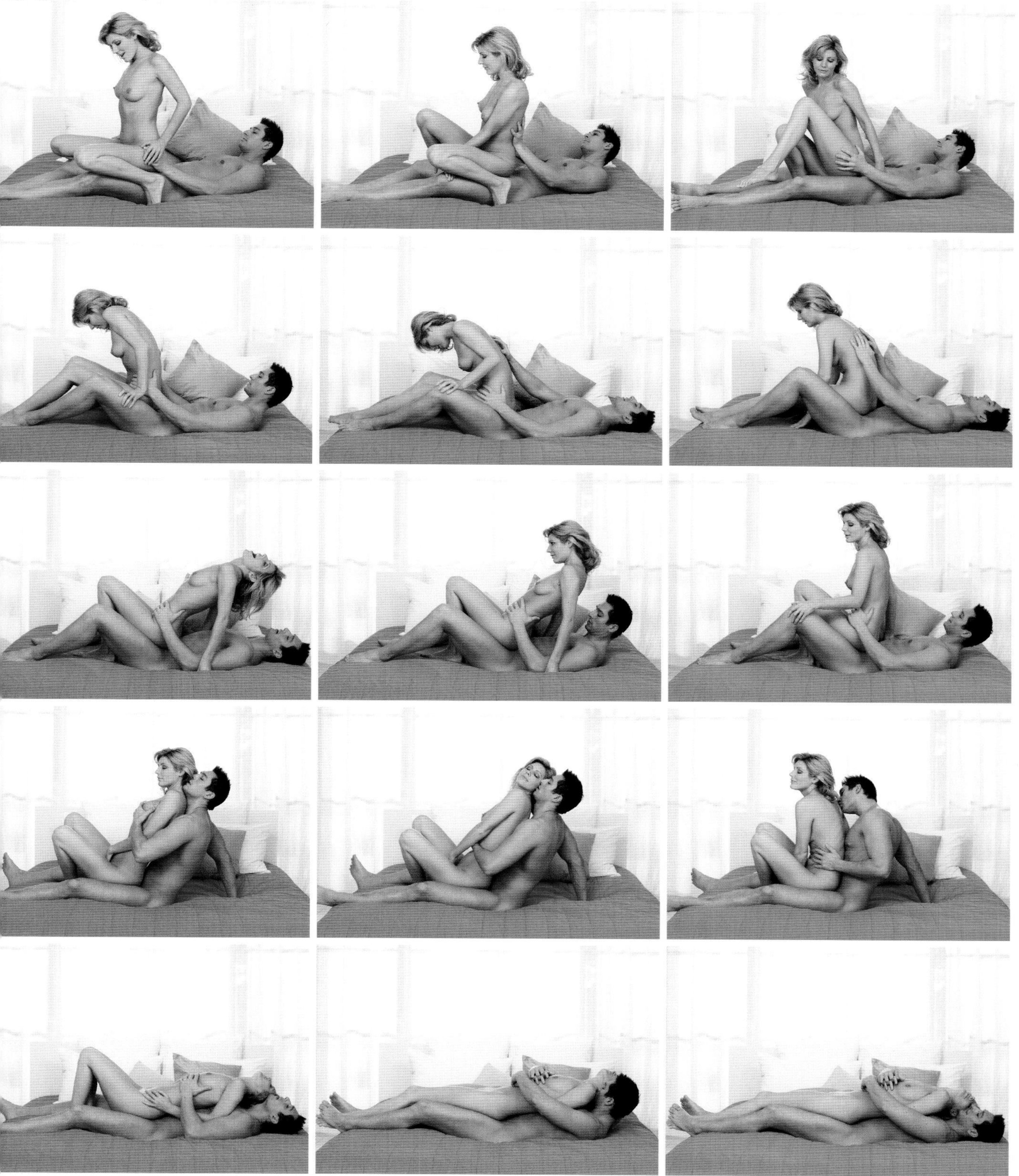

The dragon turn and Galloping horse

☆☆☆☆ Kama sensation rating

The appeal of this spicy pair of positions lies in the erotic atmosphere they create as much as the exact position of your limbs. Let the mood burn from smoldering intensity to roaring flames of passion as you both gallop toward the finishing line.

Why they work

– She's thrilled by the way he bears down hungrily as if he can't wait another moment.

– He's intoxicated by the "I want you now" body language of her wide-open legs and the way her heels pull him in deep.

– You can both close your eyes and savor the ecstasy of a deep connection, both physical and emotional.

– Moving from The Dragon Turn to Galloping Horse ups the dominance/submission stakes. She reveals her trust in him as she lets him "hold her down" at the foot and neck. He gets the aphrodisiac power of having her completely in his hands.

Turn on…

… Grip her by the neck and the ankle in Galloping Horse. The point is to play around with roles; he needs to be the boss, and she needs to submit.

Turn off…

… Don't hold the front of her neck. Despite what you may have heard about asphyxiation being erotic, anything that has the potential to cut off her air supply is dangerous and to be avoided.

1 Deep entry

He jumps on her in missionary position, and she pulls her knees up to draw him in as deeply as possible.

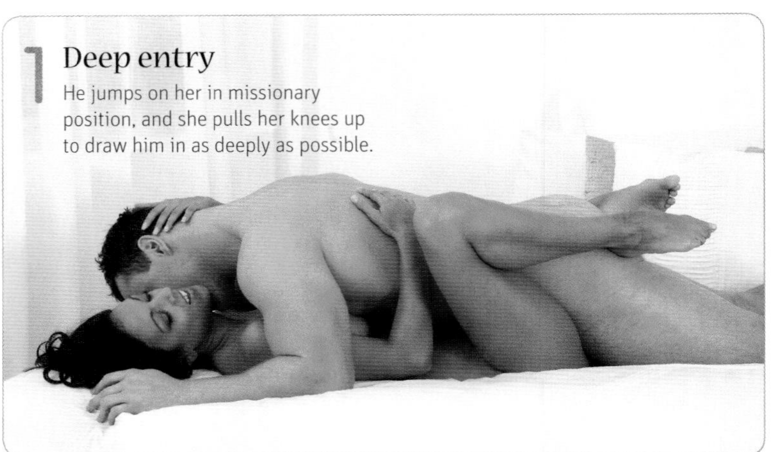

2 Heel to butt

He thrusts on all fours with her heels resting on his butt. This is The Dragon Turn.

She uses her hands and heels on his buttocks to pull him closely to her.

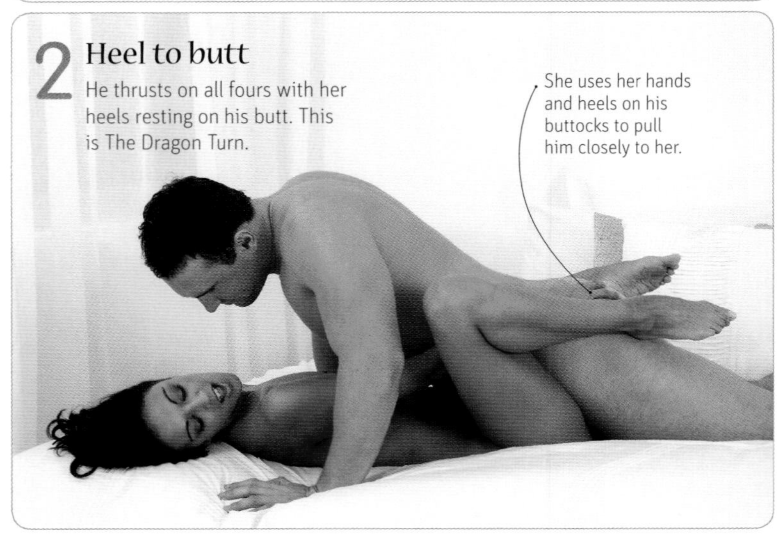

"Woman's orgasm is a series of eight upward-rising steps, then one declining." THE TAO

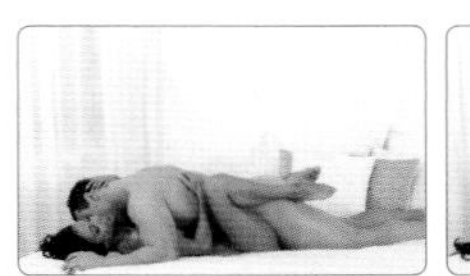

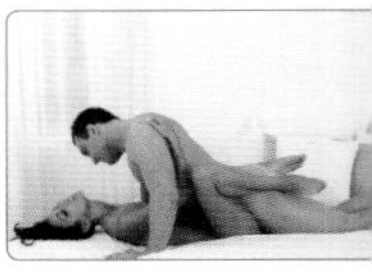

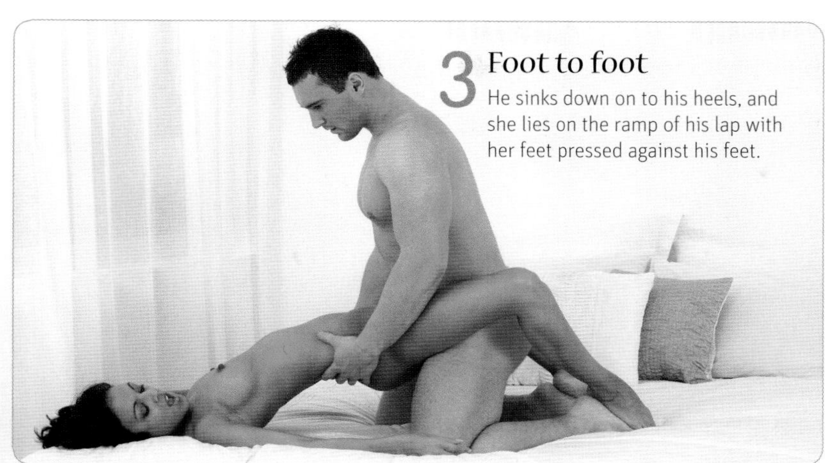

3 Foot to foot

He sinks down on to his heels, and she lies on the ramp of his lap with her feet pressed against his feet.

Taking it further

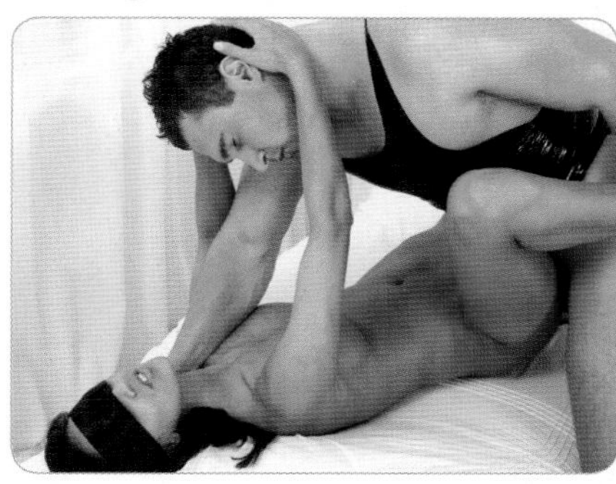

Kinky props

For extra kink value he dresses in black rubber, vinyl, or latex. She wears a blindfold to experience the ultimate in erotic surrender.

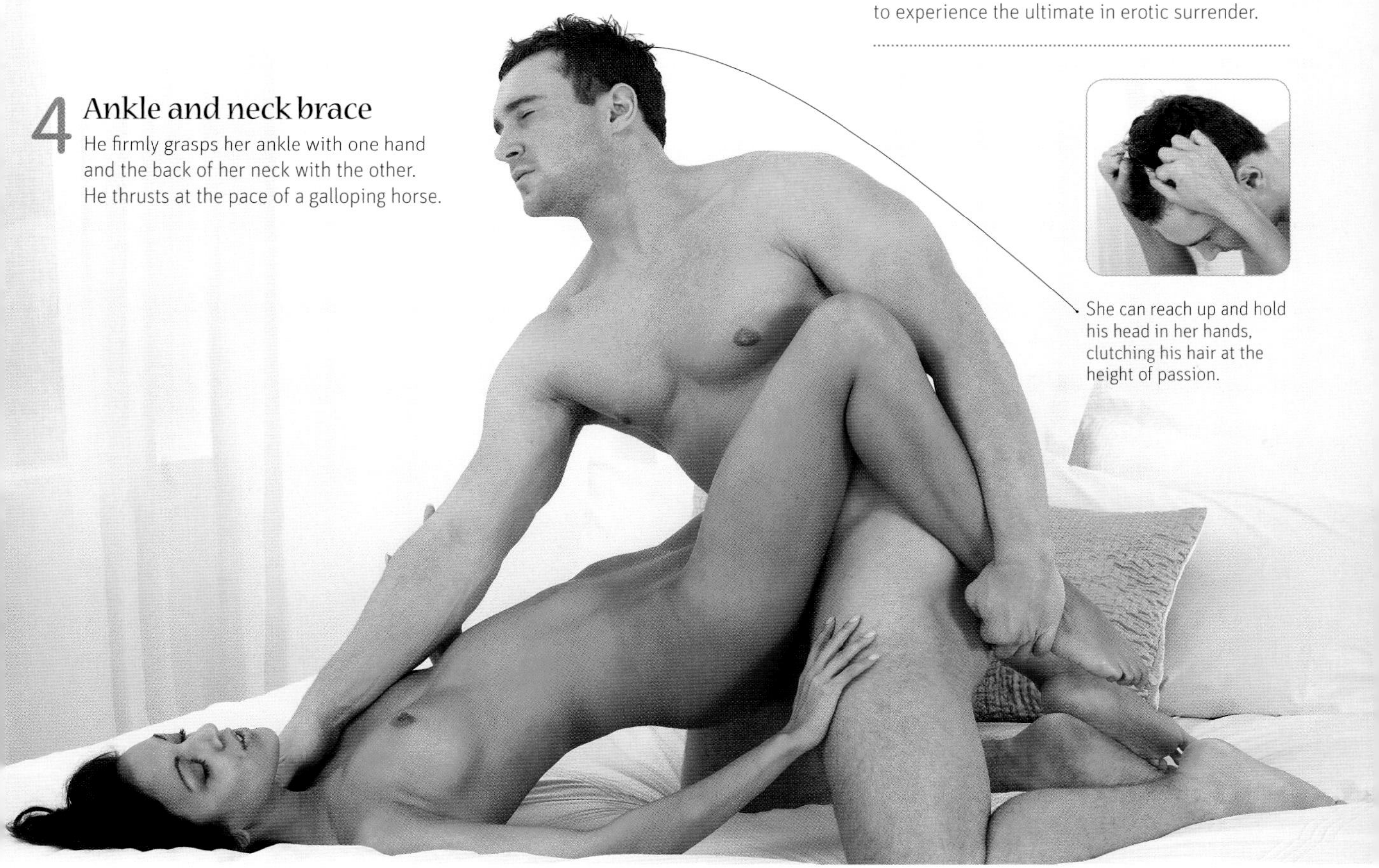

4 Ankle and neck brace

He firmly grasps her ankle with one hand and the back of her neck with the other. He thrusts at the pace of a galloping horse.

She can reach up and hold his head in her hands, clutching his hair at the height of passion.

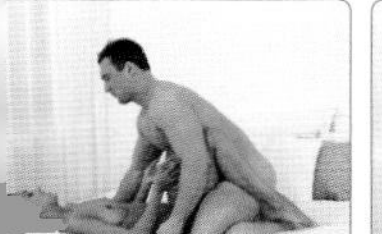
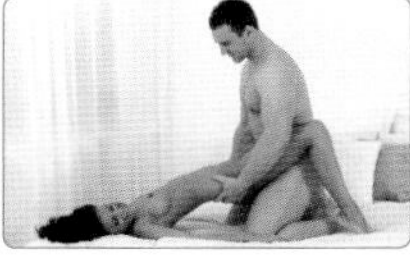
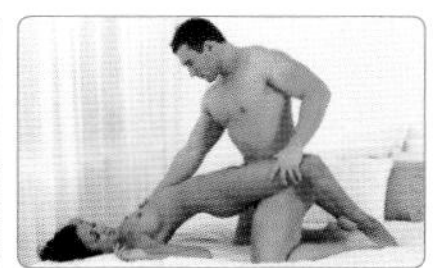
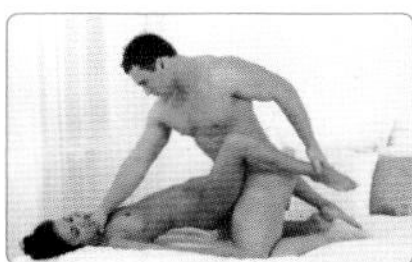
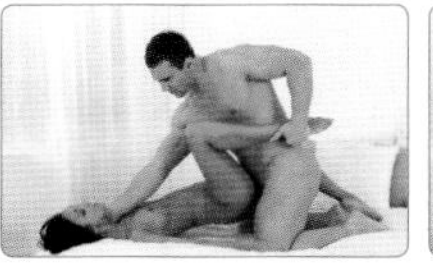
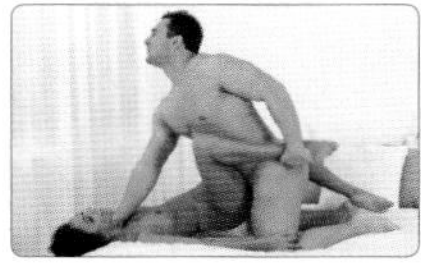

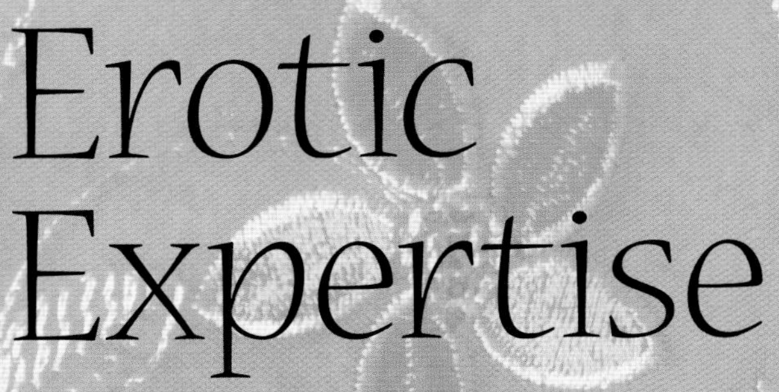

Erotic Expertise

The positions in this chapter are all scorchingly hot, deeply difficult, or wildly filthy. You'll find some of the ancient world's greatest lust-quenchers here alongside some of the greatest sexual showpieces. If watching yourselves is a turn-on, now's the time to set up a tripod and video camera.

Most of these positions require lovers to be to be low on inhibition and high on flexibility. And some depend on him being big in the biceps department. Try poses such as Suspended Congress after he's had a few sessions at the gym and Tail of the Ostrich after she's been to yoga. Alternatively, erotic expertise can mean knowing when to cheat. There's no shame in letting her hands, his back, or her ass rest against a handy wall or table top.

Finally… when you've Hung the Bow, Raced the Member, Fixed the Nail, and Spun the Top, you can lie back and take a well-deserved break. Summon the last of your energy and turn to the end of the chapter for the best in post-sex come-downs.

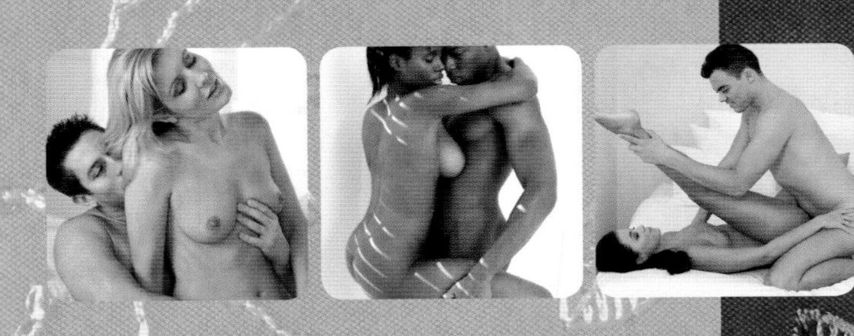

Suspended congress

☆☆ Kama sensation rating

This is wild one-night stand material. Your mission is to try the hottest, trickiest, showiest positions known to man and woman, and Suspended Congress checks all the boxes. Your aim: to end your sex session breathless, damp, and 100 percent satiated.

Why it works

– It's sex at its most energetic: she feels like a sex queen; he feels like a sex god. And it's ideal for reliving your adolescence.

– You don't need a bed; any small cubicle or empty wall space will do.

– It indulges her pick-me-up-and-hold-me-in-your-arms fantasies. And, if he pulls it off, he can bask in that I'm-so-strong feeling.

– If this is the first time you've had sex with each other, this will break the ice and make you extremely familiar with one another. The only challenge will be what boundary-breaking position to try next.

Turn on…

… Segue neatly into mid-intercourse oral sex by slithering down his body, squatting before him, and sliding your lips smoothly over his penis. You can always climb his mountain again in a minute.

Turn off…

… Don't expect to move in and out of her completely. Content yourself with jiggling her around (unless she's tiny and you're built like Arnold Schwarzenegger).

1 The push and kiss

She pushes him against a wall and leans in for a hot kiss. He leans back and lets himself be taken.

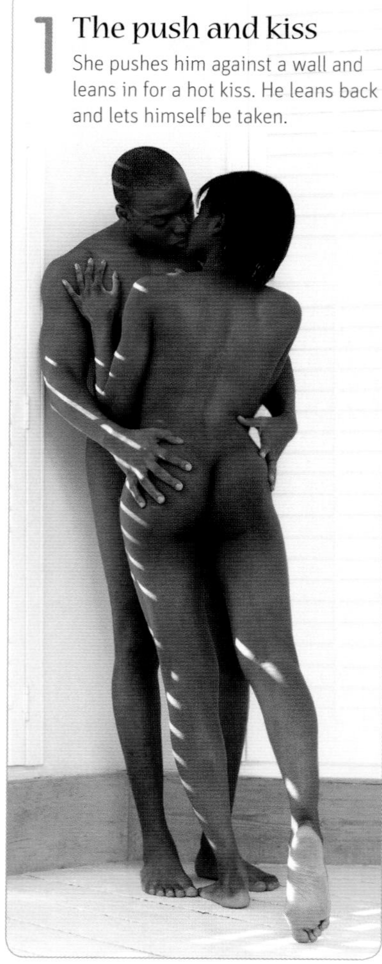

2 Thigh to thigh

She slides one of her thighs up the side of his. He supports her leg with his hand.

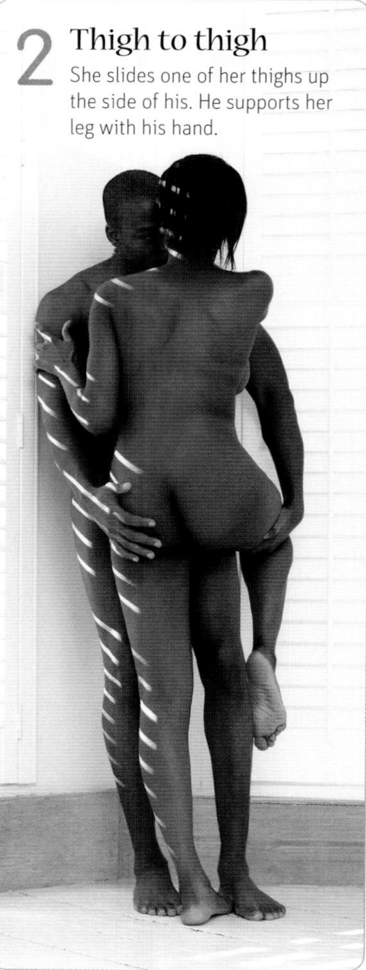

"She sits in the cage of his hands and wraps the noose of her thighs around his pelvis." KAMA SUTRA

Taking it further

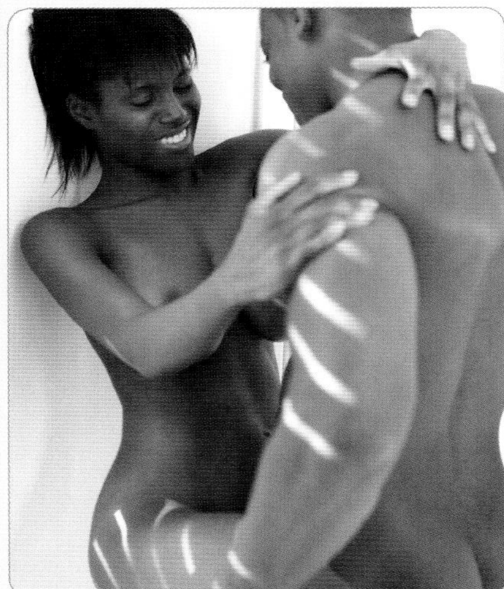

Up against the wall

Still holding her in his arms, he turns around and presses her back against the wall. This steadies you both and helps him to thrust.

3 Thigh seat

He bends and clasps her other leg in his hand, then picks her up to penetrate her in standing position. He leans back against the wall with his knees slightly bent so that she can "sit" on his thighs.

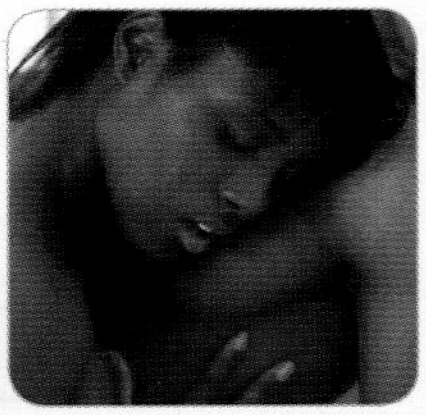

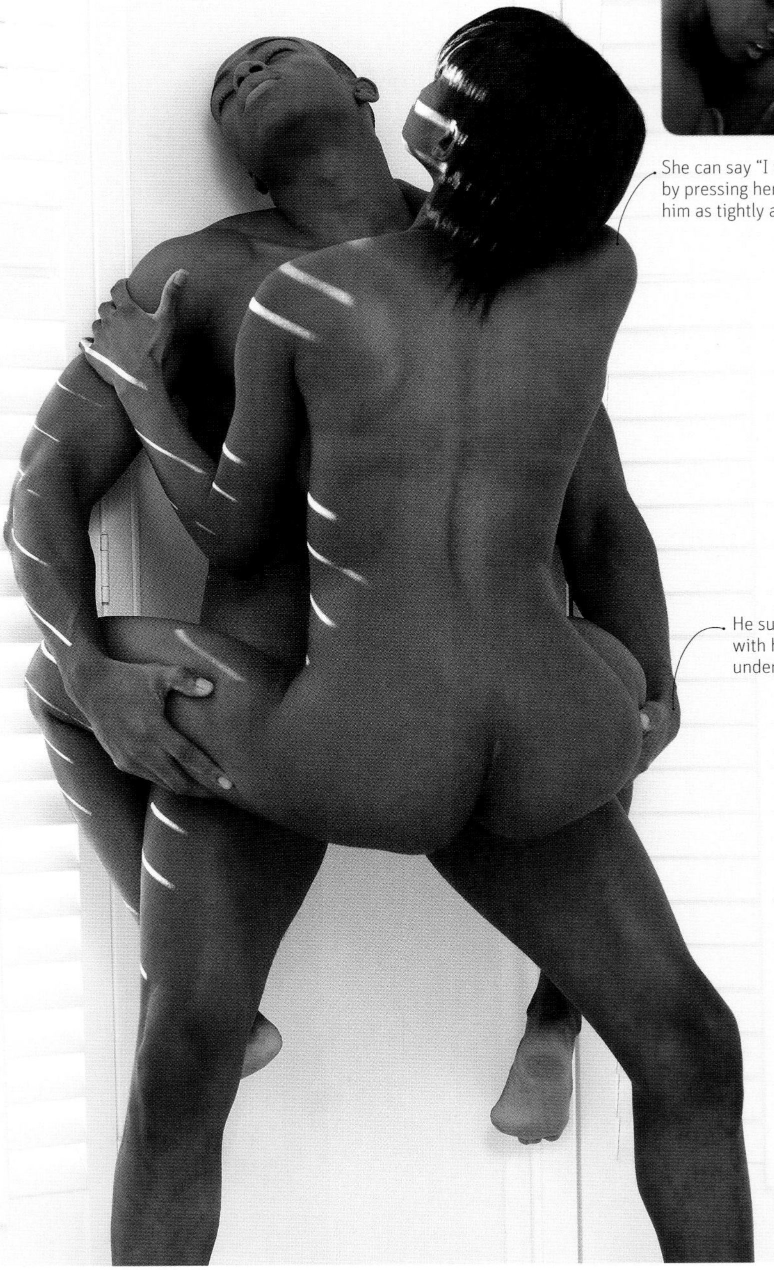

She can say "I want you" by pressing herself against him as tightly as possible.

He supports her with his hands under her thighs.

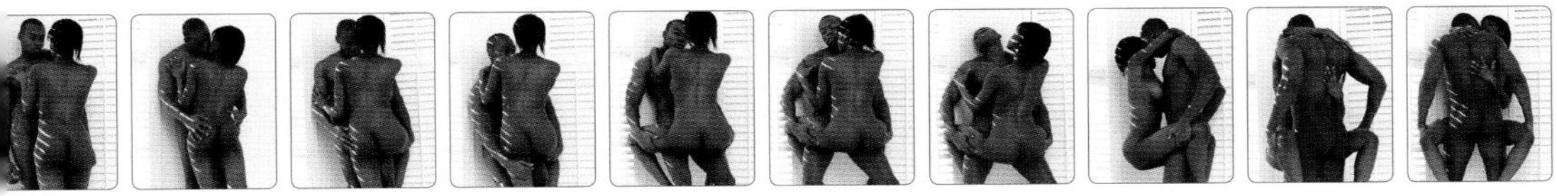

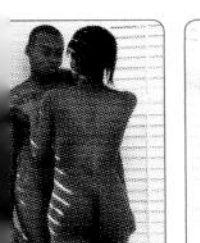
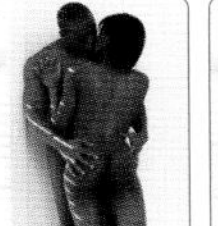
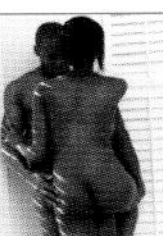
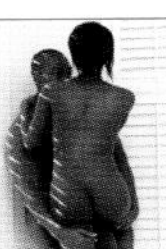
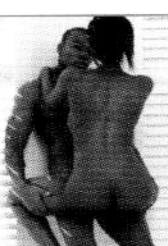
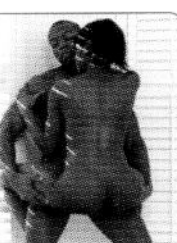
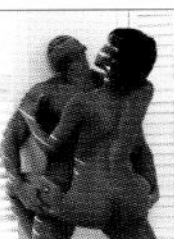
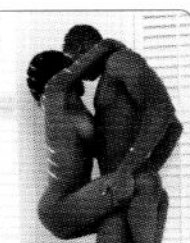
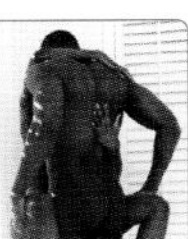
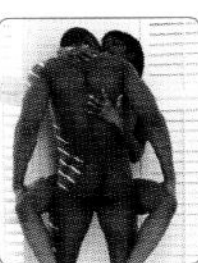

Position of equals and The snake trap

☆☆☆☆ Kama sensation rating

Don't be fooled by the easy and friendly appearance of these two positions, as they aren't what they seem. There's a seething snake pit of sensation happening right there in your laps, so cover yourselves in massage oil and writhe like serpents.

Why they works

– His proximity to her breasts gives him an erotic eyeful and a nipple-nibbling mouthful.

– A conventional in-and-out thrust is almost impossible, so you're forced into some very wiggly naughtiness.

– Things get off to a playful start as she sits in his lap, then get saucier as you move into The Snake Trap and secure each other's legs in an iron grip that says, "I'm not letting go."

– Enjoy the tussle-like nature of The Snake Trap; writhing against each other is guaranteed to rid you of sexual tension.

Turn on...

... Massage each other with a generous quantity of oil beforehand. The more slippery you are, the easier it will be for you to slide and glide against one another in snake-like bliss.

Turn off...

... Don't give up just because you don't have the quick and easy satisfaction of penile pounding. Resist the urge to pounce on top of each other. Instead, torture yourselves with anticipation for as long as you possibly can... then for a bit longer.

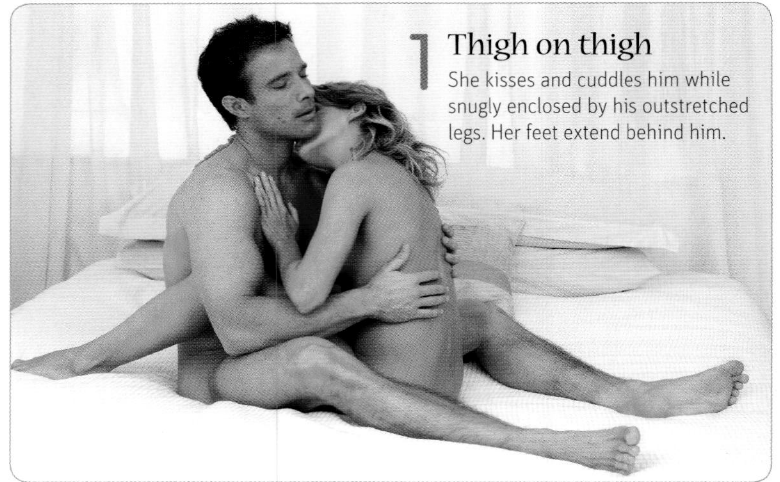

1 Thigh on thigh

She kisses and cuddles him while snugly enclosed by his outstretched legs. Her feet extend behind him.

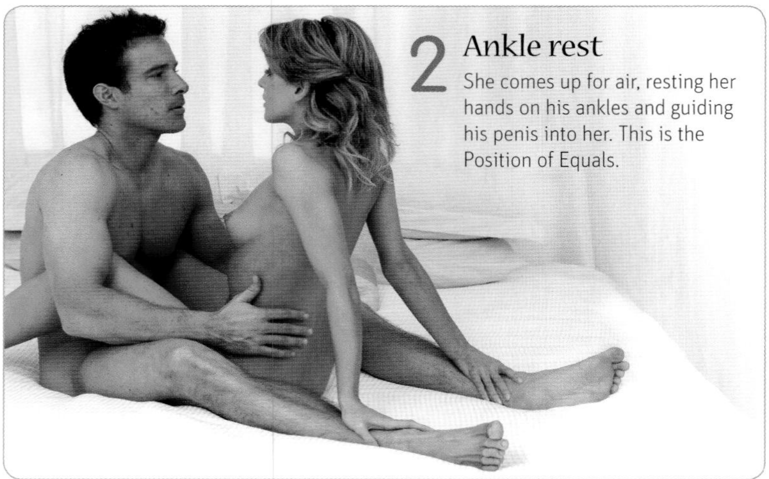

2 Ankle rest

She comes up for air, resting her hands on his ankles and guiding his penis into her. This is the Position of Equals.

"... they initiate a swaying movement, moving with little concussions, and keeping their movements in exact rhythm." THE PERFUMED GARDEN

3 Ankle grasp

He leans back with his hands on her legs. You grasp each other's ankles in The Snake Trap and wriggle against each other.

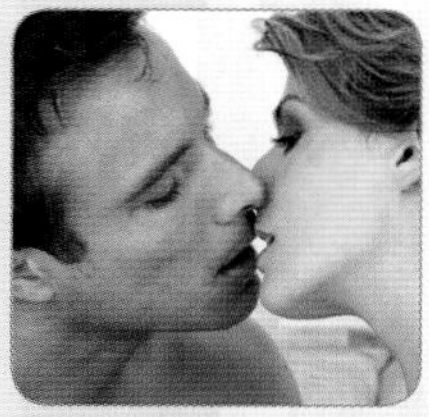

He can lean forward to excite her with a gasping, lust-fuelled kiss.

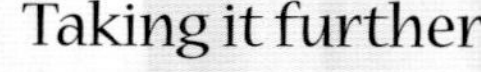

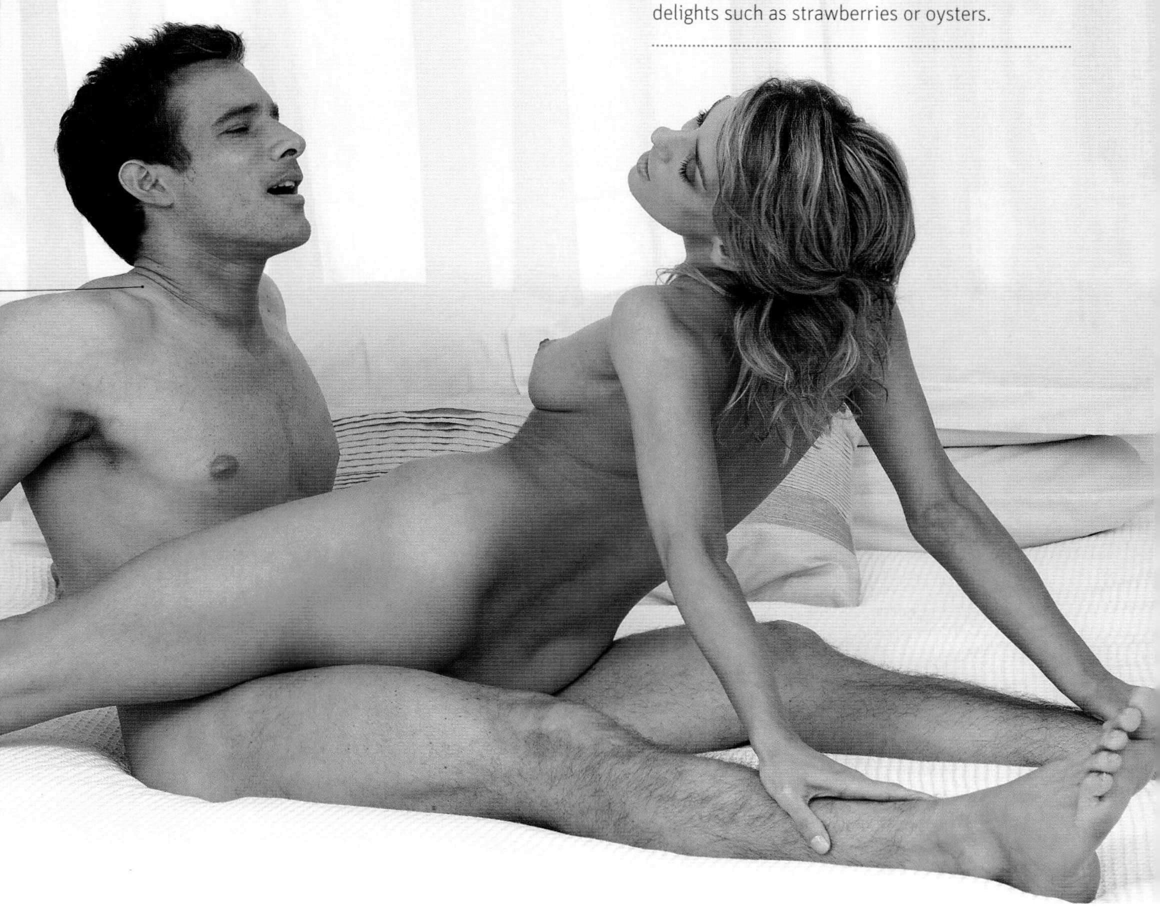

Taking it further

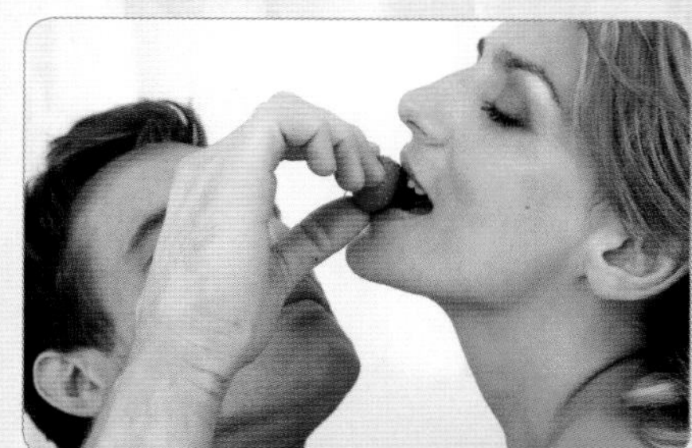

Heavenly aphrodisiacs

Take advantage of the Position of Equals by feeding each other with sensual or indulgent delights such as strawberries or oysters.

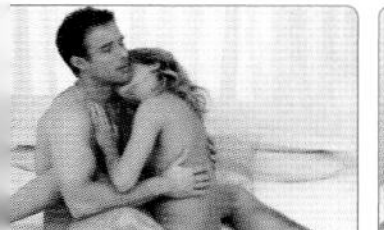
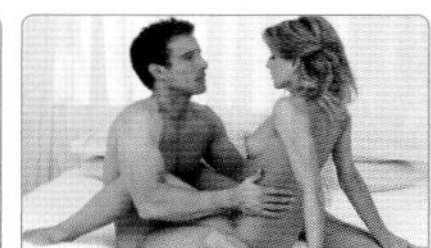
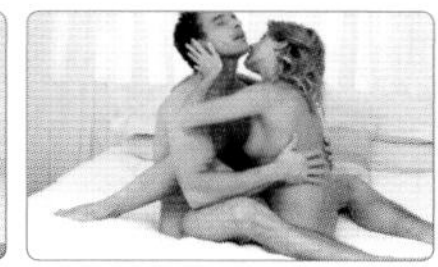
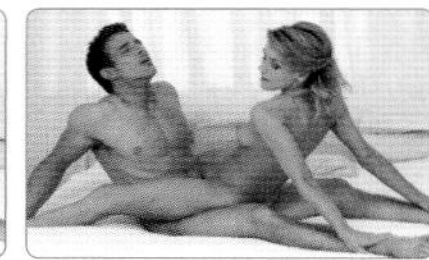
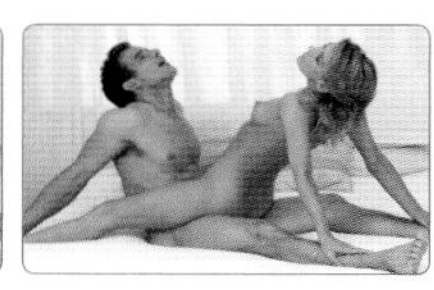

Tail of the ostrich

☆☆☆☆ Kama sensation rating

If you're one of those guys who likes to be a towering presence during sex, this is ideal. And if she likes being upside down while scaling his tower, you're a perfect match for each other. One word of caution: this is not really suitable for after-dinner frolics.

Why it works

– He can rub his shaft in parallel motion against her vulva to fill her with melting-butter sensations.

– You get to ogle each other from an entirely new angle.

– Her legs-together position creates tight ripples of pleasure for both of you.

– He can experiment with a novel sexual alternative: plunging his ostrich tail back and forth between her clasped thighs. He can either make this the main event or a racy opener. Either way, rubbing some lube on her thighs will make this his new erotic haven.

Turn on...

... Practice doing a shoulder stand before you get frisky. Lie on your back, curl your knees into your belly, and swing your hips up into the air with your hands supporting them.

Turn off...

... Depending on your individual builds and fit, you may find his penis resting snugly between her buttocks rather than in her vagina. If this is the case, you could enter by the back door instead.

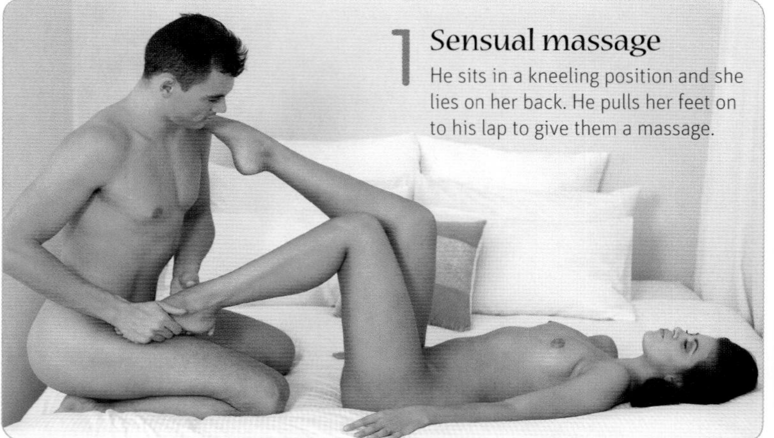

1 Sensual massage

He sits in a kneeling position and she lies on her back. He pulls her feet on to his lap to give them a massage.

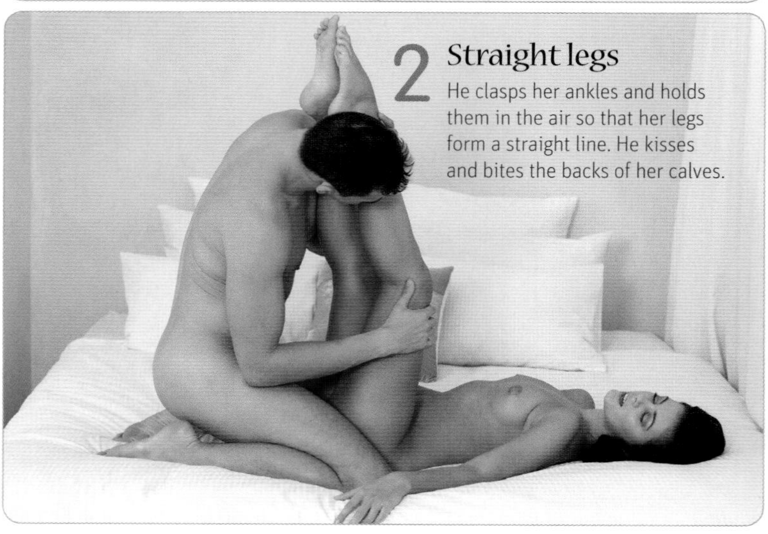

2 Straight legs

He clasps her ankles and holds them in the air so that her legs form a straight line. He kisses and bites the backs of her calves.

"He may also consider other special matings... imitating the behaviour of a dog, stag, or billygoat, the donkey's assault, the cat's pounce, the tiger's spring..." KAMA SUTRA

3 Leg hug

He hugs her legs in a tight embrace, then moves into an upright kneeling position, lifting her body with him as he goes. He penetrates her when he gets to full height.

She can put her hands on her hips or in the small of her back to push higher.

Taking it further

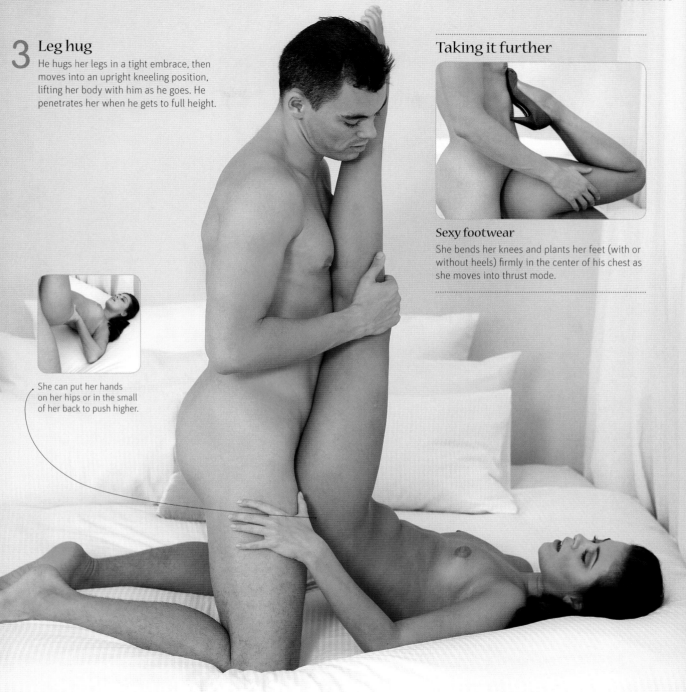

Sexy footwear

She bends her knees and plants her feet (with or without heels) firmly in the center of his chest as she moves into thrust mode.

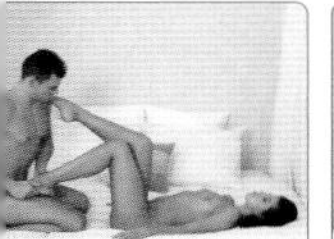
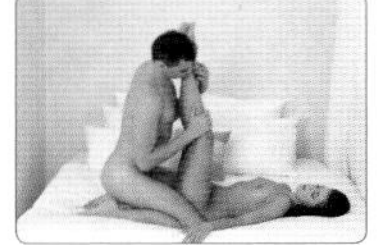
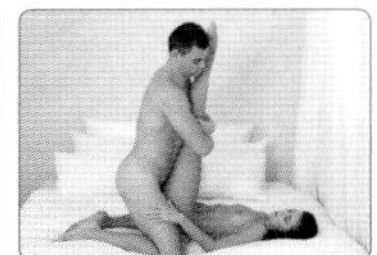
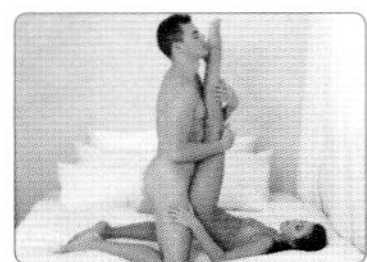
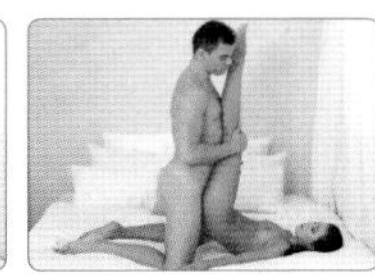

Lotus-like

☆☆☆ Kama sensation rating

Here's another bit of *Kama Sutra* acrobatics to make you hot and sweaty (even more so if you're not a world-class yogi). If you can't do a lotus position, cheat by crossing your legs; the effect is much the same. If you can manage the lotus: respect.

Why it works

– He can't plumb her depths, but the tip of his penis nudges her vaginal entrance in the most tantalizing way. This builds up your carnal appetite to the point where you're ready to devour each other.

– The barrier of her knotted legs gives you springy, bouncy sensations you won't get in any other sex position.

– You can congratulate each other on having super-advanced sex.

– It's perfect for master/slave role-playing games; with her legs sandwiched between you, there's little chance of an easy escape.

Turn on...

... Try a little tantric meditation. Gaze deeply into each other's eyes, and take long, slow tantric-inspired breaths that still your minds and unite your spirits in deep, floating harmony.

Turn off...

... Attempting the lotus position if you're not a yogi. If you can't do a lotus position sitting upright, it's even harder to achieve one on your back with a sex-hungry man on top.

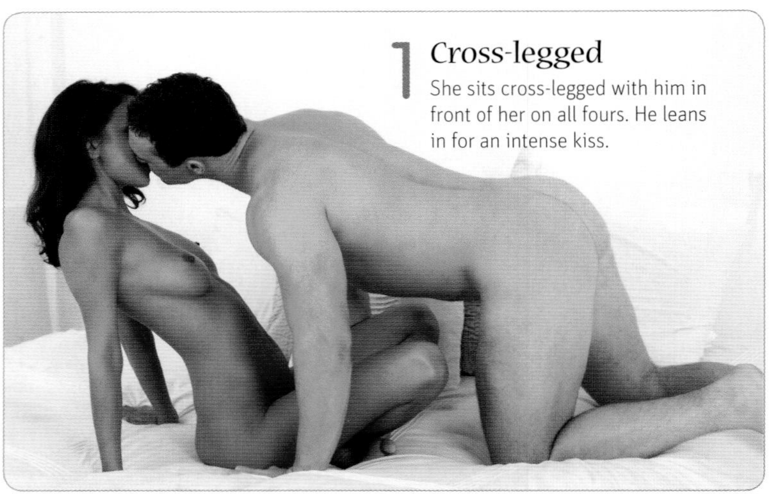

1 Cross-legged
She sits cross-legged with him in front of her on all fours. He leans in for an intense kiss.

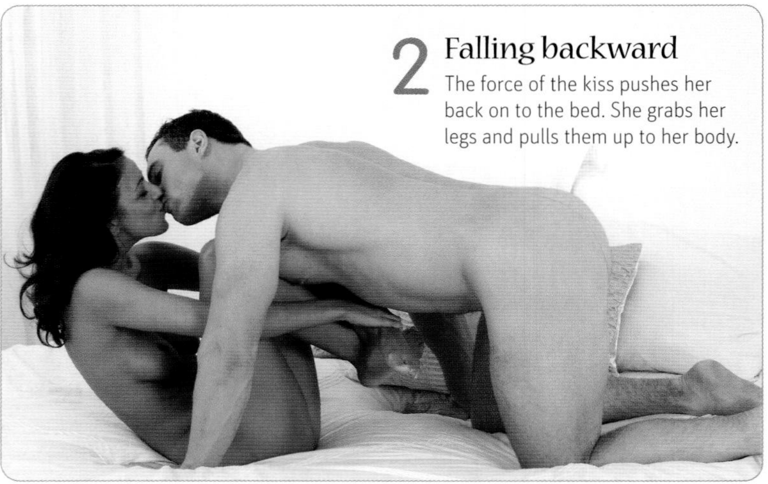

2 Falling backward
The force of the kiss pushes her back on to the bed. She grabs her legs and pulls them up to her body.

"A man who understands the heart should expand his repertoire of techniques for sexual bliss." KAMA SUTRA

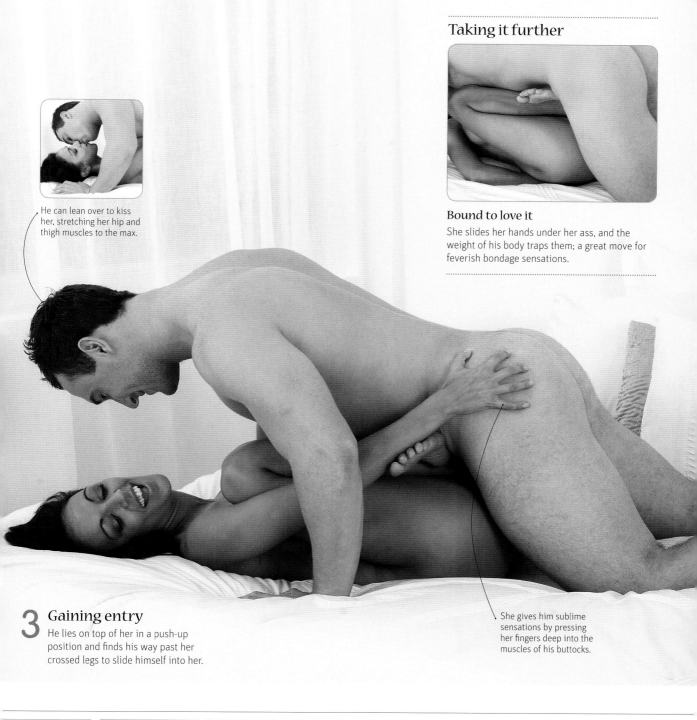

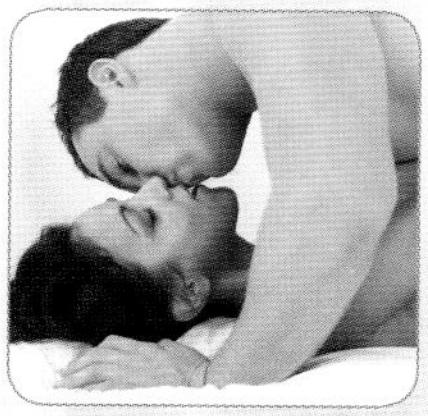

Taking it further

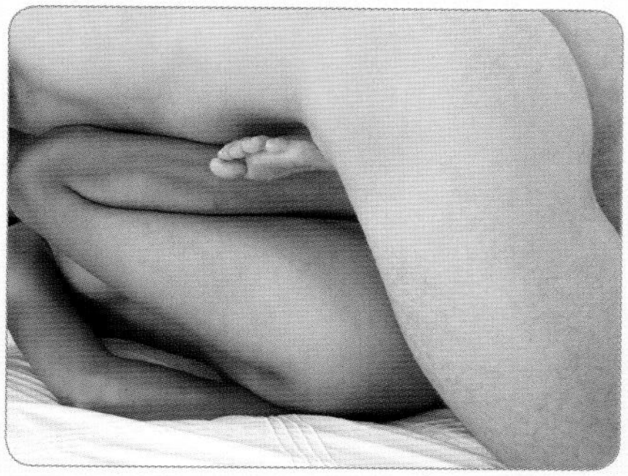

Bound to love it

She slides her hands under her ass, and the weight of his body traps them; a great move for feverish bondage sensations.

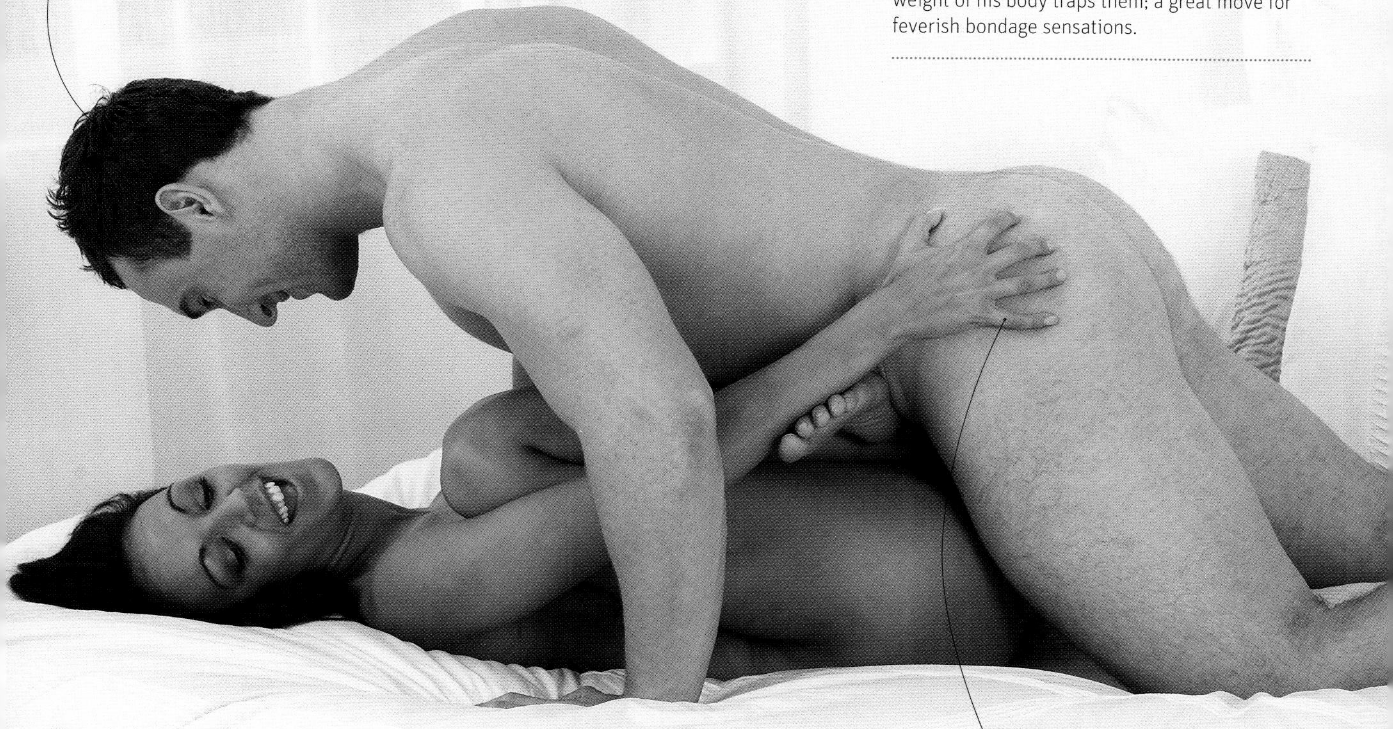

He can lean over to kiss her, stretching her hip and thigh muscles to the max.

3 Gaining entry

He lies on top of her in a push-up position and finds his way past her crossed legs to slide himself into her.

She gives him sublime sensations by pressing her fingers deep into the muscles of his buttocks.

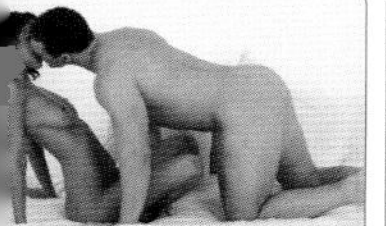
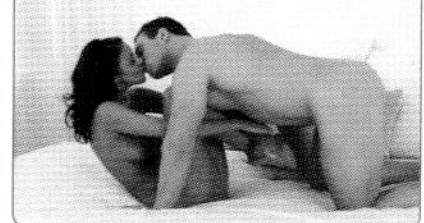
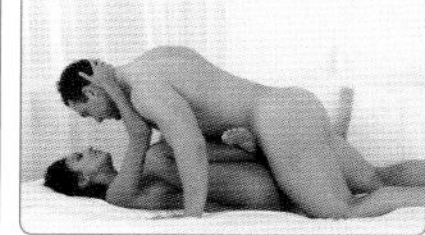
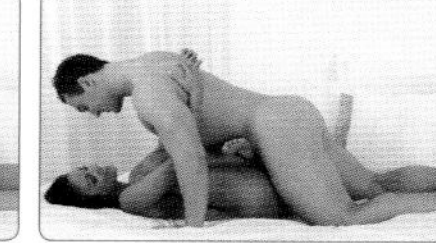
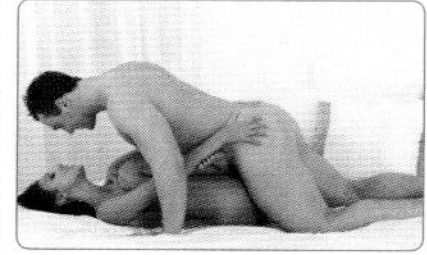

The hanging bow

Her body curves away from his at an alarming angle in this acrobatic position for flexible lovers. Before you say a nervous "No way," take a moment to consider the novelty, and the immense post-coital smugness that awaits you if you do manage to pull it off. Besides, it's guaranteed to make you the guests of honor at any sex party.

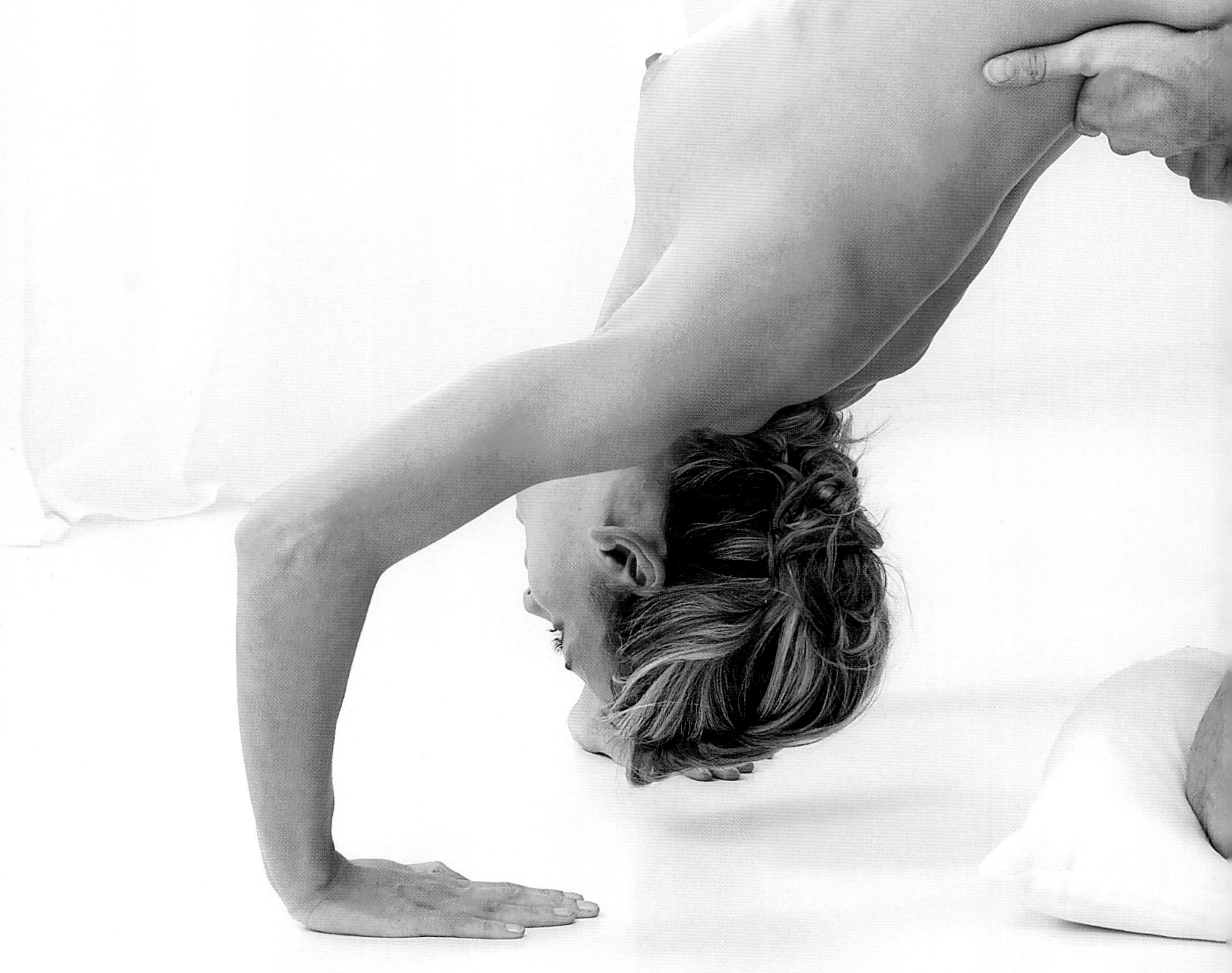

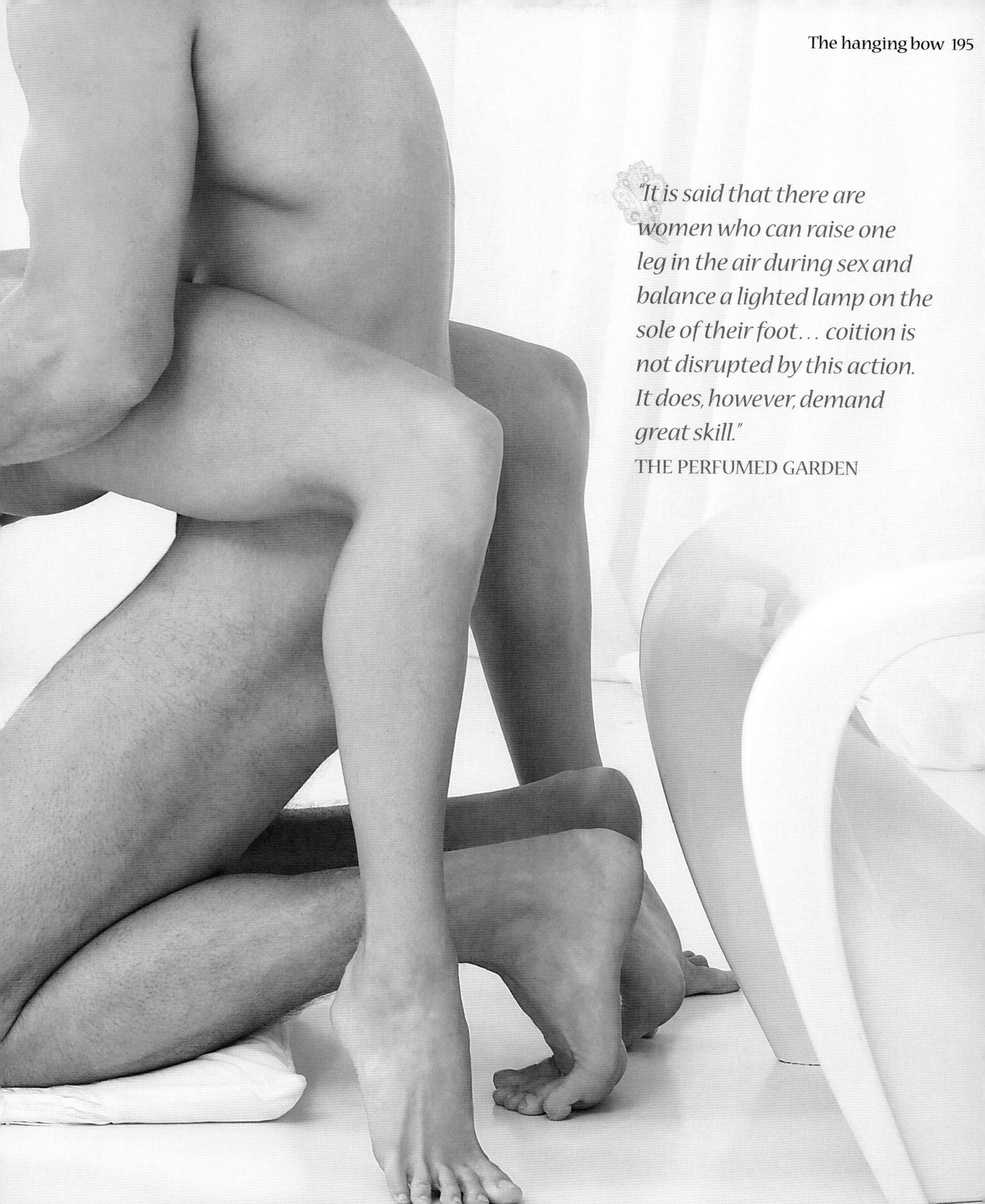

"It is said that there are women who can raise one leg in the air during sex and balance a lighted lamp on the sole of their foot... coition is not disrupted by this action. It does, however, demand great skill."

THE PERFUMED GARDEN

The hanging bow

Kama sensation rating

Why it works

– The sheer challenge teaches you high-level sexual teamwork; if you can successfully achieve The Hanging Bow, your sex life knows no bounds.

– You get an erotic buzz from the stretched athleticism of the position.

– All the blood rushes to her head, giving her an eye-popping natural high.

– Being upside-down is good for you; according to inversion devotees, it boosts circulation, relieves stress, encourages good posture, alleviates back and neck pain, reduces hair loss, and increases flexibility. Some say that daily inversion even helps you to age gracefully.

Turn on...

... Film it. Set up a video camera on a tripod or a flat surface, and capture this moment of erotic adventure. If you're worried about looking foolish, practice the moves before your shoot. And if she's worried about how she'll look upside down, a sexy corset will ensure glamor at all times.

Turn off...

... Stopping to admire your handiwork. She'll probably be able to sustain The Hanging Bow only for seconds (anything over a minute earns you sexual athlete status), so get thrusting immediately.

1 Straddle and sit

He sits on a chair, and she lowers herself down on to his lap for a kiss and slides his penis inside her.

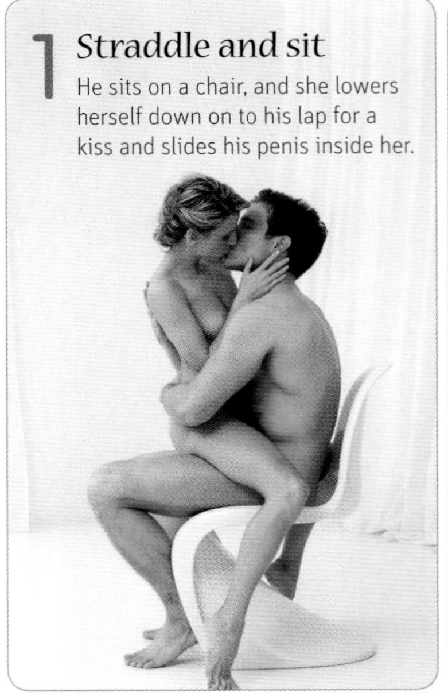

2 Leaning back

She clasps his wrists in her hands and leans back provocatively on his lap while holding his gaze.

3 Lift off

She arches her spine, letting her head fall back. He gently lowers her body down from the waist so she gets closer to the floor.

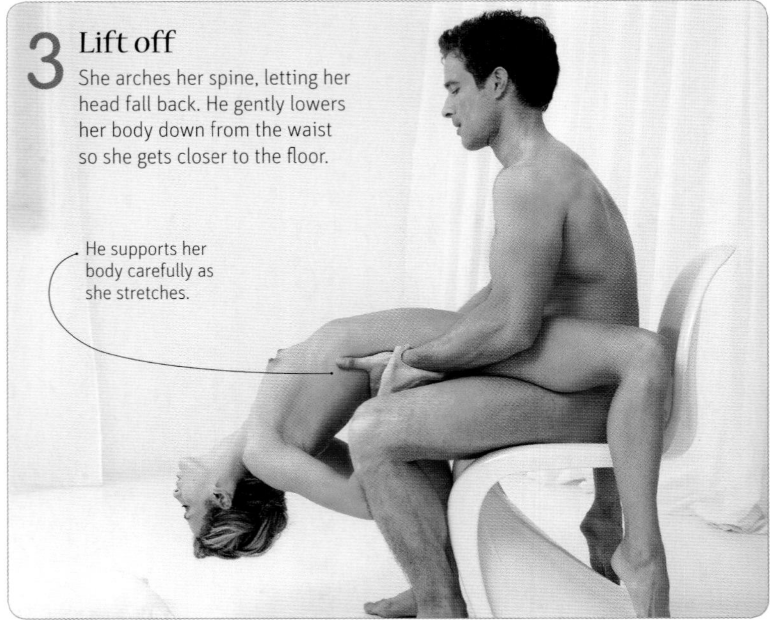

He supports her body carefully as she stretches.

"Try different ways of copulating to see which one brings you the most pleasure." THE PERFUMED GARDEN

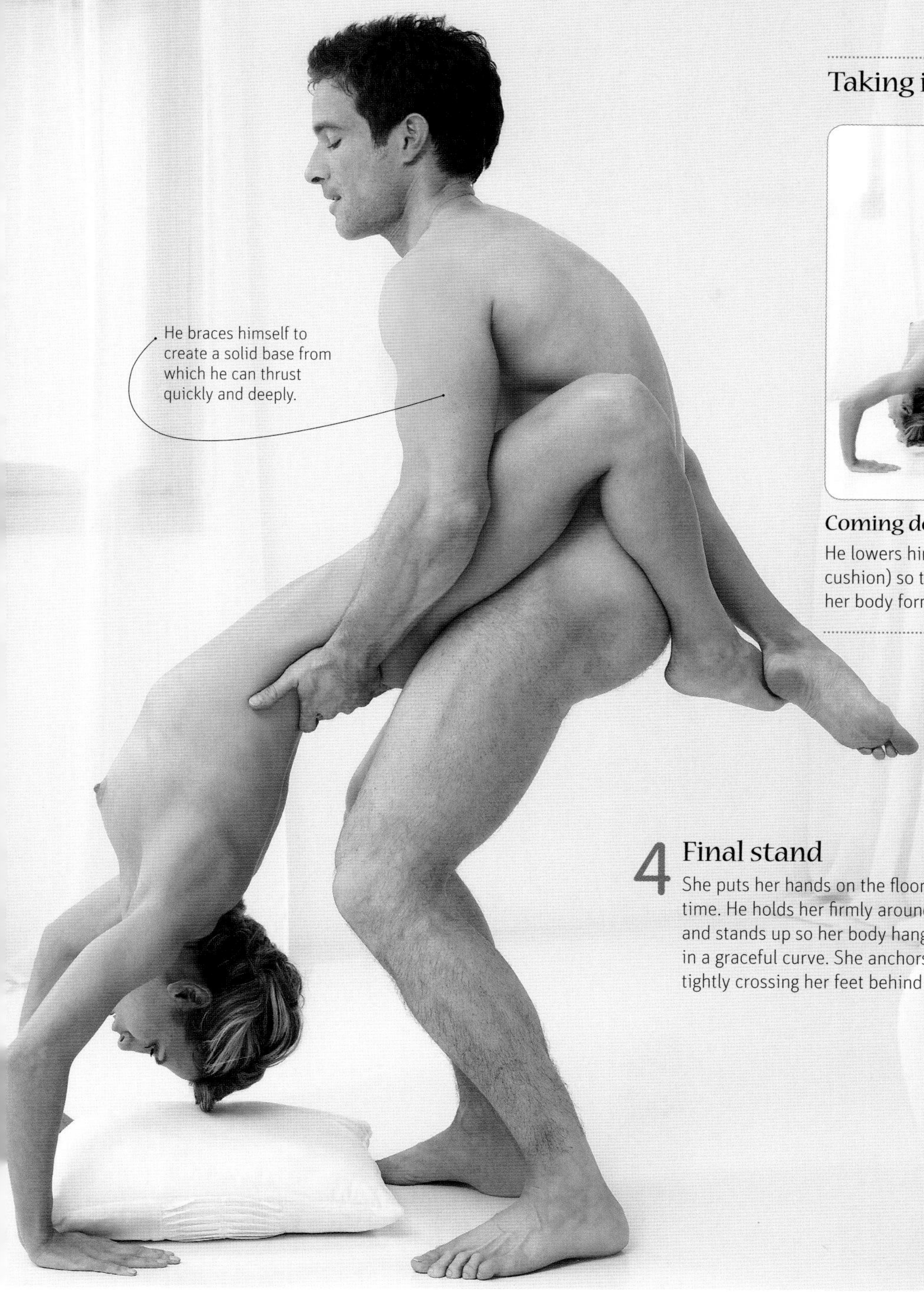

He braces himself to create a solid base from which he can thrust quickly and deeply.

Taking it further

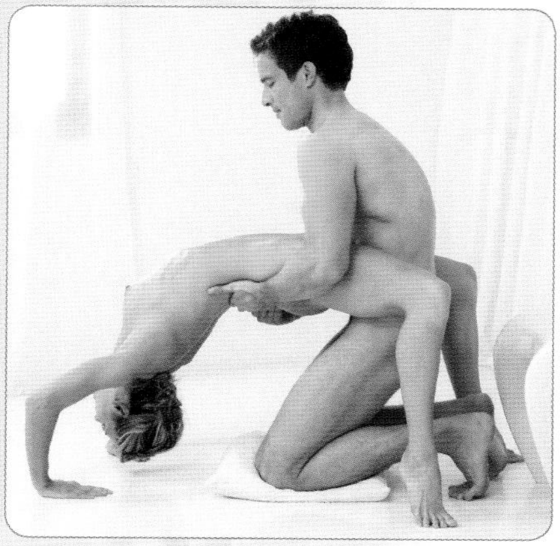

Coming down to earth

He lowers himself to the floor (or onto a handy cushion) so that he kneels between her legs and her body forms an arching bridge.

4 Final stand

She puts her hands on the floor, one at a time. He holds her firmly around the waist and stands up so her body hangs from his in a graceful curve. She anchors herself by tightly crossing her feet behind him.

If you liked this, try…

- Showing off your talents in another party piece such as Race of the Member (see page 218).
- Making an equally aesthetic curve in Drawing the Bow (see page 224).

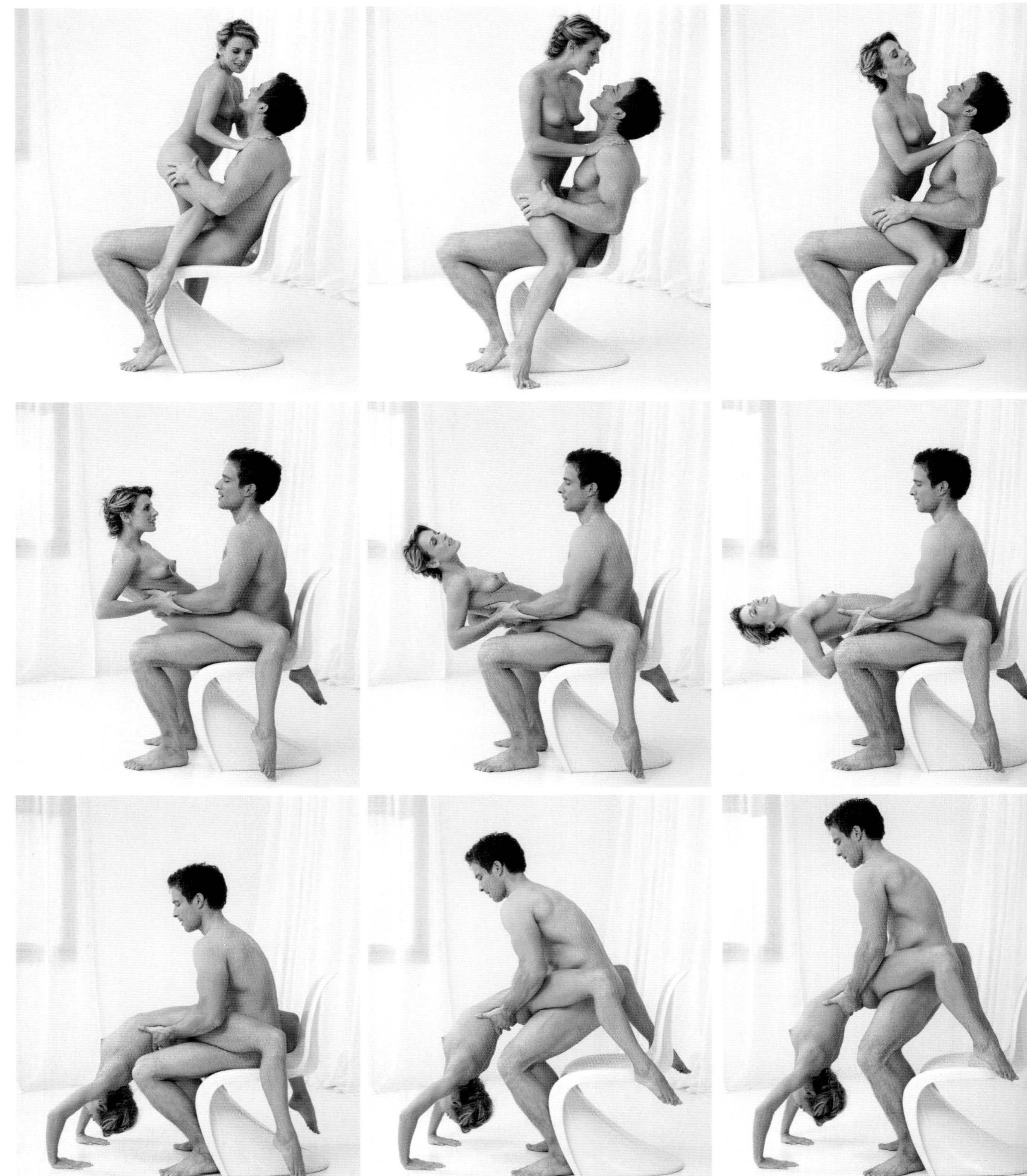

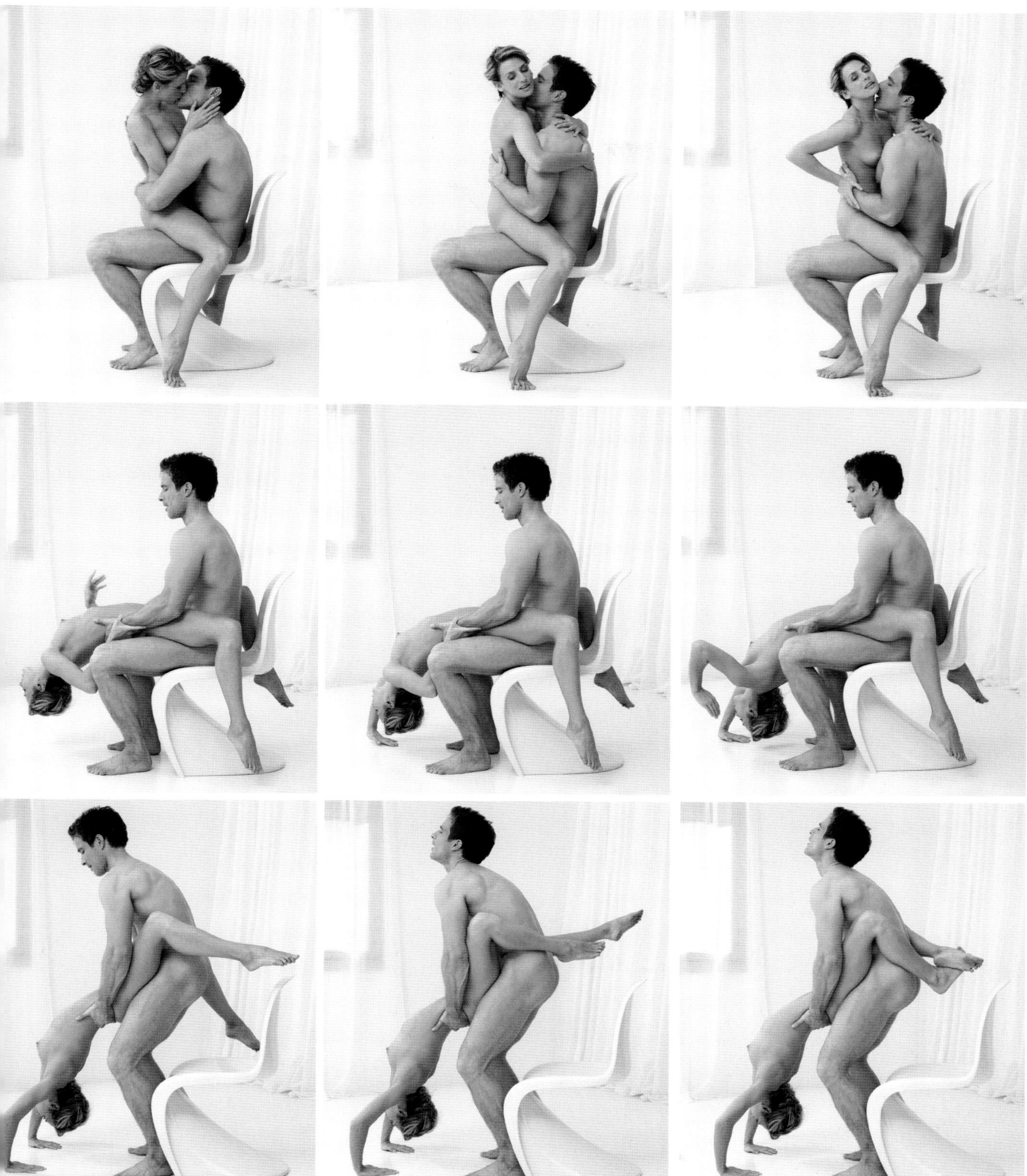

Paired feet

☆☆☆ Kama sensation rating

With its unusual angle of penetration, this is the sun lounger of sex positions: it's laid-back and custom-made for chill-out sex on a hot summer's day, preferably by the poolside. Try it while lying back and sipping a Screaming Orgasm or a Sex on the Beach.

Why it works

- She flutters and ripples her vaginal muscles to give him a swelling tide of pleasure.
- She lies back on her elbows with a come-and-get-me casualness that draws him in.
- It's great for showcasing her breasts and making him dizzy with desire.
- It's tight and compact, making it perfect for compressed lust in hammocks, sun loungers, sofas, and twin beds.
- Your movements are more flexing and wiggling than hammering and pounding. They help him to go the distance because they're subtle rather than strenuous.

Turn on...

... Choose this position if you're having sex for the third time in a row. Once you've satisfied urgent lust, you'll be in the mood for something less frenetic but equally moan-inducing.

Turn off...

... Don't sit still in this position for too long (unless you're skilled in the tantric art of near-stationary sex). Try a seesaw motion to turn up the heat.

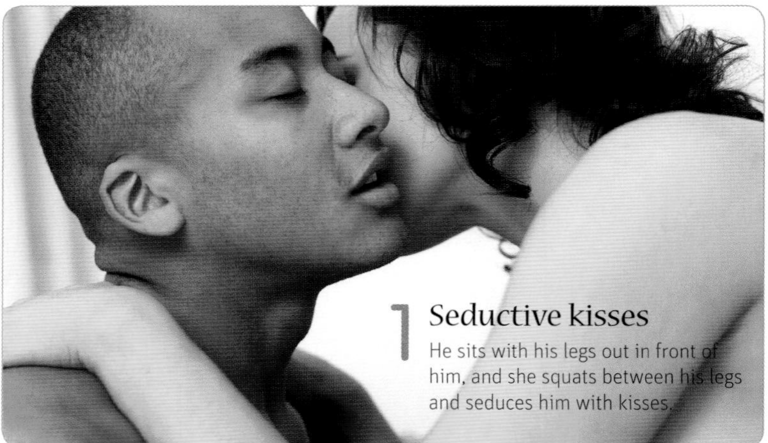

1 Seductive kisses
He sits with his legs out in front of him, and she squats between his legs and seduces him with kisses.

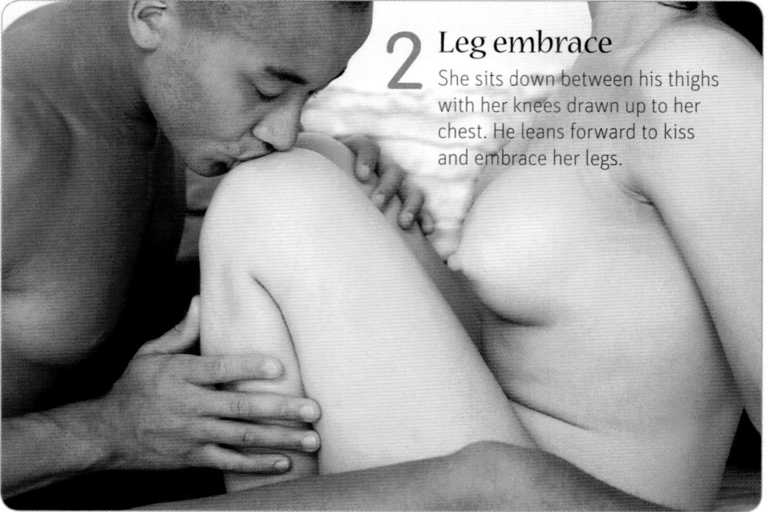

2 Leg embrace
She sits down between his thighs with her knees drawn up to her chest. He leans forward to kiss and embrace her legs.

"There are three forces of carnal desire: furious appetite, moderate desire, and slow kindling." ANANGA RANGA

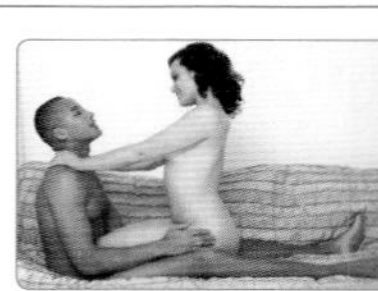

3 Elbow rest

She slides her feet over his thighs and lowers her body so that she's resting on her elbows between his feet. He shifts forward to penetrate her.

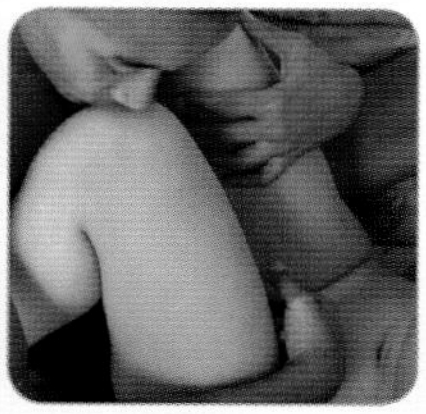

He can give her feather-light caresses along the insides of her thighs.

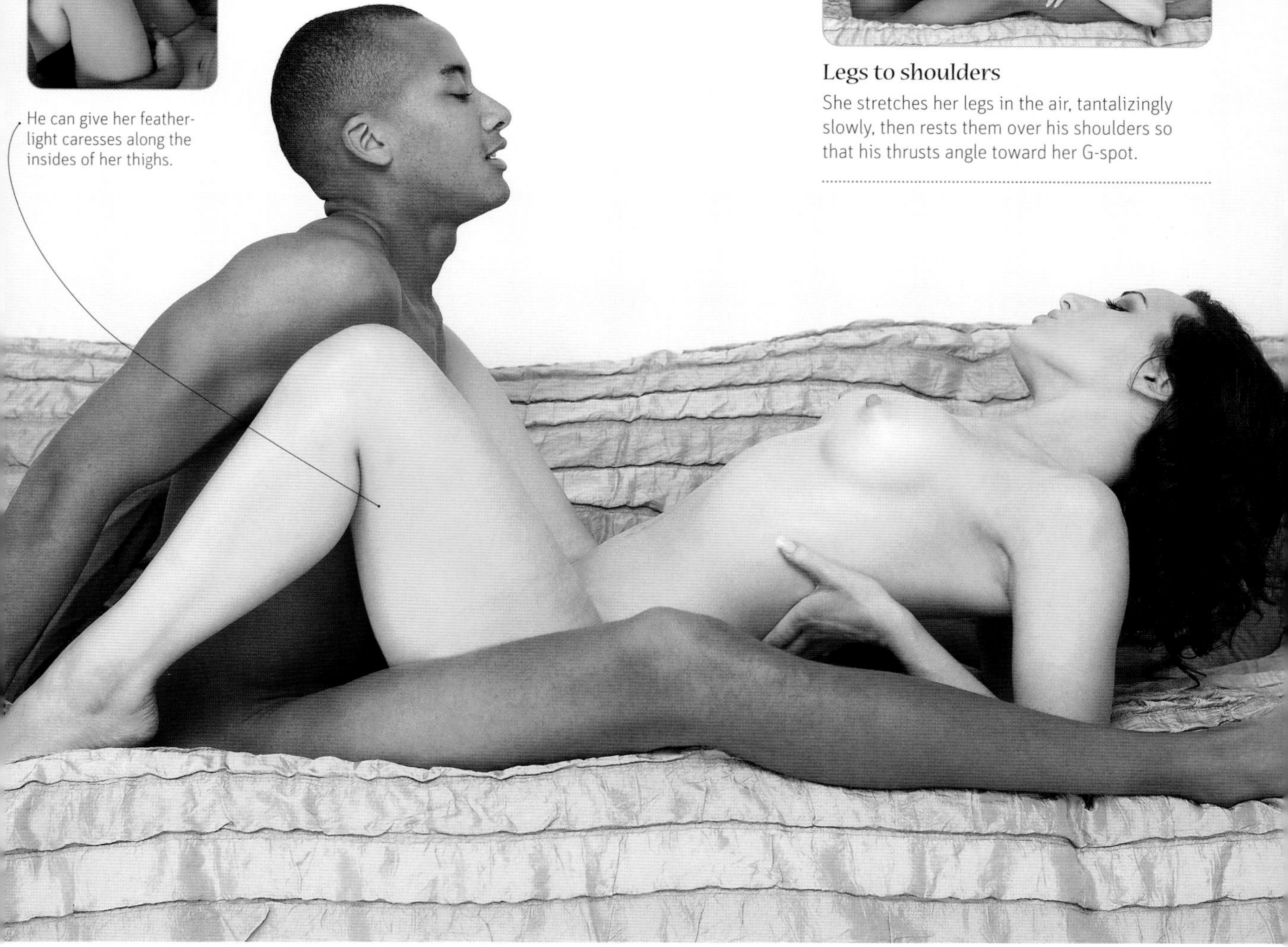

Taking it further

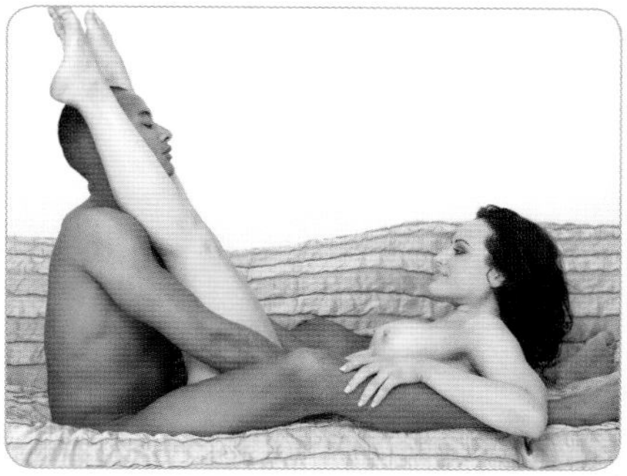

Legs to shoulders

She stretches her legs in the air, tantalizingly slowly, then rests them over his shoulders so that his thrusts angle toward her G-spot.

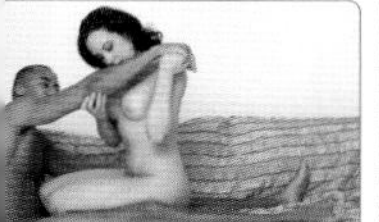
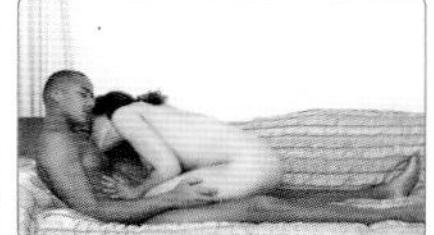
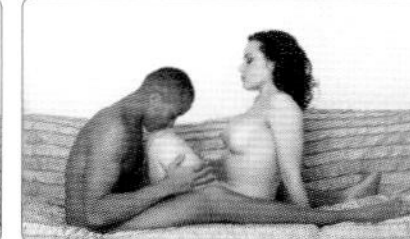
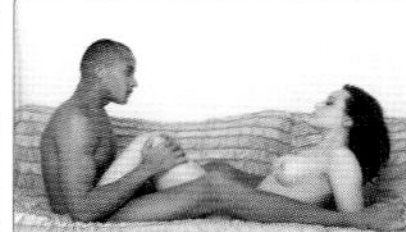
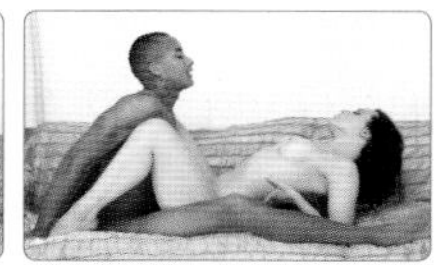

The third posture

☆☆☆☆ Kama sensation rating

It looks like she's doing a mid-air sprint, but this is actually a good position for reeling him in rather than running away from him. Do it when you want all the joy and intimacy of face-to-face lovin', but with a dash of extra slinkiness.

Why it works

– He can treat her to scintillatingly slow strokes, or he can do a sudden slam for erotic shock value.

– You're locked in erotic battle. He pushes against her thigh in an attempt to get closer. She holds firm with her leg braced against his chest. Luckily, because it feels so hot and steamy, you're both winners.

– She can tailor it to her personal flexibility rating; her leg may be anything from slightly raised to touching her chin.

– If he's a leg lover, the slinky feel of her thigh will speed him toward the finishing line.

Turn on...

... Do it to music. Choose a track that's either fast and upbeat, or slow and mellow, depending on the love mood you're in, and synchronize to the rhythm.

Turn off...

... Neglecting romantic touches. Even if you're going at it hammer and tongs, there's no rule to say you can't stop to trace the outline of her lips with your fingers or cup his face in your hands.

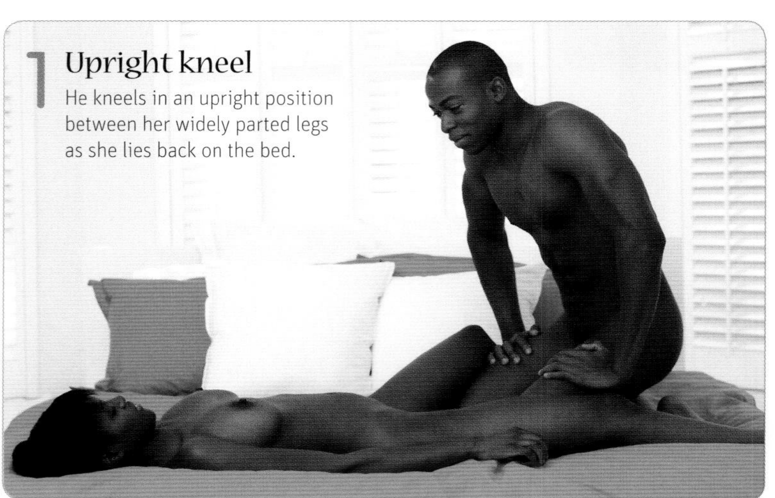

1 Upright kneel
He kneels in an upright position between her widely parted legs as she lies back on the bed.

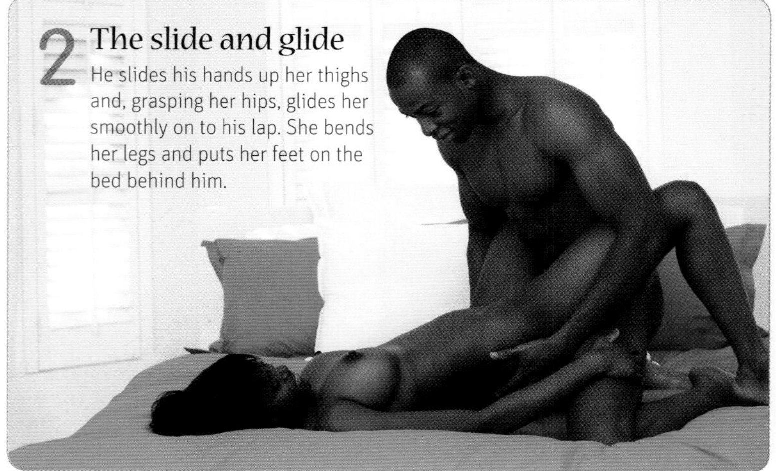

2 The slide and glide
He slides his hands up her thighs and, grasping her hips, glides her smoothly on to his lap. She bends her legs and puts her feet on the bed behind him.

"Lay the woman on the ground... put one of her legs on your shoulder and the other under your arm—then enter her." THE PERFUMED GARDEN

3 Opening up

She opens herself up to him by raising one of her legs and hooking it over his shoulder.

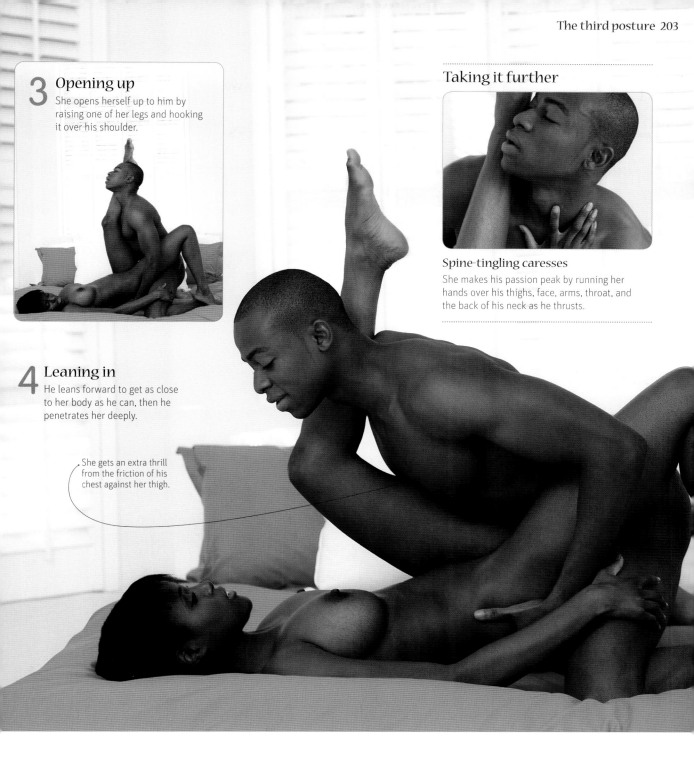

Taking it further

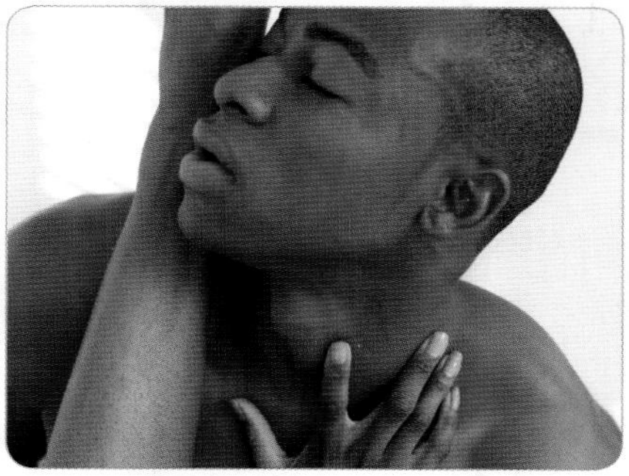

Spine-tingling caresses

She makes his passion peak by running her hands over his thighs, face, arms, throat, and the back of his neck as he thrusts.

4 Leaning in

He leans forward to get as close to her body as he can, then he penetrates her deeply.

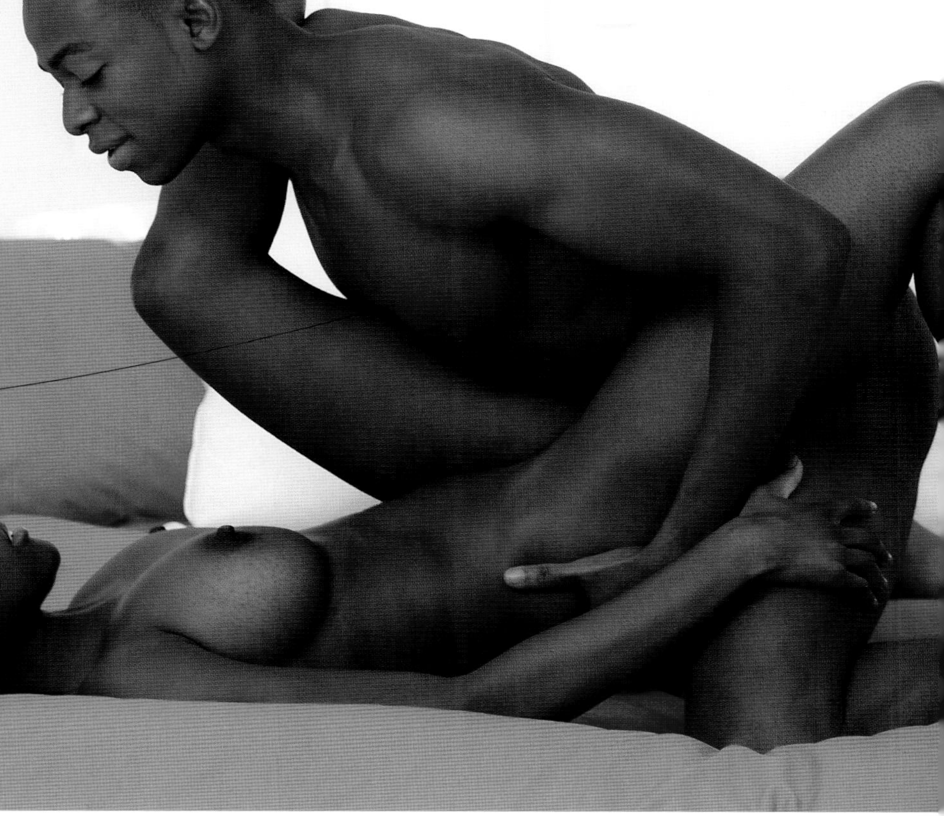

She gets an extra thrill from the friction of his chest against her thigh.

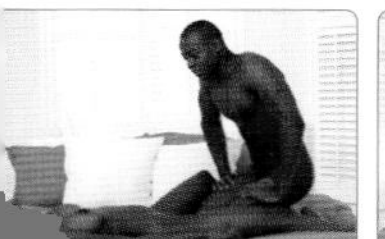
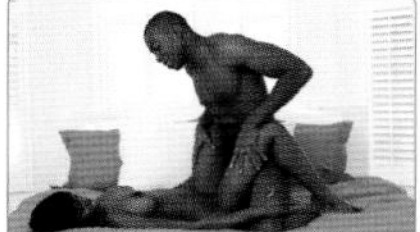
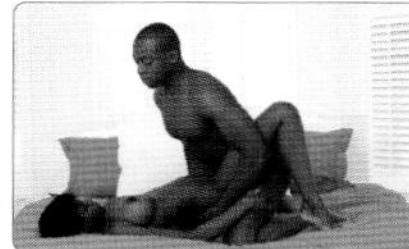
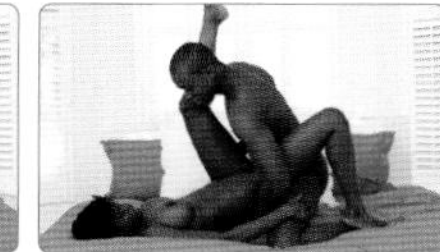
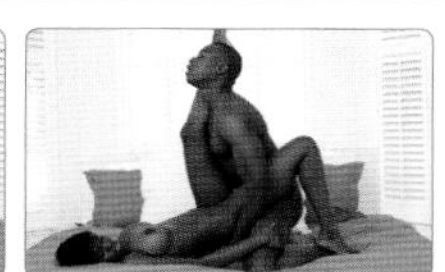
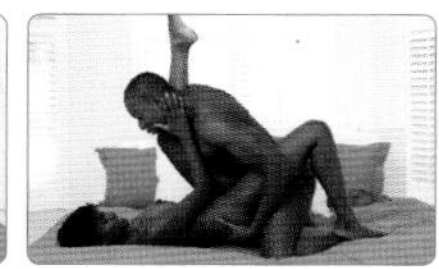

The wife of Indra

☆☆☆☆ Kama sensation rating

He kneels reverentially before her as she offers herself up in a provocative half shoulder stand. Accept her offer by grabbing her hips and plunging in. Try this position after intense foreplay, when you're both at the peak of arousal and ready for some incredible sensations.

Why it works

– Her vagina is shortened, which makes sex feel super-intense for both of you, and is an asset if he's a hare and she's an elephant (read pages 128–9 and you'll understand).

– Her half shoulder stand is one of those reveal-all poses that will make him cross-eyed with desire.

– Her feet against his chest give her powerful leverage if she wants to control the motion.

– His penis is close to her butt; if you want anal sex to feature on your sexual menu, he doesn't have to travel far. (For hygiene's sake, never follow anal sex with vaginal sex).

Turn on...

... Get her to hold her knees with her hands and pull them as close to her chest as possible; this will contract her vagina even further.

Turn off...

... Don't attempt this position before she's aroused and wet. Because her vagina is contracted, the friction of his penis will feel uncomfortable if she's not ready. A dollop of lube can smooth things out.

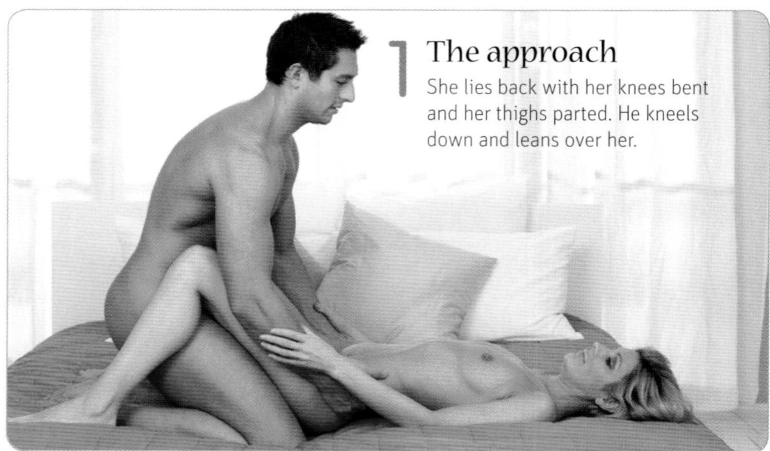

1 The approach
She lies back with her knees bent and her thighs parted. He kneels down and leans over her.

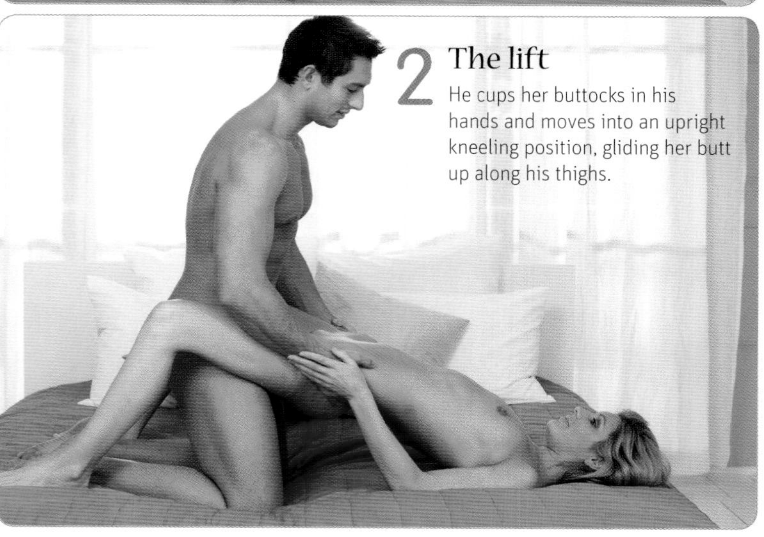

2 The lift
He cups her buttocks in his hands and moves into an upright kneeling position, gliding her butt up along his thighs.

"This position is useful in the case of the highest congress."

KAMA SUTRA

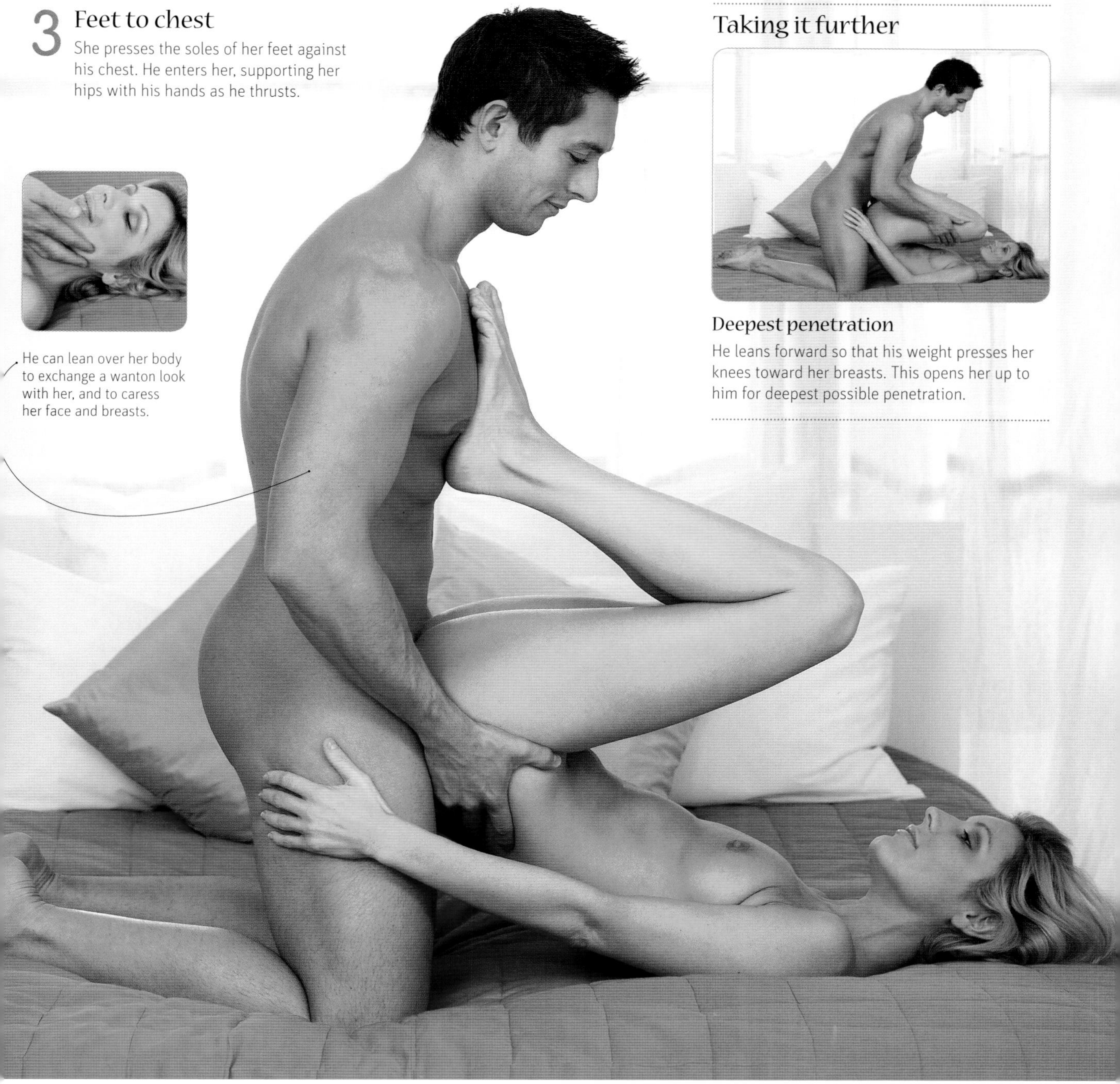

3 Feet to chest

She presses the soles of her feet against his chest. He enters her, supporting her hips with his hands as he thrusts.

He can lean over her body to exchange a wanton look with her, and to caress her face and breasts.

Taking it further

Deepest penetration

He leans forward so that his weight presses her knees toward her breasts. This opens her up to him for deepest possible penetration.

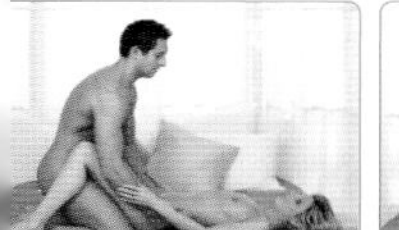
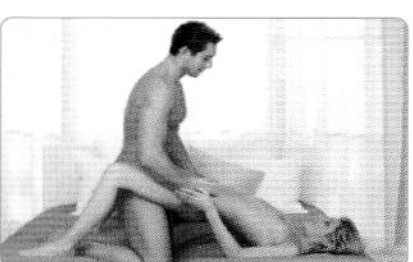
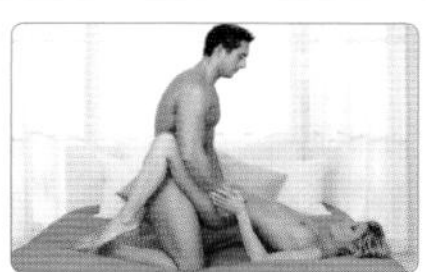
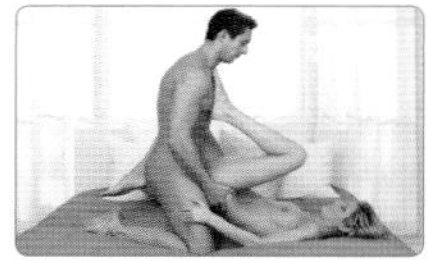
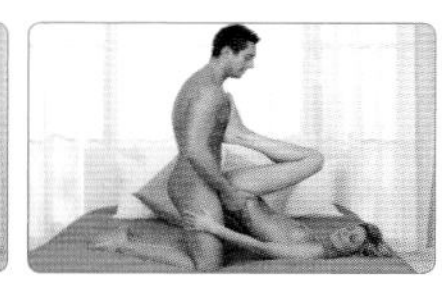

Crying out

☆☆☆ Kama sensation rating

It looks as easy as sitting down and having a kiss, but it's actually one of the most difficult sex positions of the East. The sitting-down smooch is the simple bit—the challenge is for him to pick her up and swing her from side to side on his shaft.

Why it works

- The pendulum-like movements on his penis will potentially send him into orbit.
- The unusual plane of motion puts satisfying pressure on the side walls of her vagina.
- It shamelessly indulges all your me-Tarzan, you-Jane fantasies.
- She loves being at the mercy of his lust.
- If you can't manage the side-to-side swing, you can melt into blissful eye-gazing, hold-each-other-tight sex.
- You're just a couple of easy movements away from cowgirl position, if you need it.

Turn on...

... Try it while sitting in a jacuzzi. Not only does it feel wickedly decadent, but it's also easier to get the sexy side-to-side motion going.

Turn off...

... Don't add this one to your repertoire if she's physically bigger than him, wears the pants in the relationship, doesn't like being manhandled or picked up, or wants an easy orgasm.

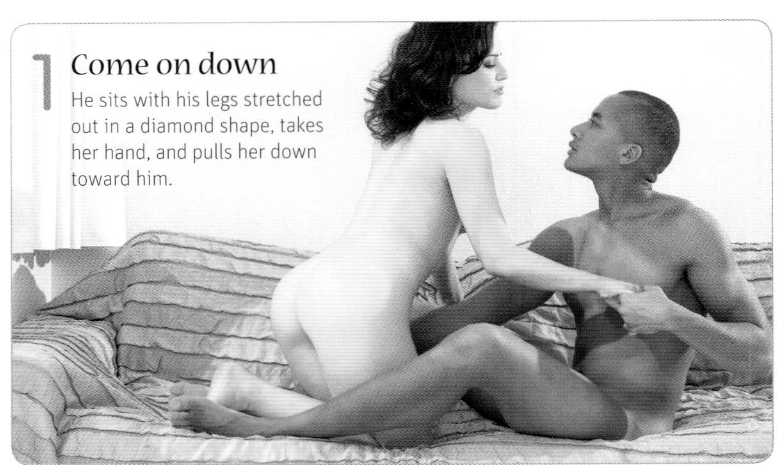

1 Come on down
He sits with his legs stretched out in a diamond shape, takes her hand, and pulls her down toward him.

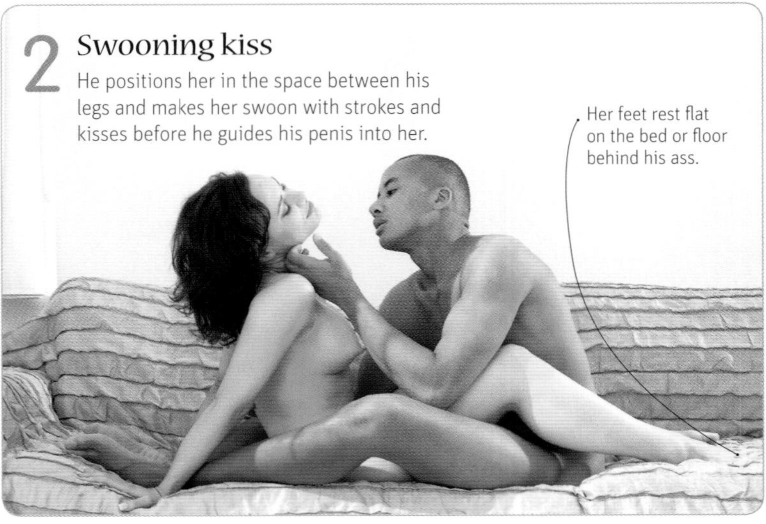

2 Swooning kiss
He positions her in the space between his legs and makes her swoon with strokes and kisses before he guides his penis into her.

Her feet rest flat on the bed or floor behind his ass.

"He raises her by passing both her legs over his arms at the elbow, and moves her about from left to right... until the supreme moment arrives." ANANGA RANGA

3 The pick-up

In a quick dominant gesture, he hooks his arms under her knees, holds her body firmly, picks her up, and moves her from side to side.

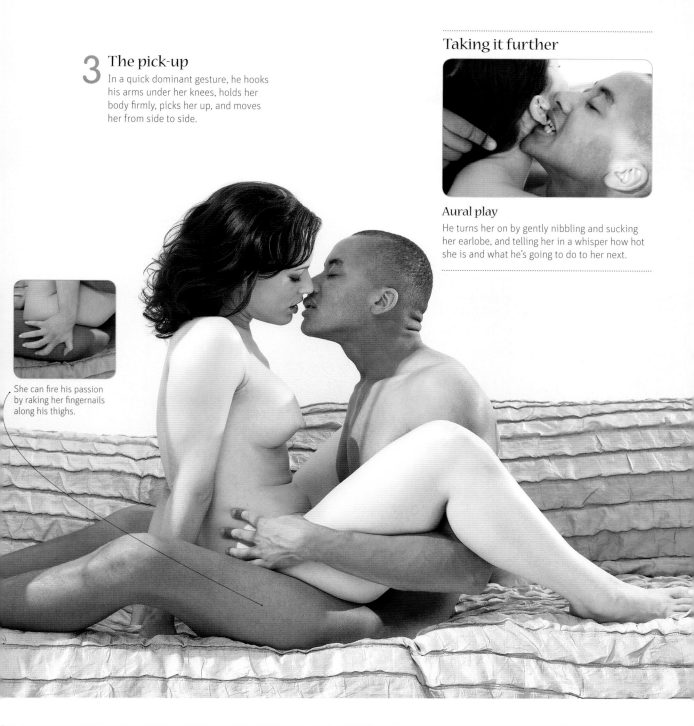

She can fire his passion by raking her fingernails along his thighs.

Taking it further

Aural play

He turns her on by gently nibbling and sucking her earlobe, and telling her in a whisper how hot she is and what he's going to do to her next.

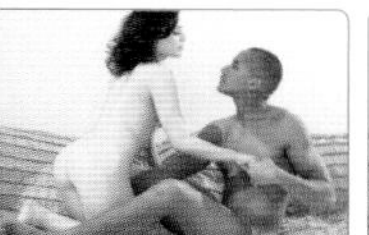
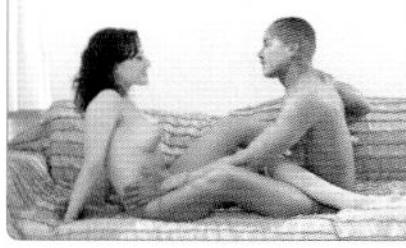
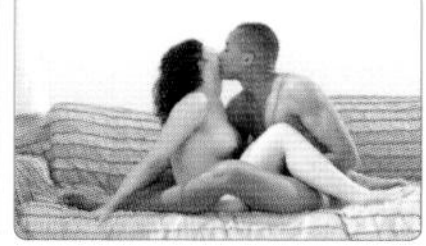
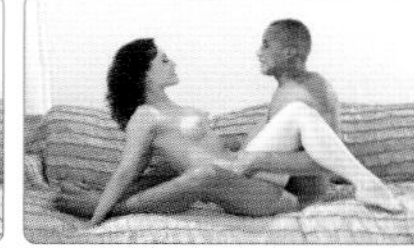
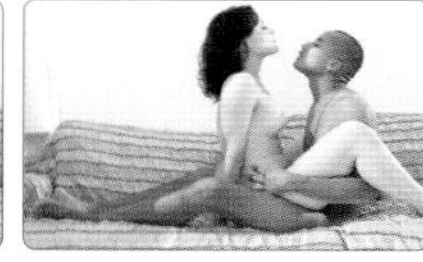
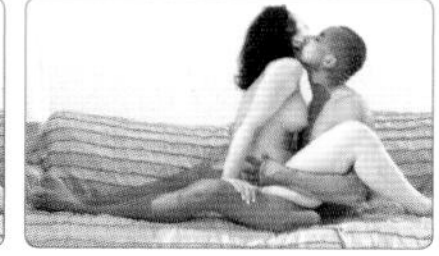

Congress of the cow

☆☆☆☆ Kama sensation rating

Made for indecent amounts of lust and lechery, this position is ideal as part of a teasing role play. She bends over to "pick something up," he sidles up behind her and, oops, before you know it, her skirt's around her waist and his pants are hugging his ankles.

Why it works

– The deep rush when he first penetrates will make you both gasp with pleasure.

– Anal sex is an option; it feels sinfully wicked in this position.

– You're left to focus on your own pleasure because you're not face-to-face, which is a definite plus if you usually devote all your attention to your lover's needs.

– He can treat her to a hot back rub that includes surprise visits to her perineum, plus some hanky-panky buttock spanking.

– If she hasn't yet discovered her G-spot, now's a great opportunity.

Turn on...

... Make this position triple X-rated by giving her oral sex beforehand. Ask her to bend over with her hands on her knees, then kneel behind her and press your face and tongue against her hot spots.

Turn off...

... Your thigh muscles may feel overstretched when you bend over. If so, walk your hands forward until they're as far away from your feet as possible.

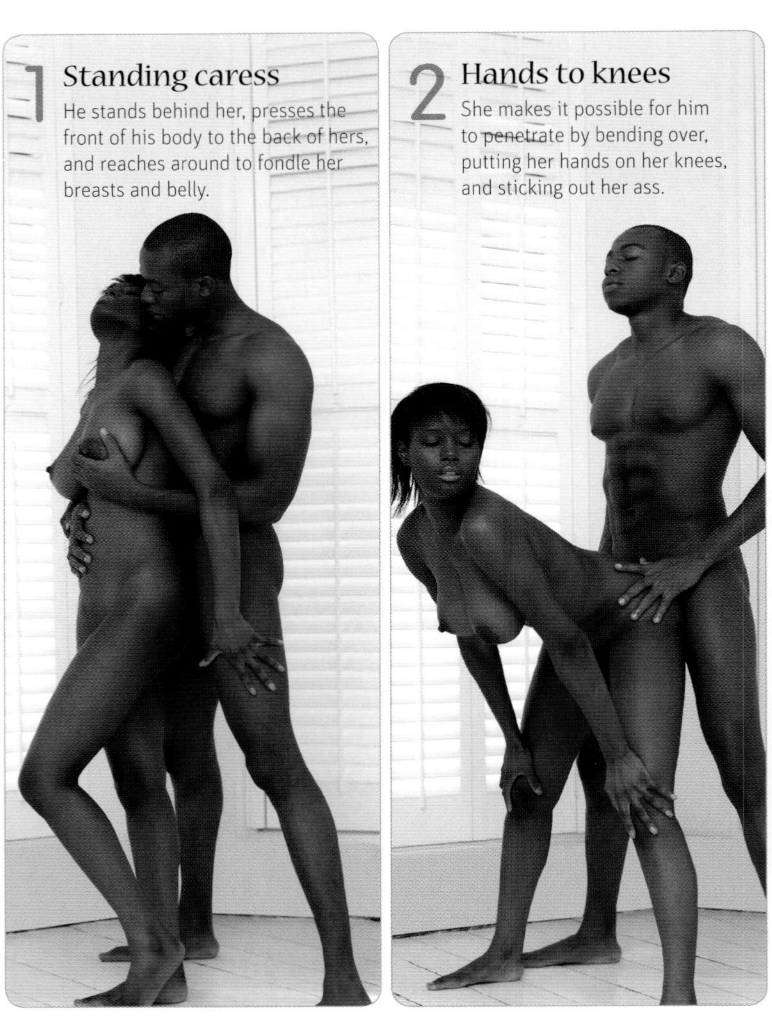

1 Standing caress
He stands behind her, presses the front of his body to the back of hers, and reaches around to fondle her breasts and belly.

2 Hands to knees
She makes it possible for him to penetrate by bending over, putting her hands on her knees, and sticking out her ass.

"At the time of Congress of a Cow, the acts that are normally done on the bosom should be done on the back." KAMA SUTRA

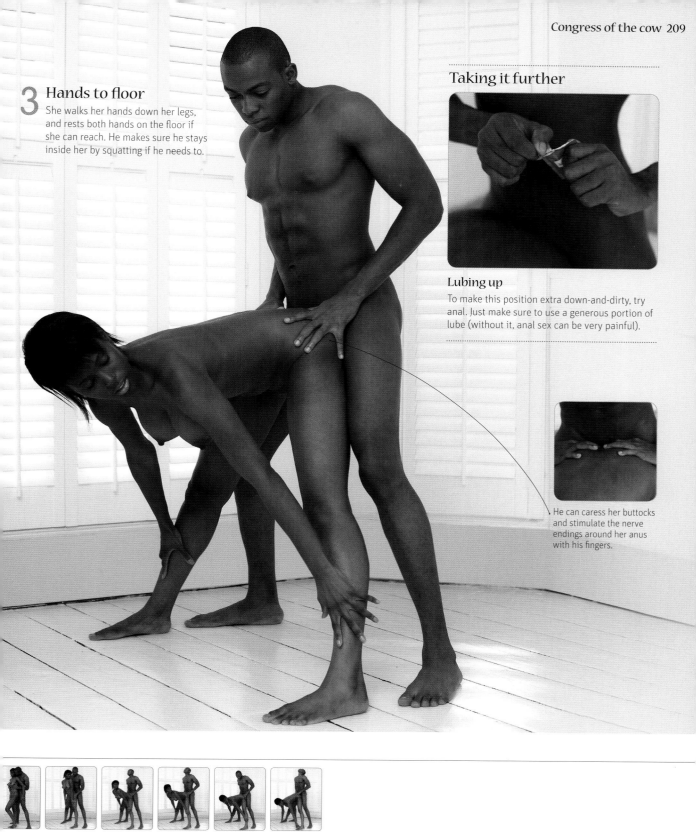

3 Hands to floor

She walks her hands down her legs, and rests both hands on the floor if she can reach. He makes sure he stays inside her by squatting if he needs to.

Taking it further

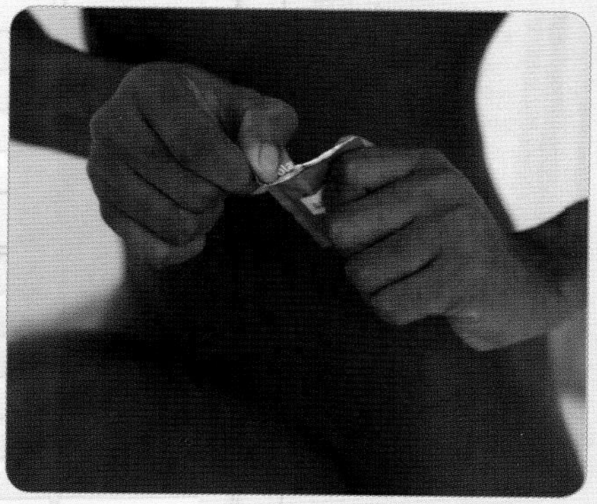

Lubing up

To make this position extra down-and-dirty, try anal. Just make sure to use a generous portion of lube (without it, anal sex can be very painful).

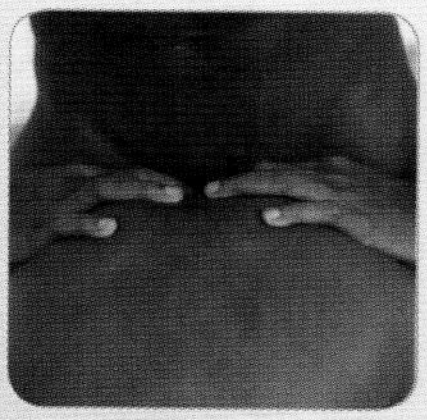

He can caress her buttocks and stimulate the nerve endings around her anus with his fingers.

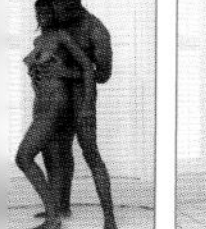
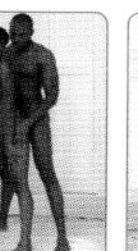
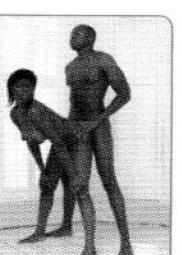
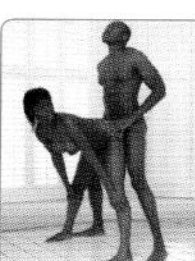
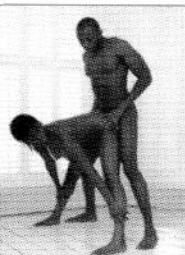
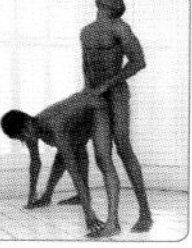

The fitter in

It's the epitome of Eastern eroticism: slow, sensual, elegant, artistic, and spiritual. Rather than worrying about when, where, or how your orgasm is coming, just submit to the mystical mood. Gaze into each other's eyes, concentrate on the glorious sensuality of skin-on-skin contact, and feel that sexual energy racing up through your chakras.

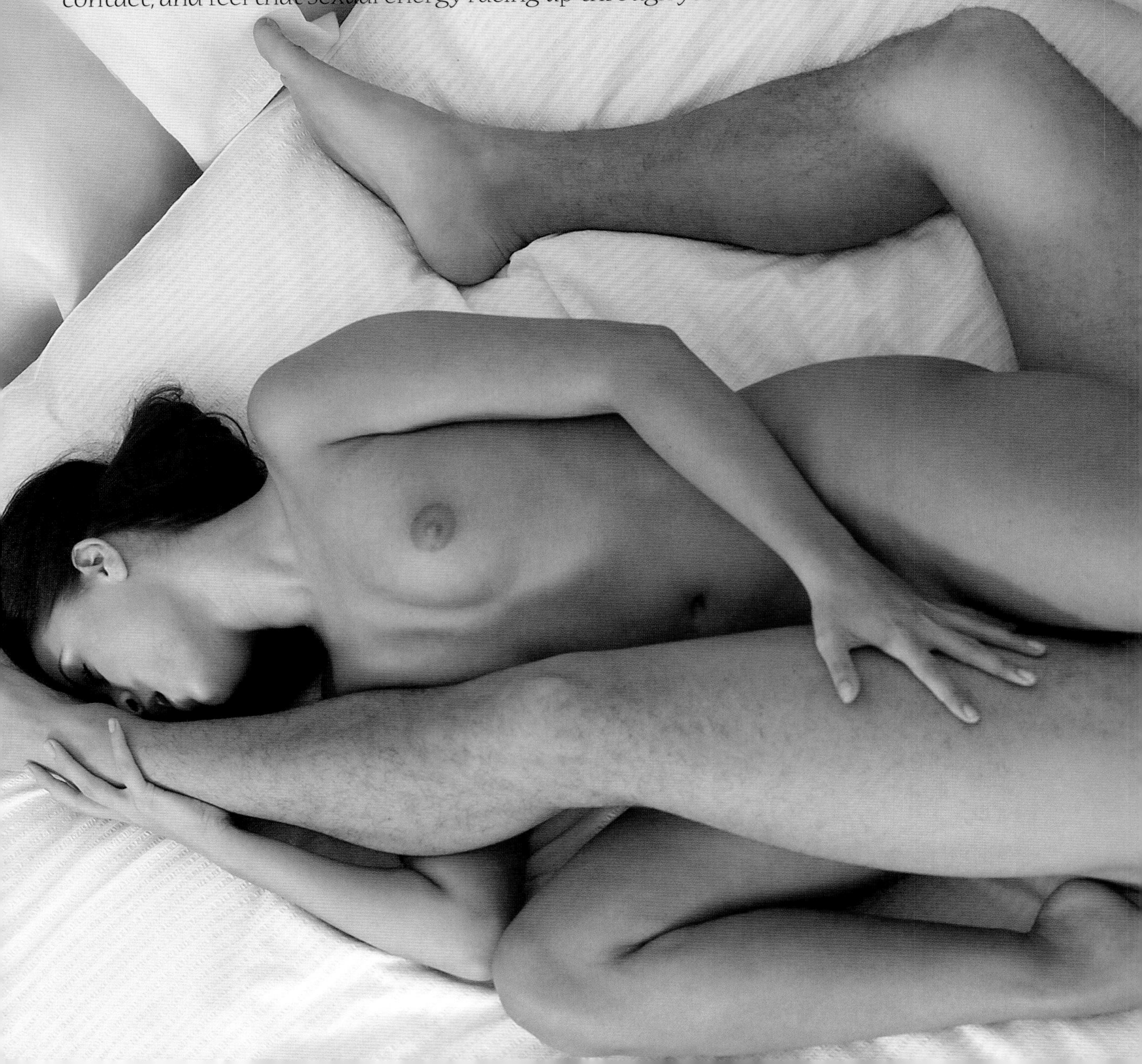

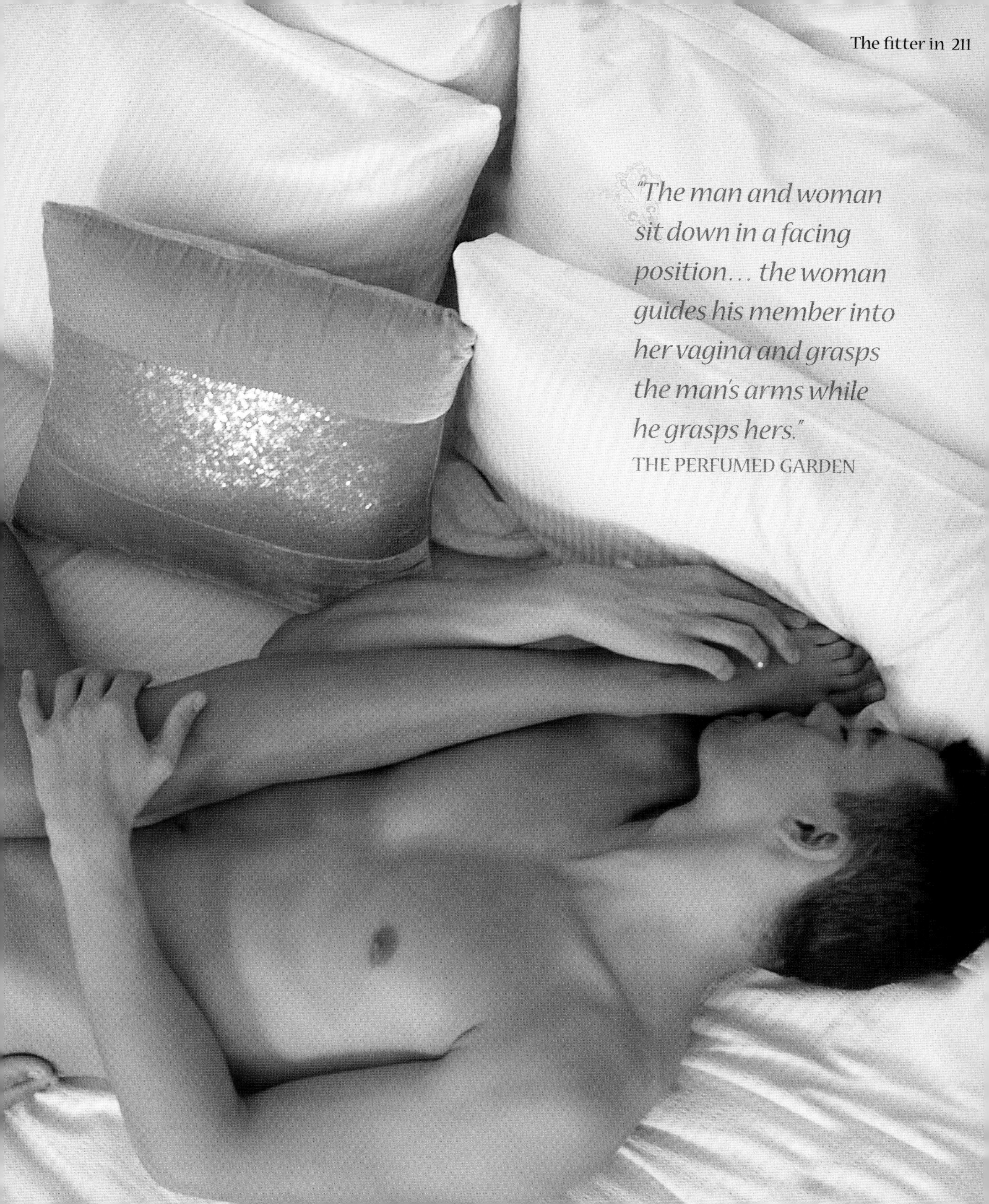

"The man and woman sit down in a facing position… the woman guides his member into her vagina and grasps the man's arms while he grasps hers."
THE PERFUMED GARDEN

The fitter in

☆☆☆☆☆

Kama sensation rating

Why it works

– Neither of you is in charge, which makes for great equal-opportunity sex and erotic cooperation.

– You have to rock against each other in a seesaw motion, which breaks the pattern of in–out thrusting which you're probably accustomed to (or even dependent on). Suddenly, sex takes on a new sensual and subtle dimension.

– When you're having a peak sex moment, enhance it by leaning so close that your lips are just a hair's breadth apart. Now all you have to do is exhale simultaneously and let your breath mingle… exquisite.

– Once penetration has been achieved, there are lots of variations, build-ups, modifications, escape routes, and get-out clauses. Take your pick, or just move with the moment.

Turn on…

… Rely on tried-and-trusted arousal boosters to turbocharge your lust. Try sucking each other's fingers, talking dirty, and moaning wantonly.

Turn off…

… Trying to figure out whose thigh should go on top of whose. If you can achieve penetration at all amidst the tangle of legs, you're doing well.

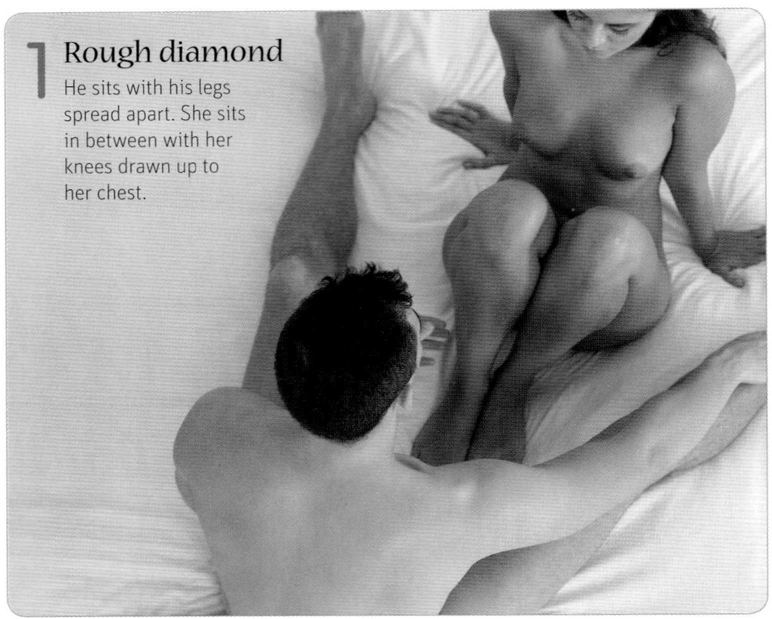

1 Rough diamond

He sits with his legs spread apart. She sits in between with her knees drawn up to her chest.

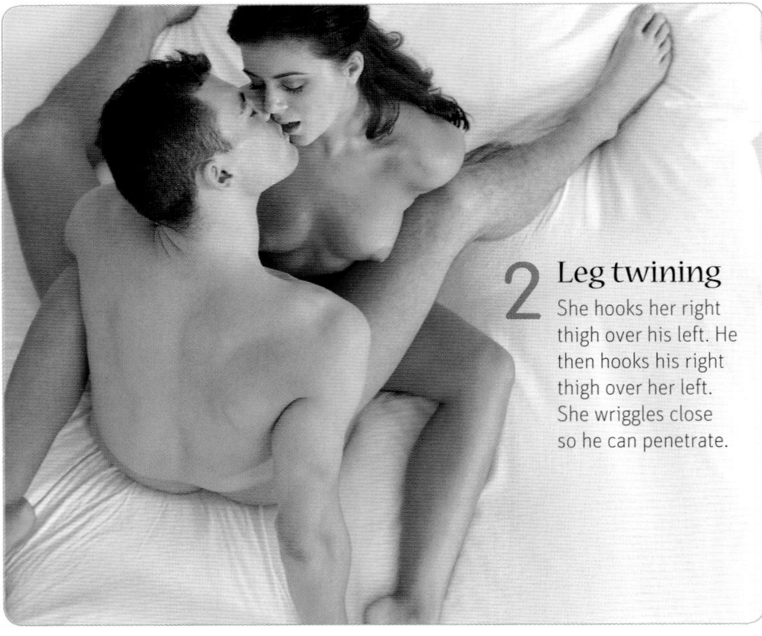

2 Leg twining

She hooks her right thigh over his left. He then hooks his right thigh over her left. She wriggles close so he can penetrate.

"They indulge in a seesaw motion, taking turns to lean backward and forward, ensuring that their movements are coordinated." THE PERFUMED GARDEN

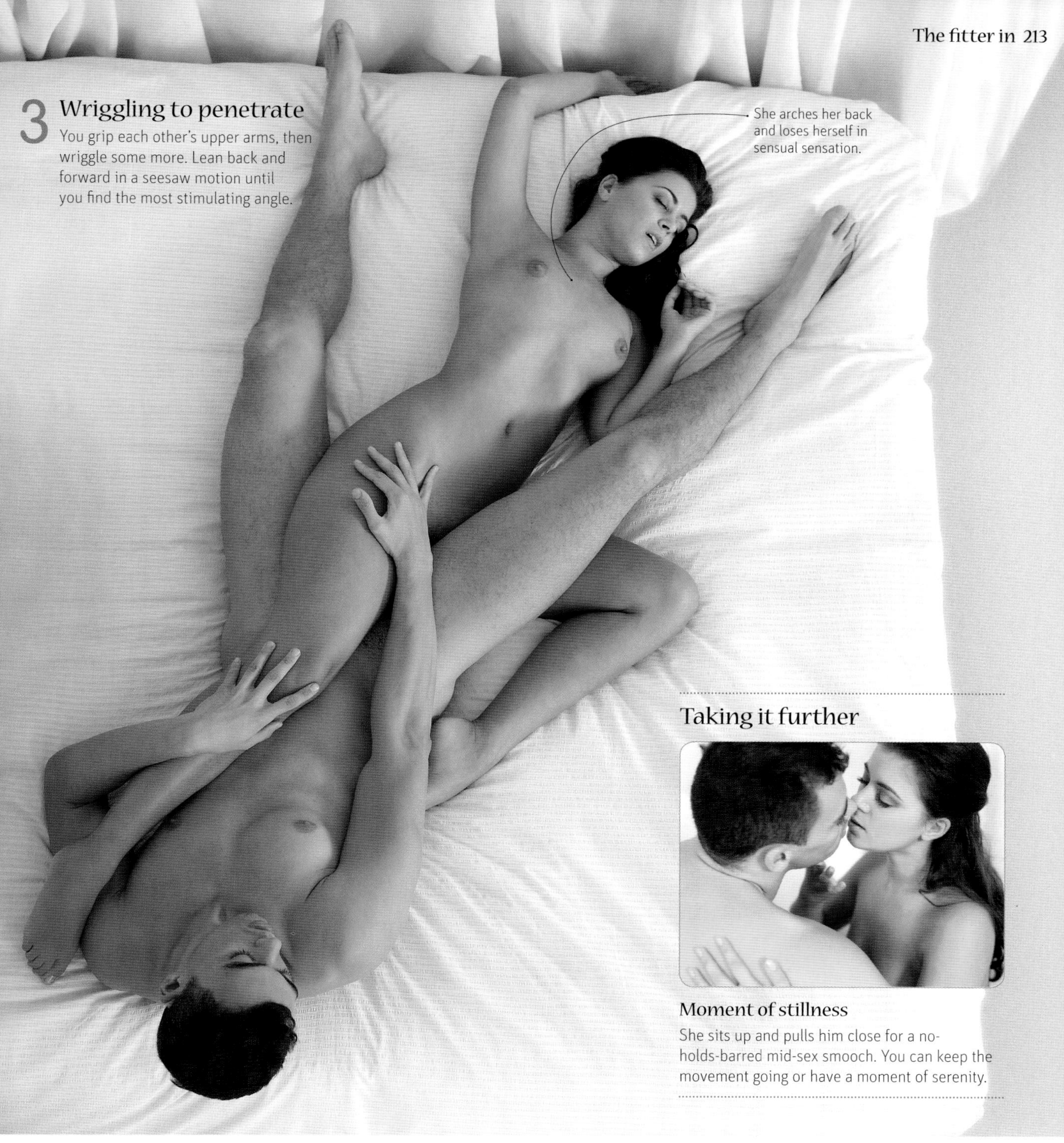

3 Wriggling to penetrate

You grip each other's upper arms, then wriggle some more. Lean back and forward in a seesaw motion until you find the most stimulating angle.

She arches her back and loses herself in sensual sensation.

Taking it further

Moment of stillness

She sits up and pulls him close for a no-holds-barred mid-sex smooch. You can keep the movement going or have a moment of serenity.

If you liked this, try…

- The equally dignified Alternate Movement of Piercing (see page 118).
- Heating things up by slipping into the Pressed Position (see page 150).

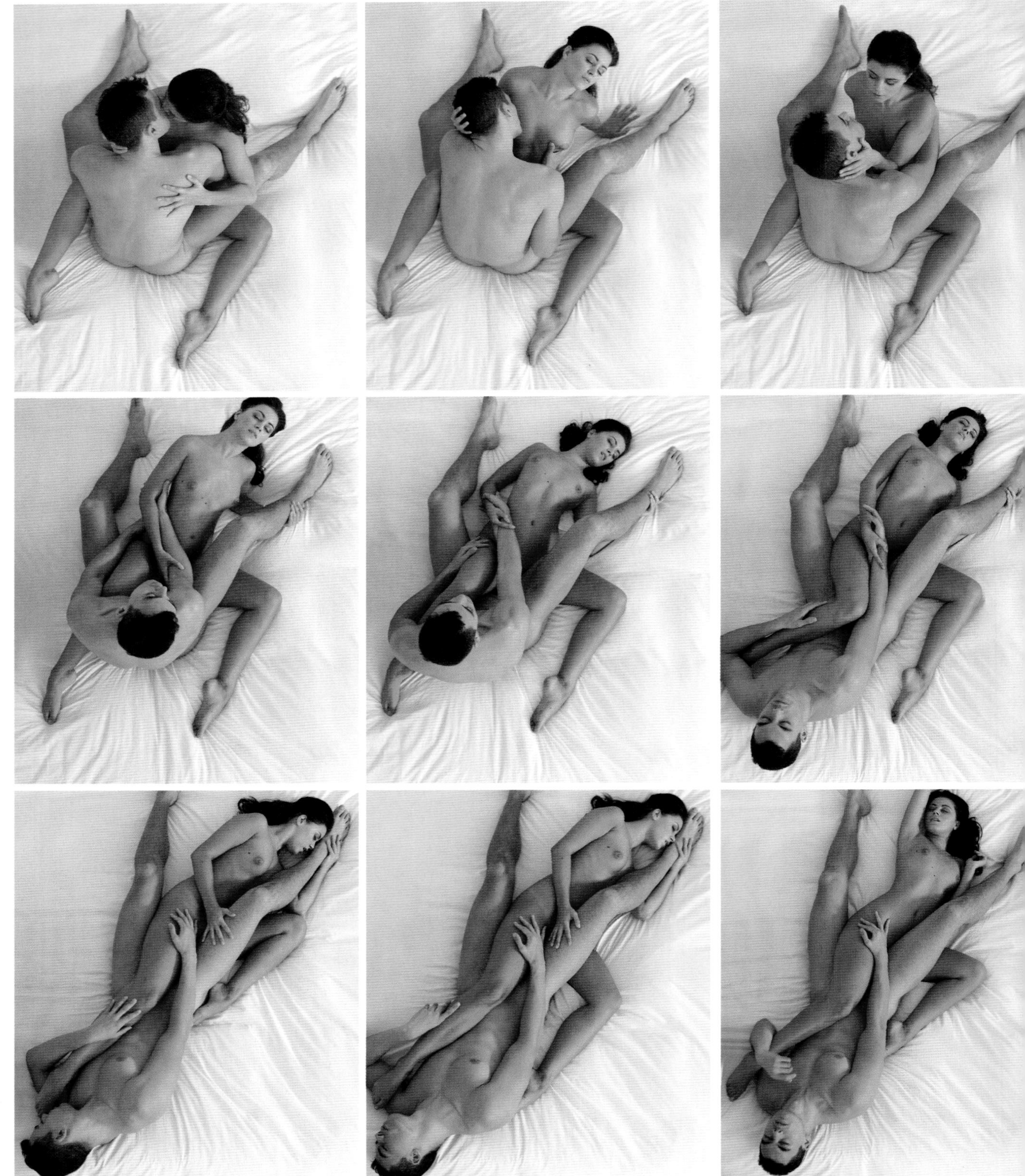

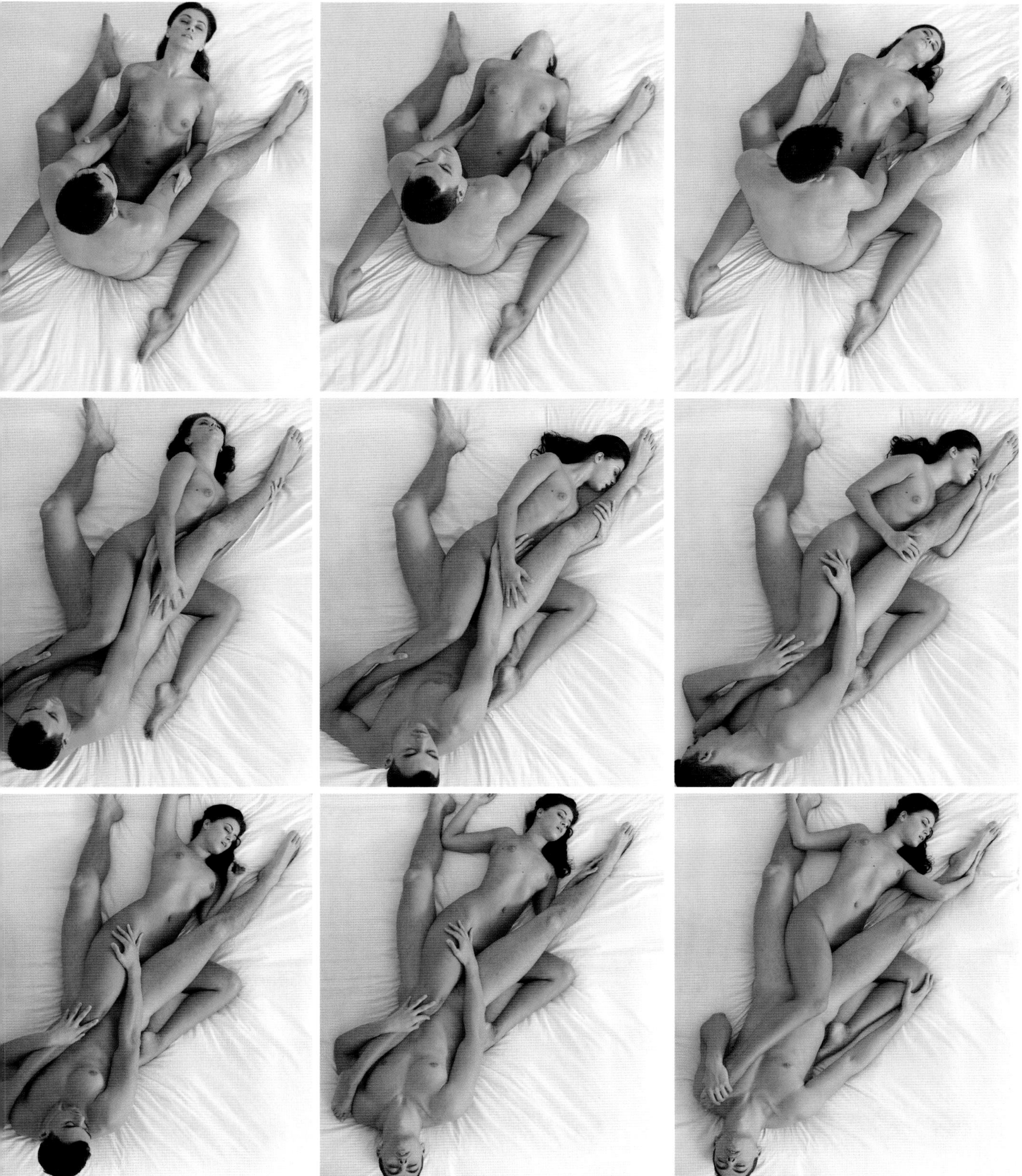

The seventh and The eighth postures

☆☆☆ Kama sensation rating

Put some champagne on ice before you try these two elegant positions. She starts on her side with one foot pointing ballet-style to the ceiling. Getting her legs into a position where he can actually penetrate can be a tall order; you may welcome that postcoital drink.

Why they work

– He can swirl and grind his hips using her raised leg as a handy support pole.

– If she can hold the on-her-side scissors position, you'll have a dramatic new angle of entry under your belt.

– With her legs knotted under her in The Eighth Posture she's all his for the taking, fulfilling his carnal cravings for dominance.

– You can snatch some quick playtime in the missionary position between The Seventh and Eighth Postures, which is perfect for some speed-thrusting that'll keep the lead in his pencil.

Turn on...

... Grab a stack of pillows to push under her ass when she's in The Eighth Posture. Raising her pelvis will be your best shot at deep penetration.

Turn off...

... Don't choose these two positions if you're looking for a wild romp in the sack. Your bits don't slot effortlessly together, so it can be difficult to feel consumed by wild passion.

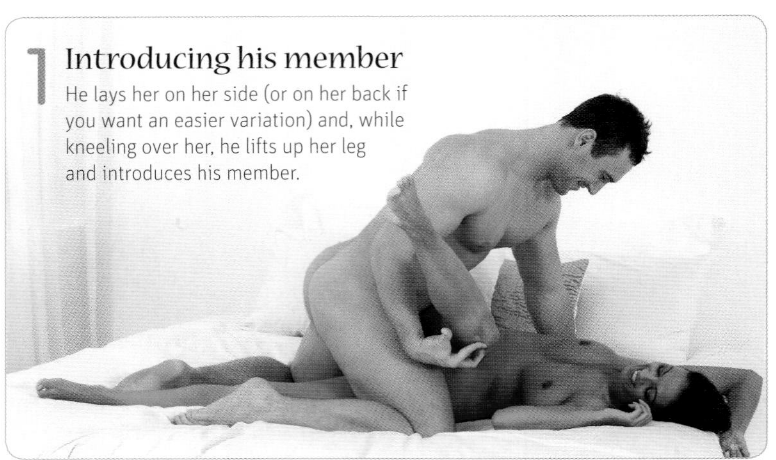

1 Introducing his member
He lays her on her side (or on her back if you want an easier variation) and, while kneeling over her, he lifts up her leg and introduces his member.

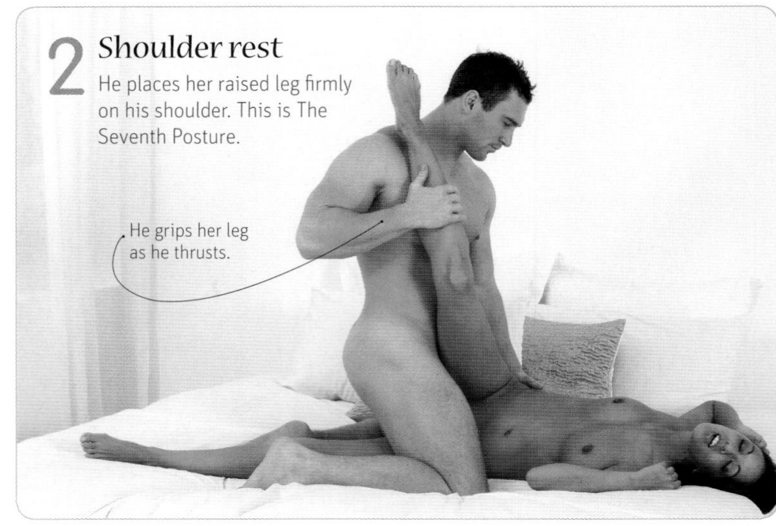

2 Shoulder rest
He places her raised leg firmly on his shoulder. This is The Seventh Posture.

He grips her leg as he thrusts.

"Straddle her like a cavalier on horseback, staying on your knees, while her legs are under her thighs." THE PERFUMED GARDEN

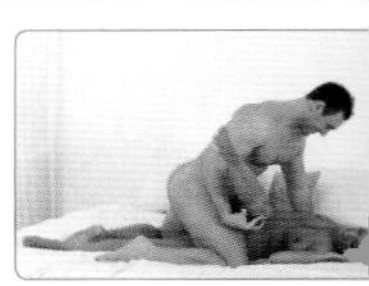

3 Moving freely

You both relax into a straightforward missionary position for some easy and satisfying thrusting.

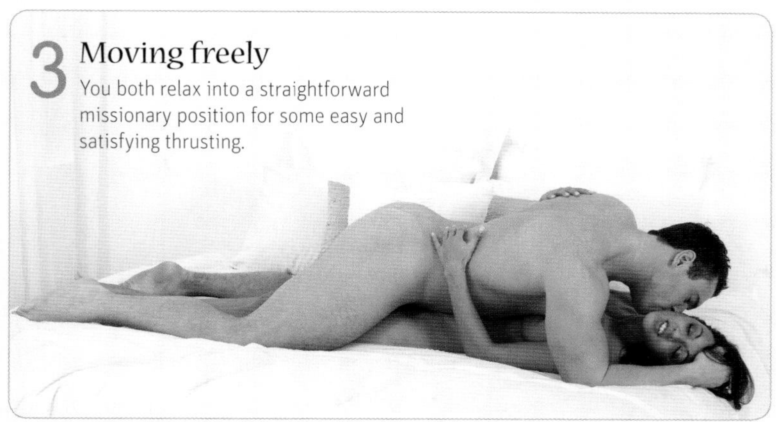

Taking it further

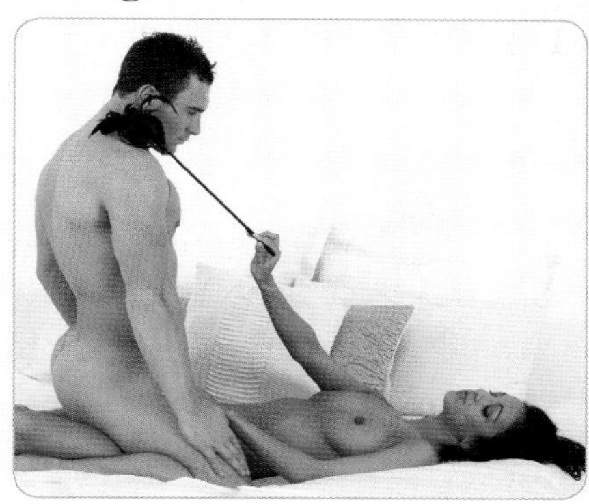

Feathery flicks

Her legs may be locked in position, but her hands aren't: she tickles and teases him with a feathery wand or a peacock feather.

4 Leg cross

He kneels upright astride her, and she twines her legs into a cross-legged or a lotus position. This is The Eighth Posture.

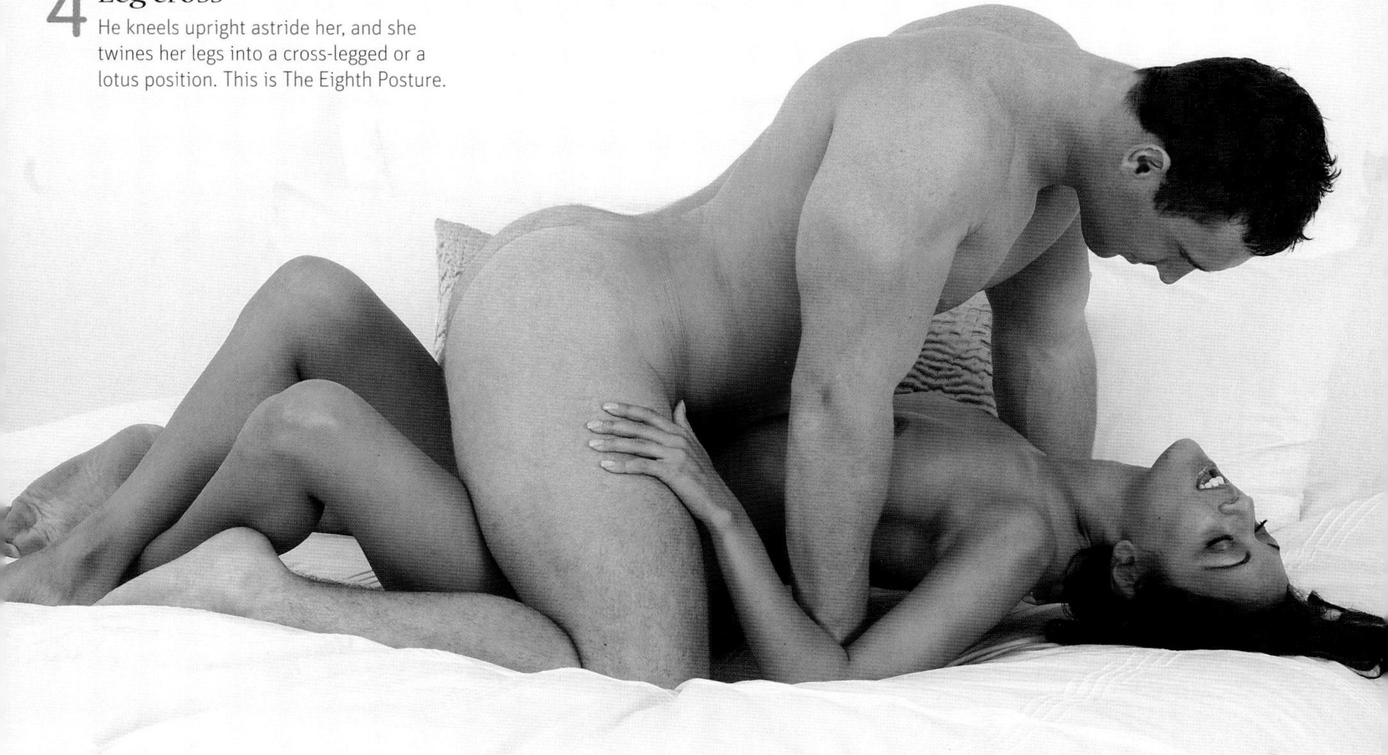

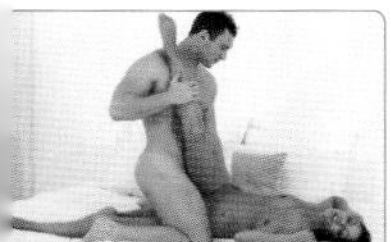
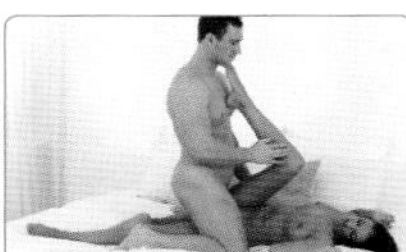
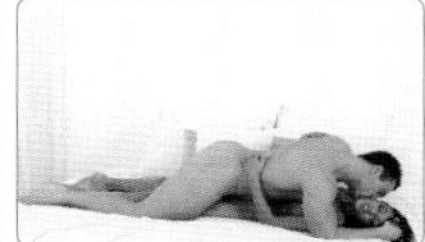
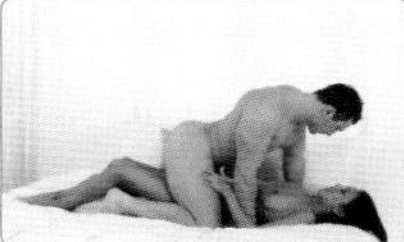
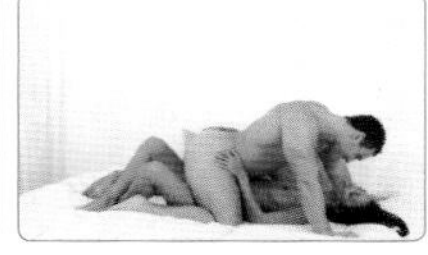

Race of the member

☆☆☆☆ Kama sensation rating

She saddles up and takes the reins before riding him fast to the finishing line in this horsey-yet-saucy position. Choose Race of the Member when he's got a stallion-sized penis; slipping it back through his thighs does a great job of minimizing the beast.

Why it works

– The shallow entry of his penis focuses all the erotic sensation into a small but sensitive area (his glans and just inside her vaginal entrance) with explosive results.

– She can make tiny bobbing movements that feel exquisite, she can slide slowly up and down his shaft, or she can hammer away like a power tool.

– She's on top and in charge of the moves, and you both love it.

– He experiences a more feminine side of sex; it's not often he penetrates her on his back with his knees by his chest.

Turn on...

... Put a cushion or pillow under his head. As well making him more comfortable, his head is better angled to catch a view of the action going on above.

Turn off...

... Don't carry on if your legs are giving way. Or, as *The Perfumed Garden* says: "She may put her knees on the floor, in which case the man moves her with his thighs while she grips his shoulders."

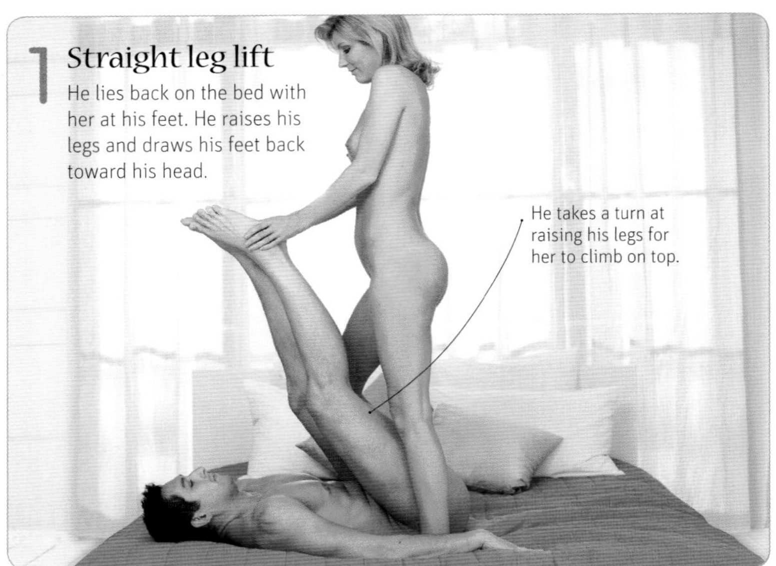

1 Straight leg lift
He lies back on the bed with her at his feet. He raises his legs and draws his feet back toward his head.

He takes a turn at raising his legs for her to climb on top.

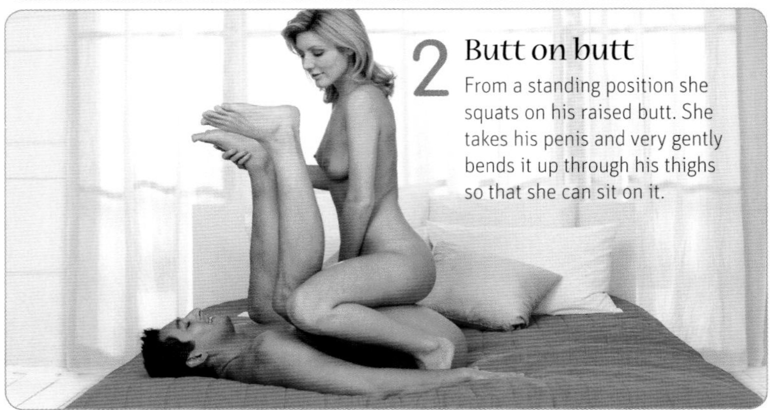

2 Butt on butt
From a standing position she squats on his raised butt. She takes his penis and very gently bends it up through his thighs so that she can sit on it.

"She stays seated, as if on horseback, the saddle being represented by his knees and his stomach." THE PERFUMED GARDEN

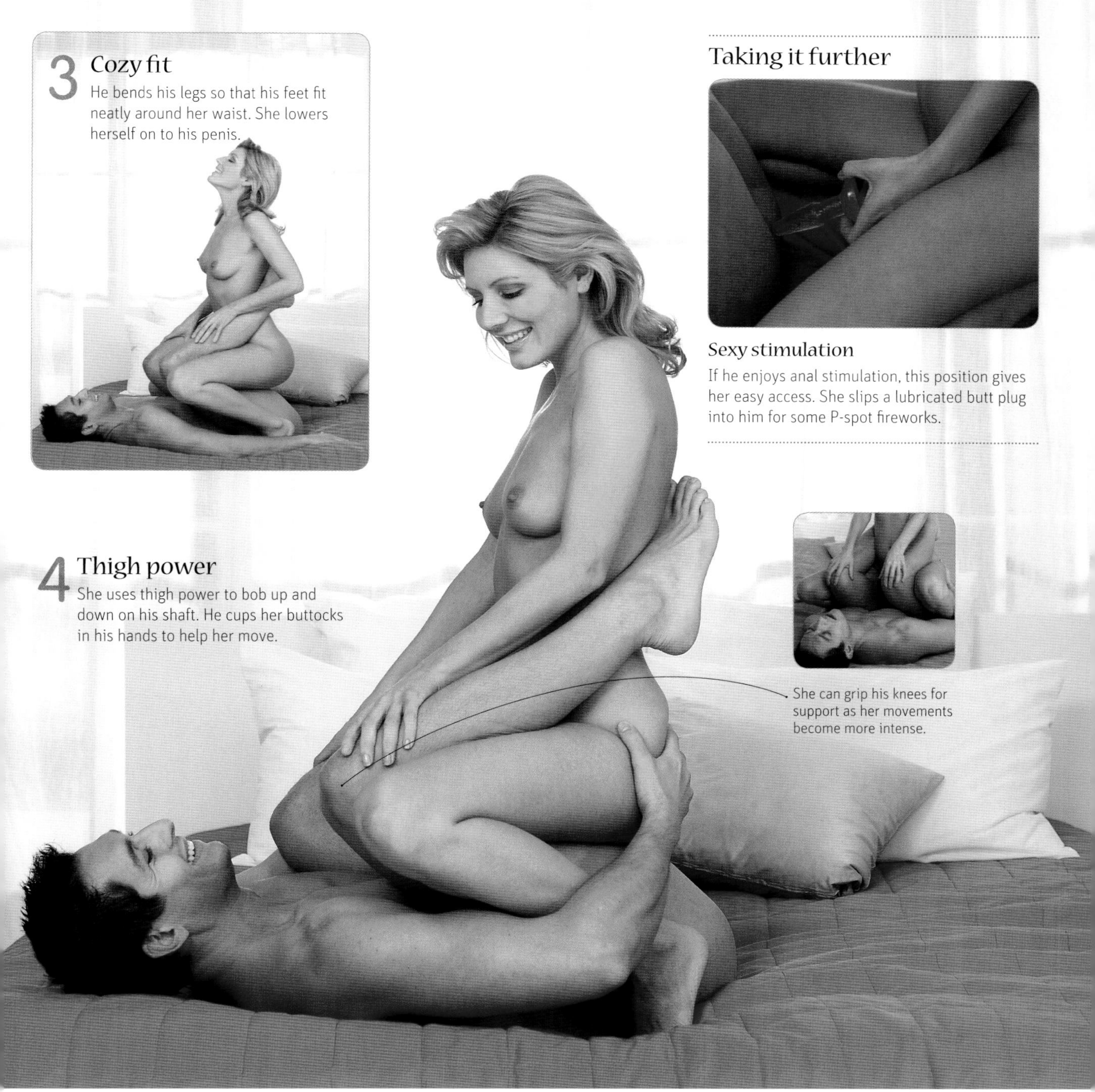

3 Cozy fit

He bends his legs so that his feet fit neatly around her waist. She lowers herself on to his penis.

4 Thigh power

She uses thigh power to bob up and down on his shaft. He cups her buttocks in his hands to help her move.

She can grip his knees for support as her movements become more intense.

Taking it further

Sexy stimulation

If he enjoys anal stimulation, this position gives her easy access. She slips a lubricated butt plug into him for some P-spot fireworks.

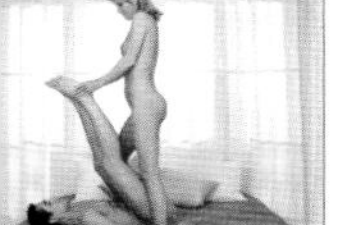
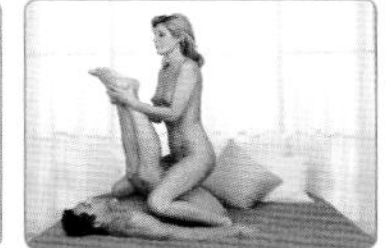
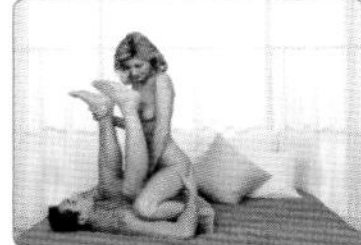
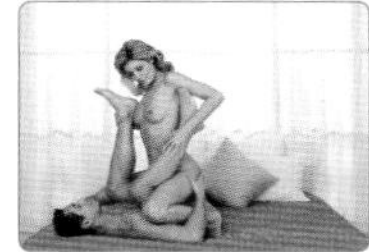
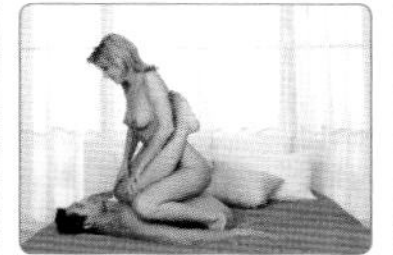
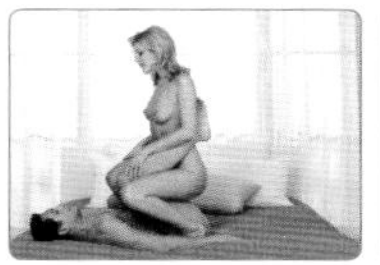
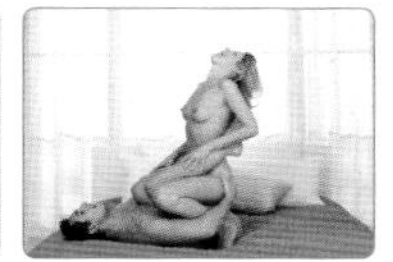

Ascending

☆☆☆ Kama sensation rating

She takes her rightful place on his throne in this queenly position. Try weaving it into a monarch-and-servant role play in which he addresses her reverentially as "Ma'am" or "Your majesty" while she gazes down regally. A fur-lined robe is optional.

Why it works

– It delivers high-impact sensations at the moment when you first impale yourself; close your eyes and relish them.

– She can move around to change the angle of entry. This way his penis hits her hot spots.

– His penis stays deep inside her as she moves; the result is an all-over internal massage that makes him glow.

– She can get the benefit of full penetration while she sits still and pays undivided attention to her clitoris.

– He loves the combination of woman-on-top sexiness and cross-legged demureness.

Turn on...

... Put your hand behind you and caress his balls. And if his anus is accessible, circle it gently then firmly with a wet fingertip.

Turn off...

... Don't lie back and do nothing if you're starting to feel understimulated (even if she is the queen). Ramp things up by touching her breasts or clitoris. Or pull her legs apart so you can take in the view.

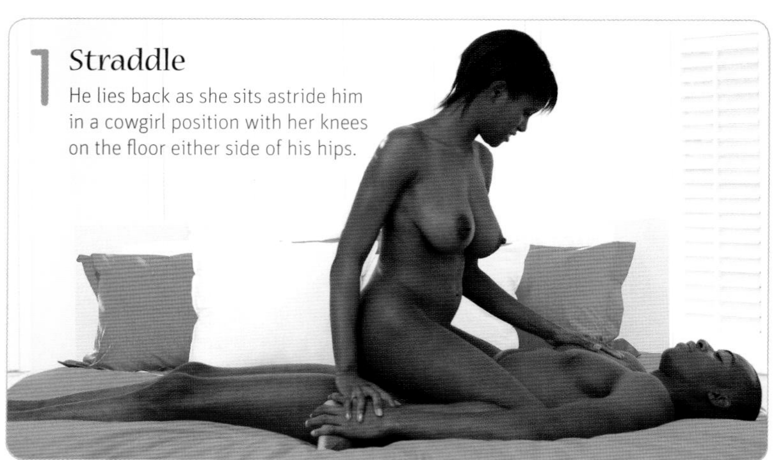

1 Straddle
He lies back as she sits astride him in a cowgirl position with her knees on the floor either side of his hips.

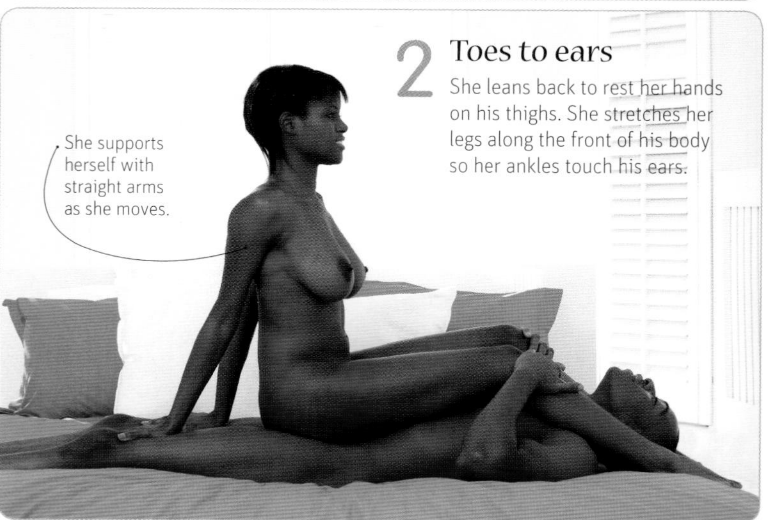

She supports herself with straight arms as she moves.

2 Toes to ears
She leans back to rest her hands on his thighs. She stretches her legs along the front of his body so her ankles touch his ears.

"When she has not been satisfied... she makes her husband lie upon his back and sits cross-legged on his thighs... she derives great comfort from this process." ANANGA RANGA

Taking it further

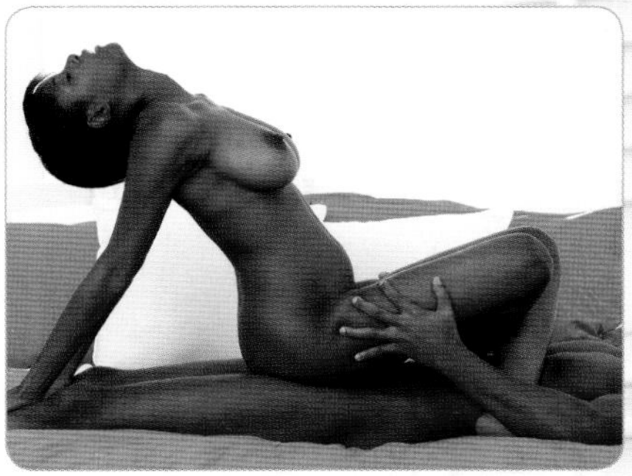

Voluptuous hip thrusting

To up the intensity, she leans back, takes her weight on her hands, and moves her hips up and down in slow, voluptuous movements.

3 Leg bend

After guiding his penis inside her, she bends first one leg, then the other, into a cross-legged position.

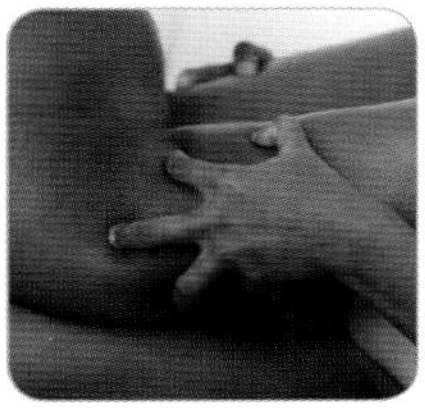

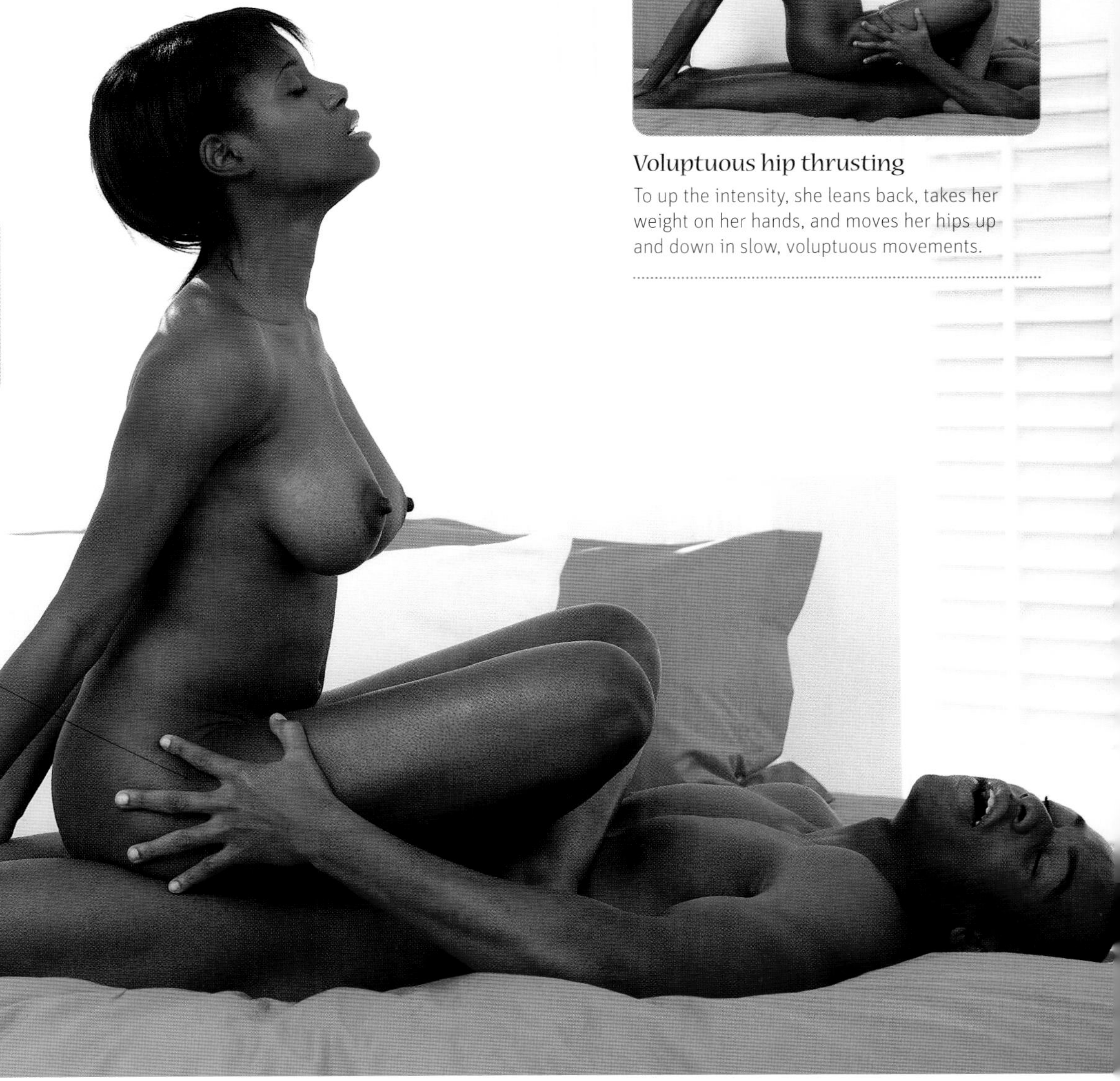

He can grab her thighs to push her back and forth for extra stimulation.

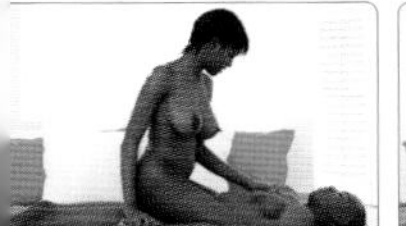
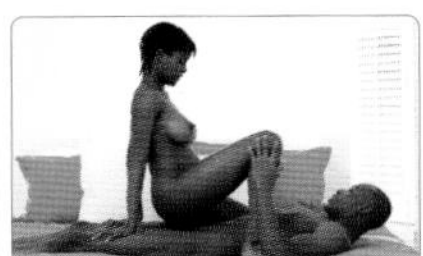
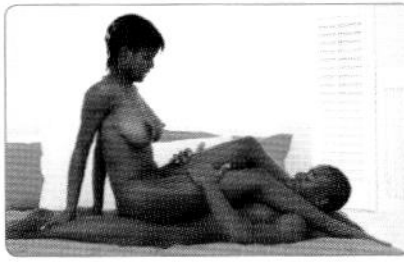
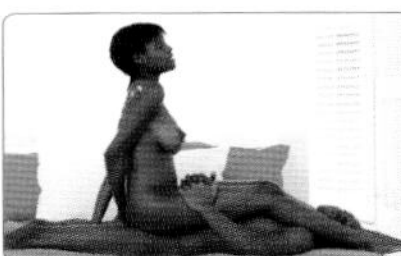
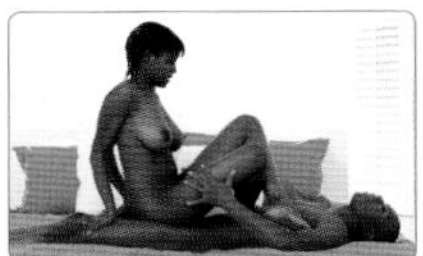
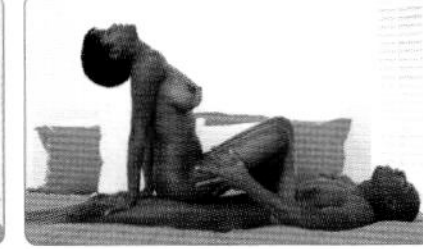

Fixing the nail and The crab's position

☆☆☆☆ Kama sensation rating

Enter sex heaven for foot fetishists. Not only will he love being brought to heel by her foot on his forehead, he's also in prime toe-sucking position. And, when you're both entering climax territory, she can drop her foot and get into The Crab's Position for rapid thrusting.

Why they work

- Her foot on his forehead draws his eye down to the lush view below.
- Toe sucking can fast-forward her arousal.
- Dropping into Crab's Position provides the excitement of some free-form thrusting.
- He can hang on to her knees as he flies off his handle.
- Fixing the Nail is made for playful, giggle-your-way-to-orgasm sex. And it's frivolous enough to be a good inhibition-buster.
- His movements are slow and considered; great for a slow-burning start to sex.

Turn on...

... Pounce on her when she's just returned from her Pilates or yoga class. Her leg muscles will still be warm, relaxed, and easily stretchable.

Turn off...

... Don't get carried away and kick him in the face. Some sex injuries, such as bites and scratches, can be an erotic reminder of last night's naughtiness; not the case with a black eye, though.

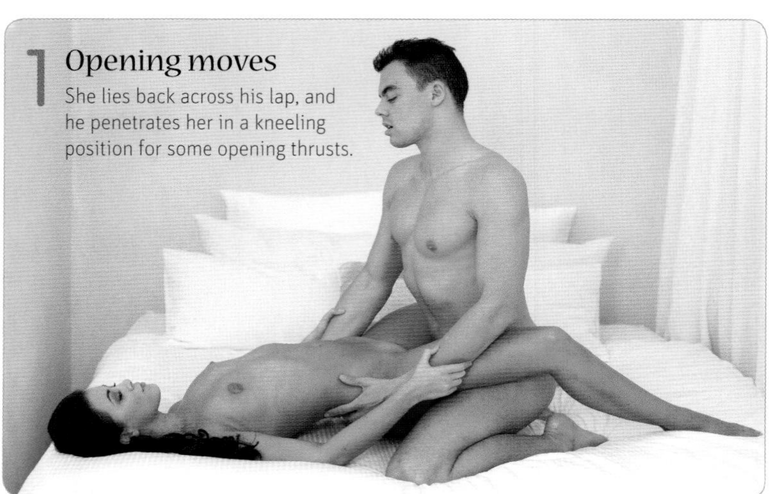

1 Opening moves
She lies back across his lap, and he penetrates her in a kneeling position for some opening thrusts.

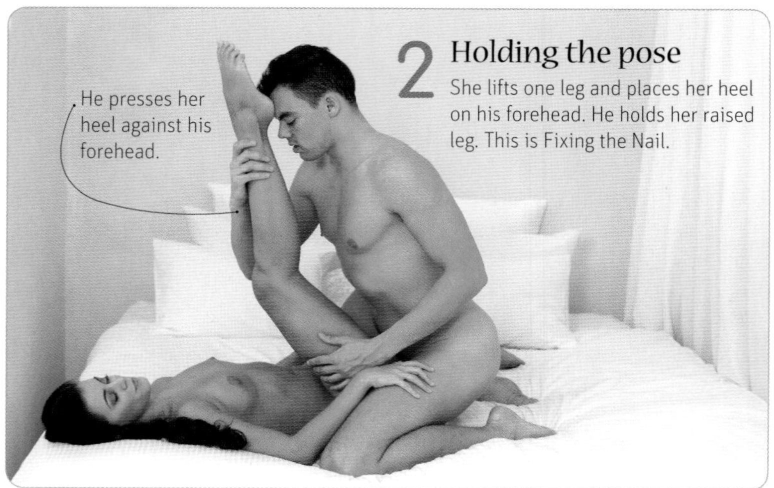

2 Holding the pose
She lifts one leg and places her heel on his forehead. He holds her raised leg. This is Fixing the Nail.

He presses her heel against his forehead.

"When one of her legs is placed on his head and the other stretched out, it is called Fixing of a Nail. It is learned only by practice." KAMA SUTRA

3 Knees to belly

She lowers her raised leg and brings both knees near her belly. He moves freely inside her. This is The Crab's Position.

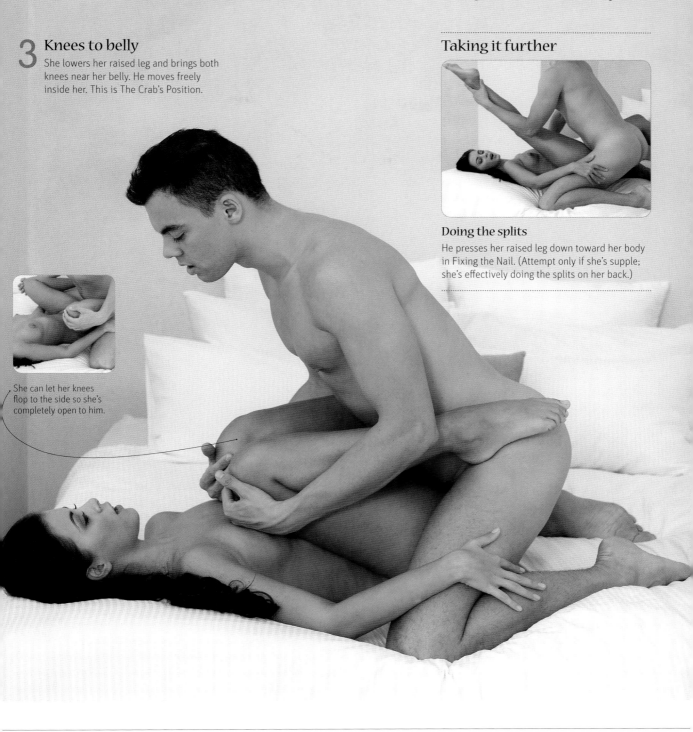

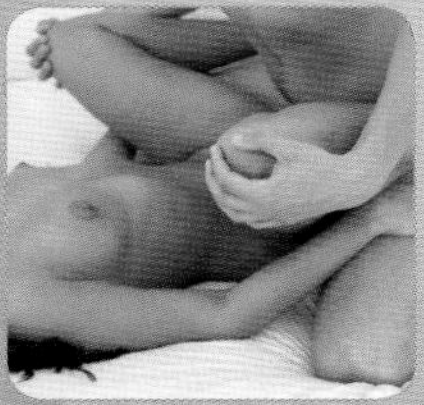

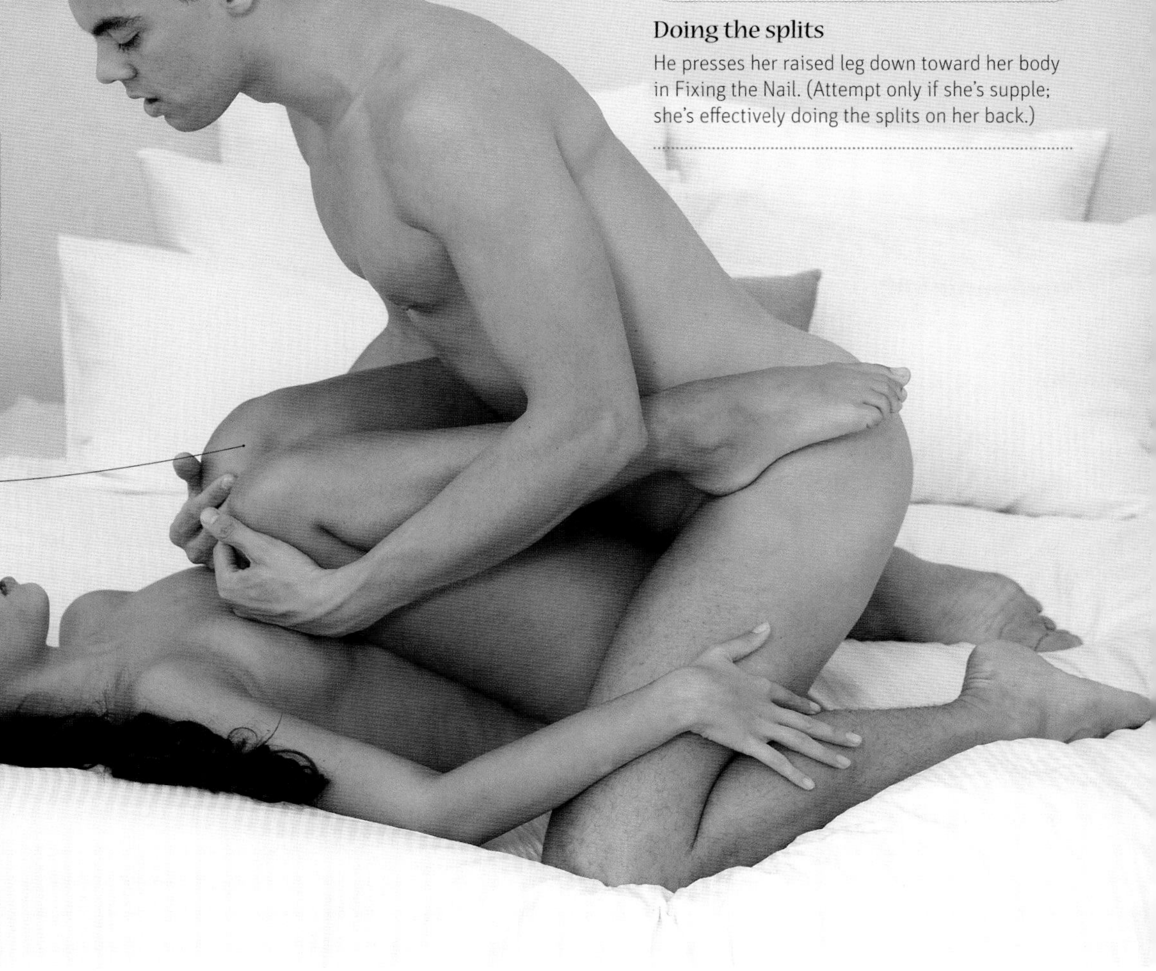

She can let her knees flop to the side so she's completely open to him.

Taking it further

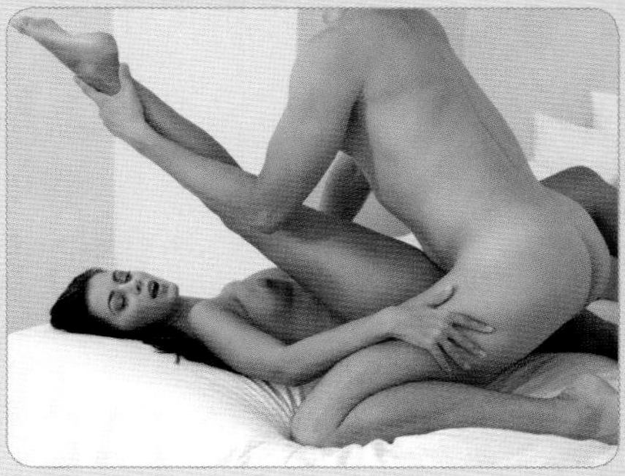

Doing the splits

He presses her raised leg down toward her body in Fixing the Nail. (Attempt only if she's supple; she's effectively doing the splits on her back.)

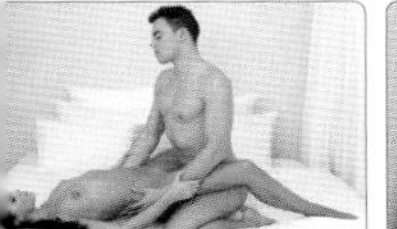
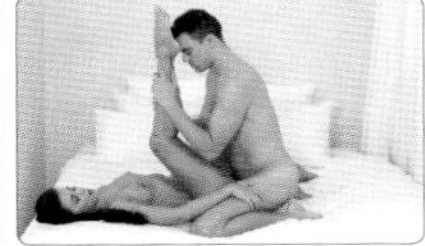
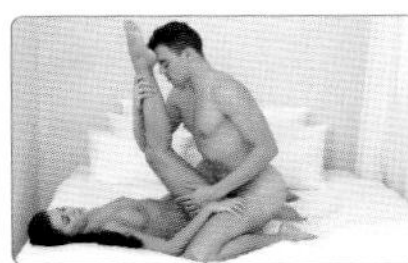
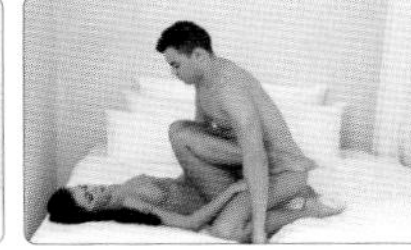
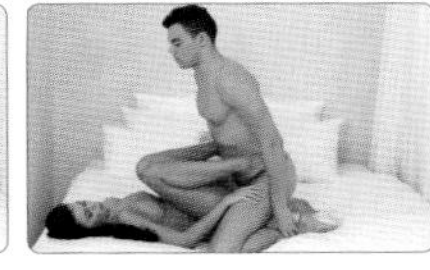
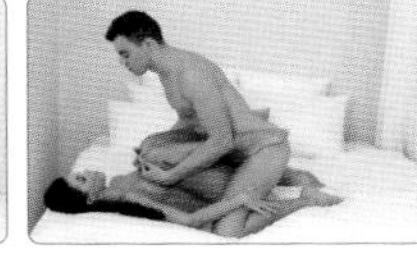

Drawing the bow

☆☆☆☆ Kama sensation rating

Draw back your bow and prepare to fire your love arrow. This archery-inspired position isn't one you'd just happen to fall into, so it's good for impressing new lovers. Mix it up with other *Kama Sutra* innovations to show how very creative you are on the mattress springs.

Why it works

– It's the laid-back option for rear-entry sex; it's easier to focus on the glorious G-spot sensations building up on the front wall of her vagina because she's lying down.

– He's in a prime ass-groping position.

– She loves feeling penetrated to the core with this unusual angle of entry.

– He gets all the deep-entry pleasure of a man-on-top position, but with a quarter of the effort; good for lazy Sunday sex.

– It's good for romps on the living-room floor when you have the house to yourself and can make as much noise as you want to.

Turn on...

... Pull her body down hard on to you and then grind against her. Try to penetrate her a little more deeply on each grind.

Turn off...

... Neglecting sensuality. Stay in touch with melting caresses. She can press her fingertips into the soles of his feet, squeeze and pinch his toes, and smooth her thumbs along his calf muscles.

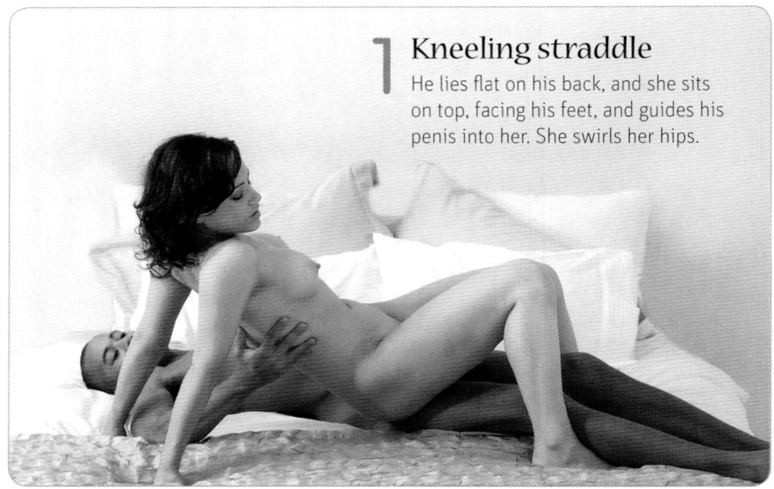

1 Kneeling straddle
He lies flat on his back, and she sits on top, facing his feet, and guides his penis into her. She swirls her hips.

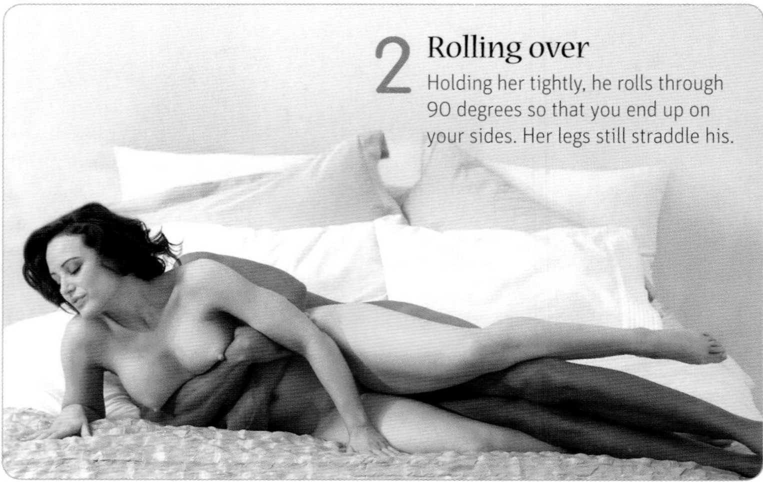

2 Rolling over
Holding her tightly, he rolls through 90 degrees so that you end up on your sides. Her legs still straddle his.

"She grasps his feet and pulls them toward her; in this way the man's body becomes a bow to which she is the arrow." THE PERFUMED GARDEN

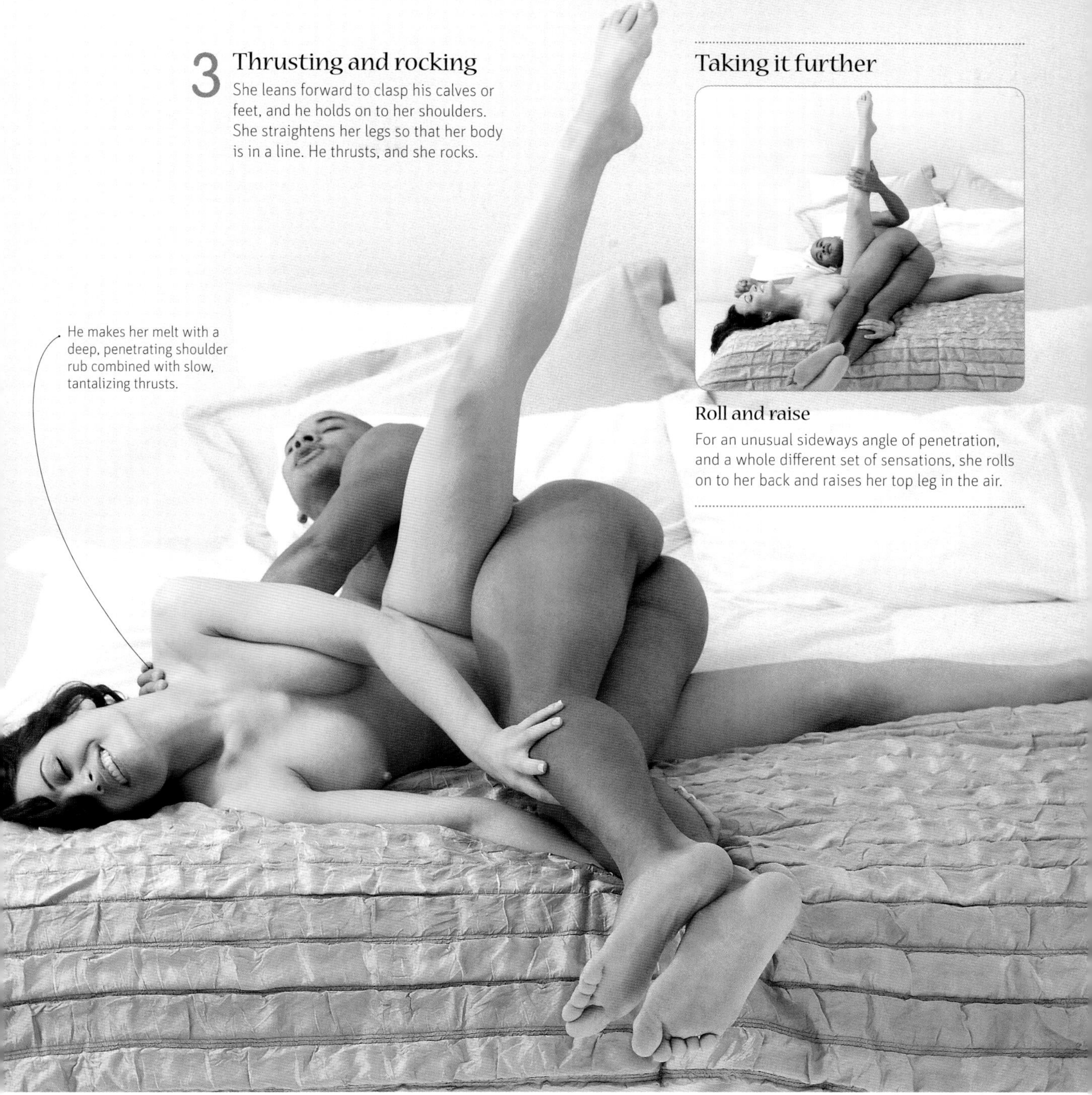

3 Thrusting and rocking

She leans forward to clasp his calves or feet, and he holds on to her shoulders. She straightens her legs so that her body is in a line. He thrusts, and she rocks.

He makes her melt with a deep, penetrating shoulder rub combined with slow, tantalizing thrusts.

Taking it further

Roll and raise

For an unusual sideways angle of penetration, and a whole different set of sensations, she rolls on to her back and raises her top leg in the air.

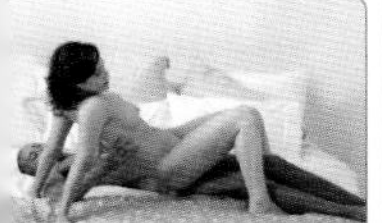
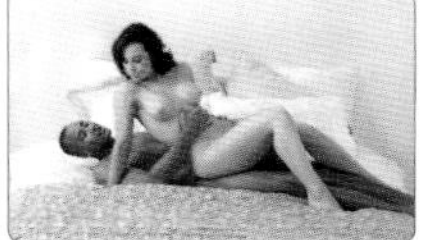
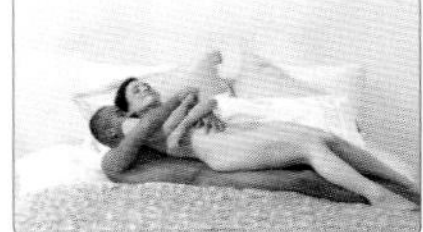
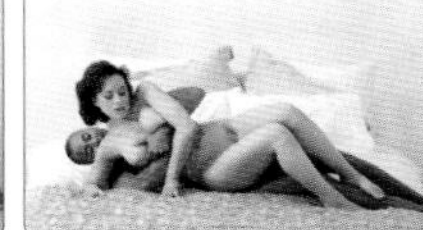
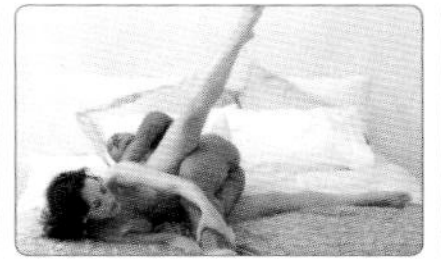
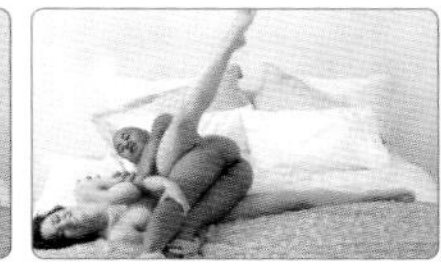

The top

Can't decide whether you're in the mood for face-to-face loving or a bit of rear-entry? Or perhaps side-on sex would flick your switch? No problem: The Top meets all three of these entry requirements. It's an all-singing, all-dancing multi-tasking sex position in which she spins around on the well-oiled pole of his penis.

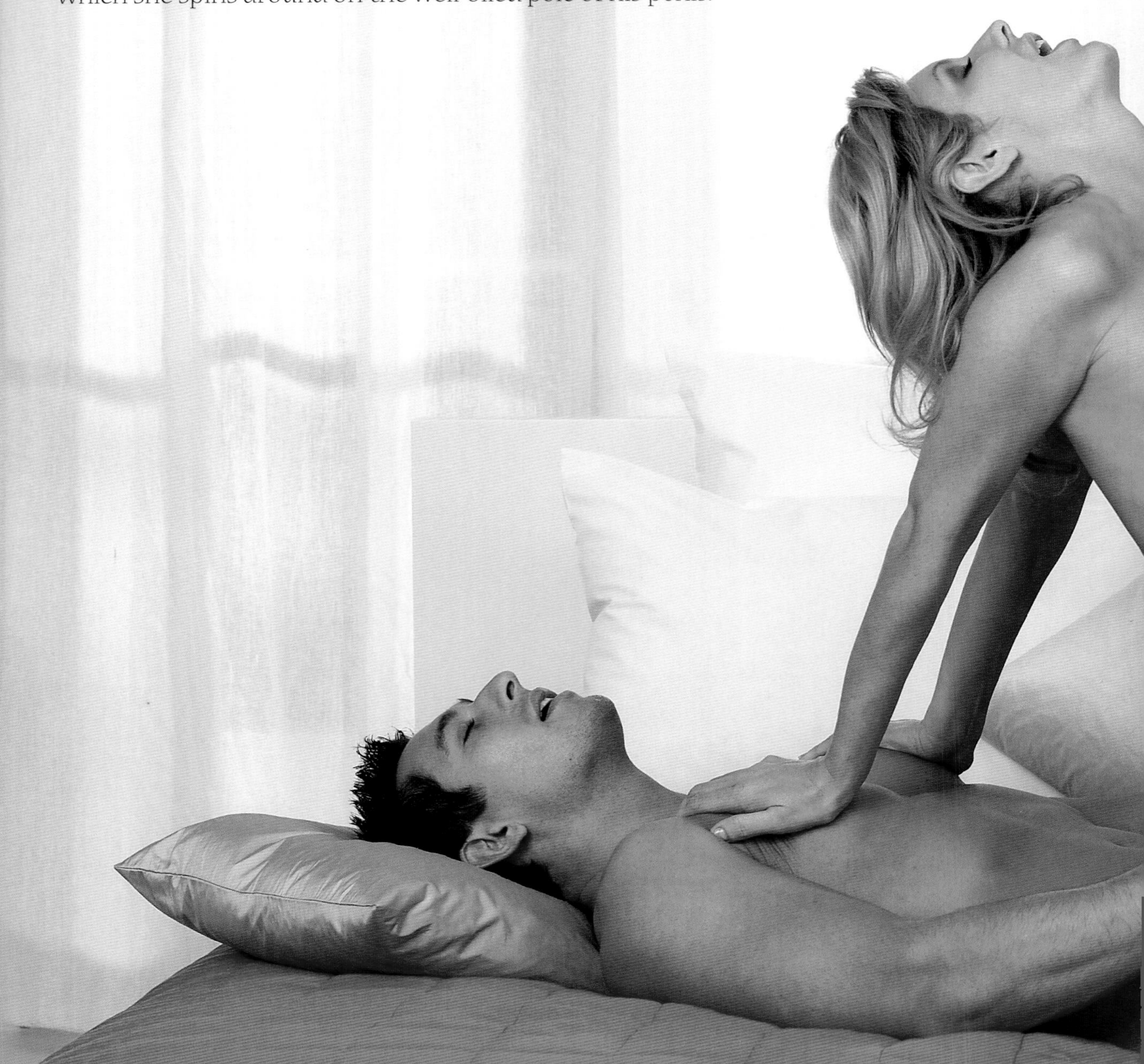

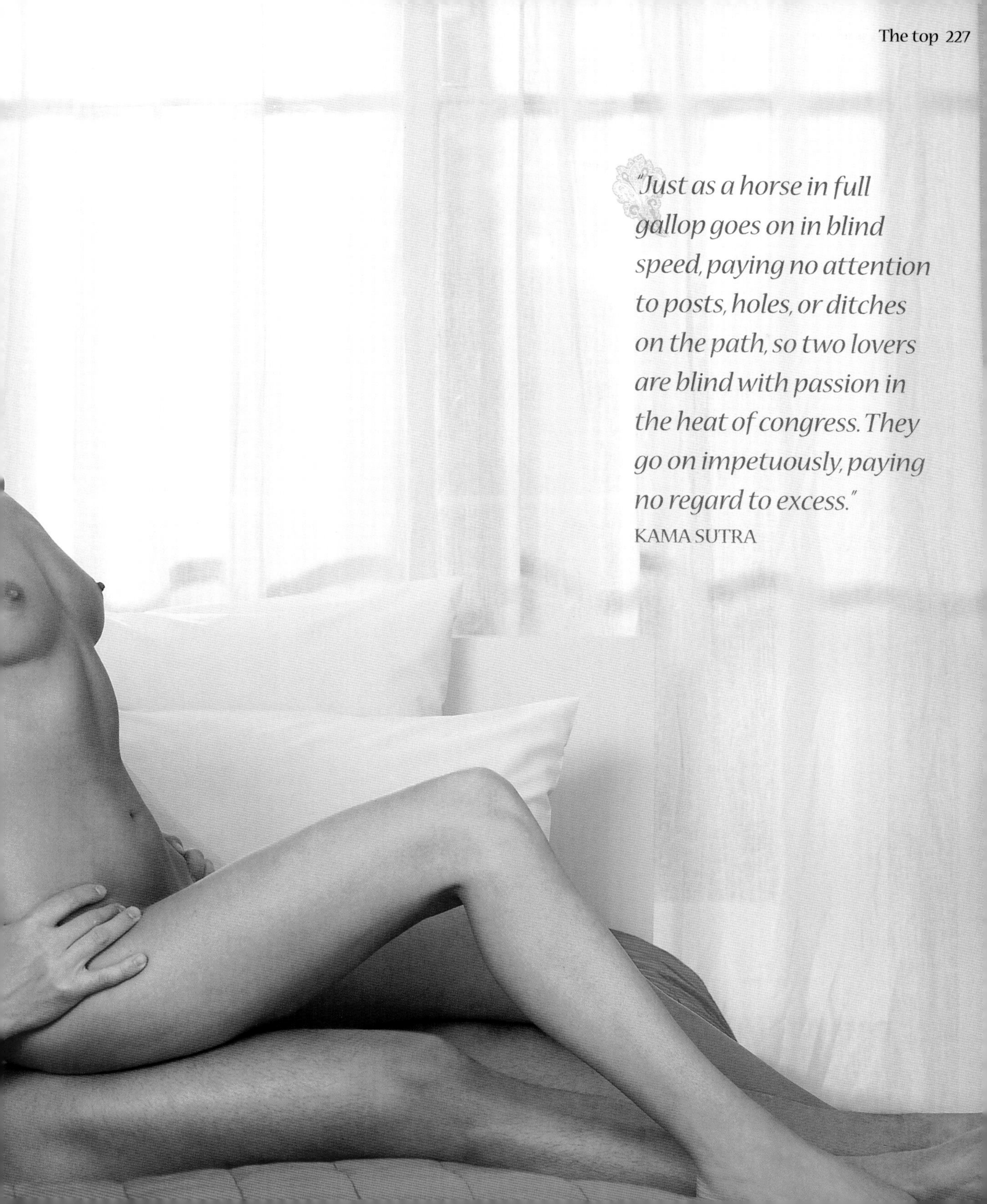

"Just as a horse in full gallop goes on in blind speed, paying no attention to posts, holes, or ditches on the path, so two lovers are blind with passion in the heat of congress. They go on impetuously, paying no regard to excess."

KAMA SUTRA

The top

☆☆☆

Kama sensation rating

Why it works

– It gives her freedom to try out a range of moves: up and down, side to side, around and around, back and forth, and anything else she can think of.

– She can easily slip her hand between her legs.

– It's the partner position to Turning. So, if she completes the maneuver, she can ask him for payment in kind.

– He gets to do all his favorite things: lie back, watch her at her sexiest, and fondle whichever of her pleasure zones happen to be within reach at the time.

– It's a journey with many stop-off points. When she finds an angle that she enjoys, she simply stops to make the most of it. Facing north and south will be familiar, but the angles in between provide novel sensations.

Turn on...

... Enjoy the performance aspect of The Top. Treat it as the horizontal equivalent of a lap dance. You can even dress accordingly.

Turn off...

... Don't get so carried away that you damage him. If you start to slip off, the base of his penis will take the strain. Ask him to keep his hands firmly on your butt for support.

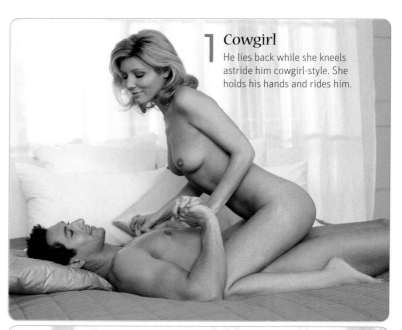

1 Cowgirl
He lies back while she kneels astride him cowgirl-style. She holds his hands and rides him.

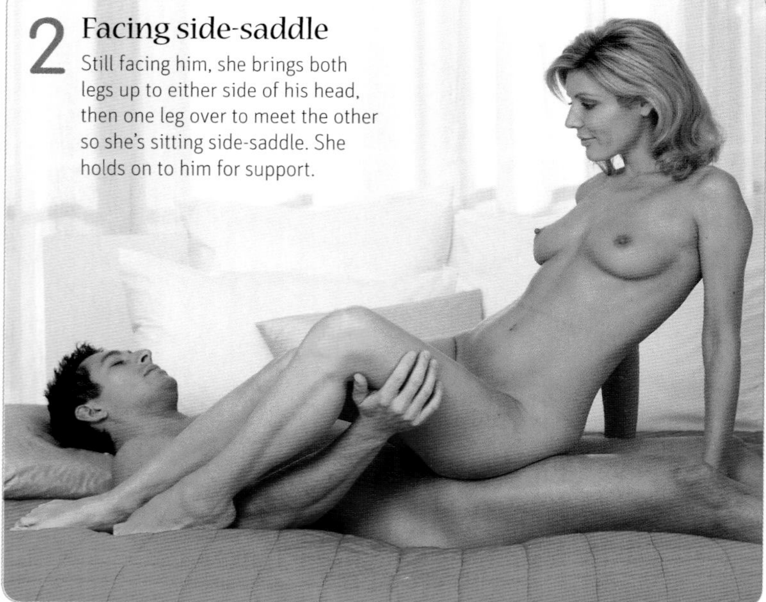

2 Facing side-saddle
Still facing him, she brings both legs up to either side of his head, then one leg over to meet the other so she's sitting side-saddle. She holds on to him for support.

"For people joined in sexual bliss, passion dictates what happens. The emotions and fantasies that arise during sex are as irregular as dreams." KAMA SUTRA

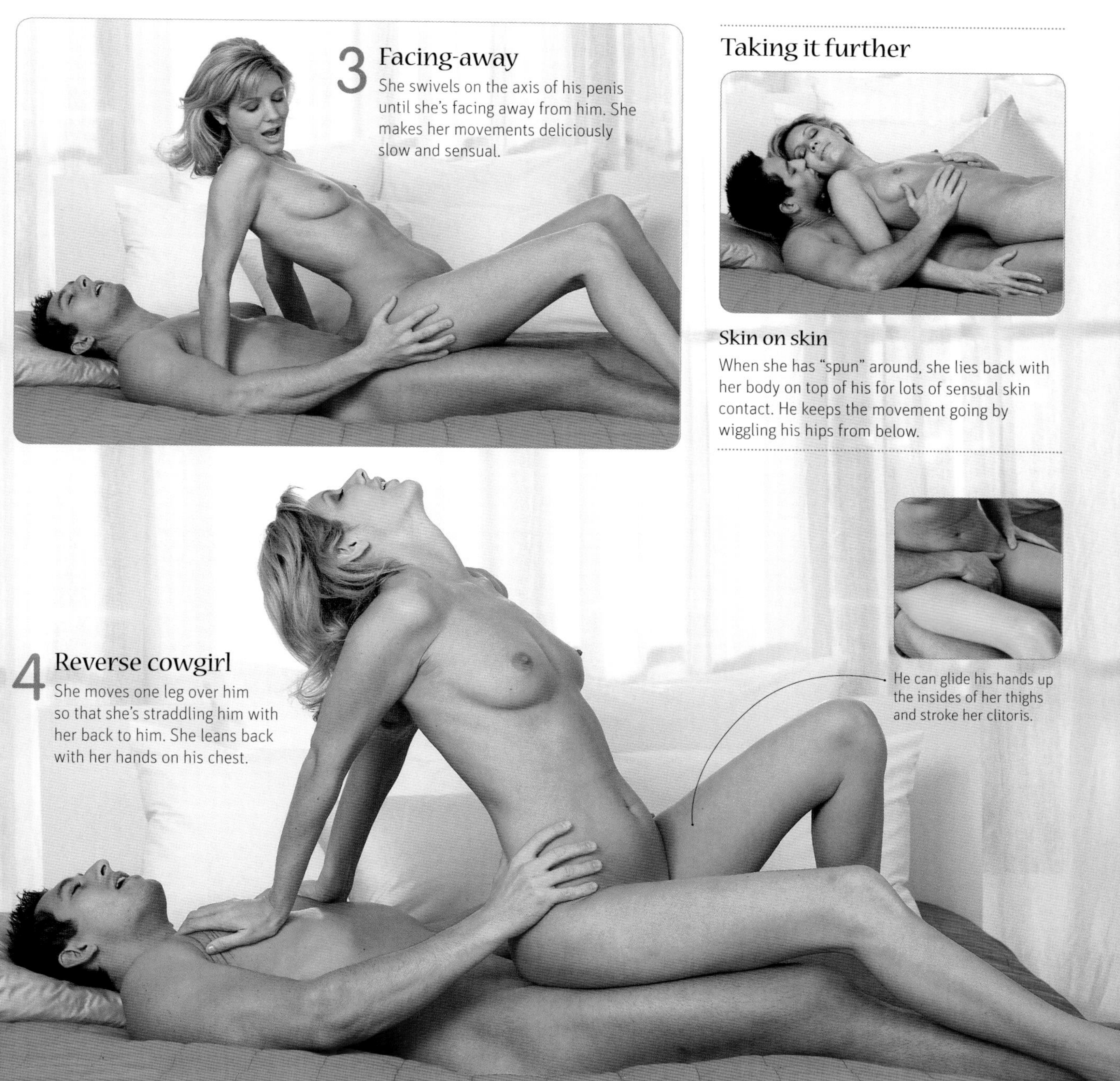

3 Facing-away

She swivels on the axis of his penis until she's facing away from him. She makes her movements deliciously slow and sensual.

Taking it further

Skin on skin

When she has "spun" around, she lies back with her body on top of his for lots of sensual skin contact. He keeps the movement going by wiggling his hips from below.

He can glide his hands up the insides of her thighs and stroke her clitoris.

4 Reverse cowgirl

She moves one leg over him so that she's straddling him with her back to him. She leans back with her hands on his chest.

If you liked this, try…

- Getting him to reciprocate in Turning (see page 160).
- Pair of Tongs for the ultimate woman-on-top sexiness (see page 78).

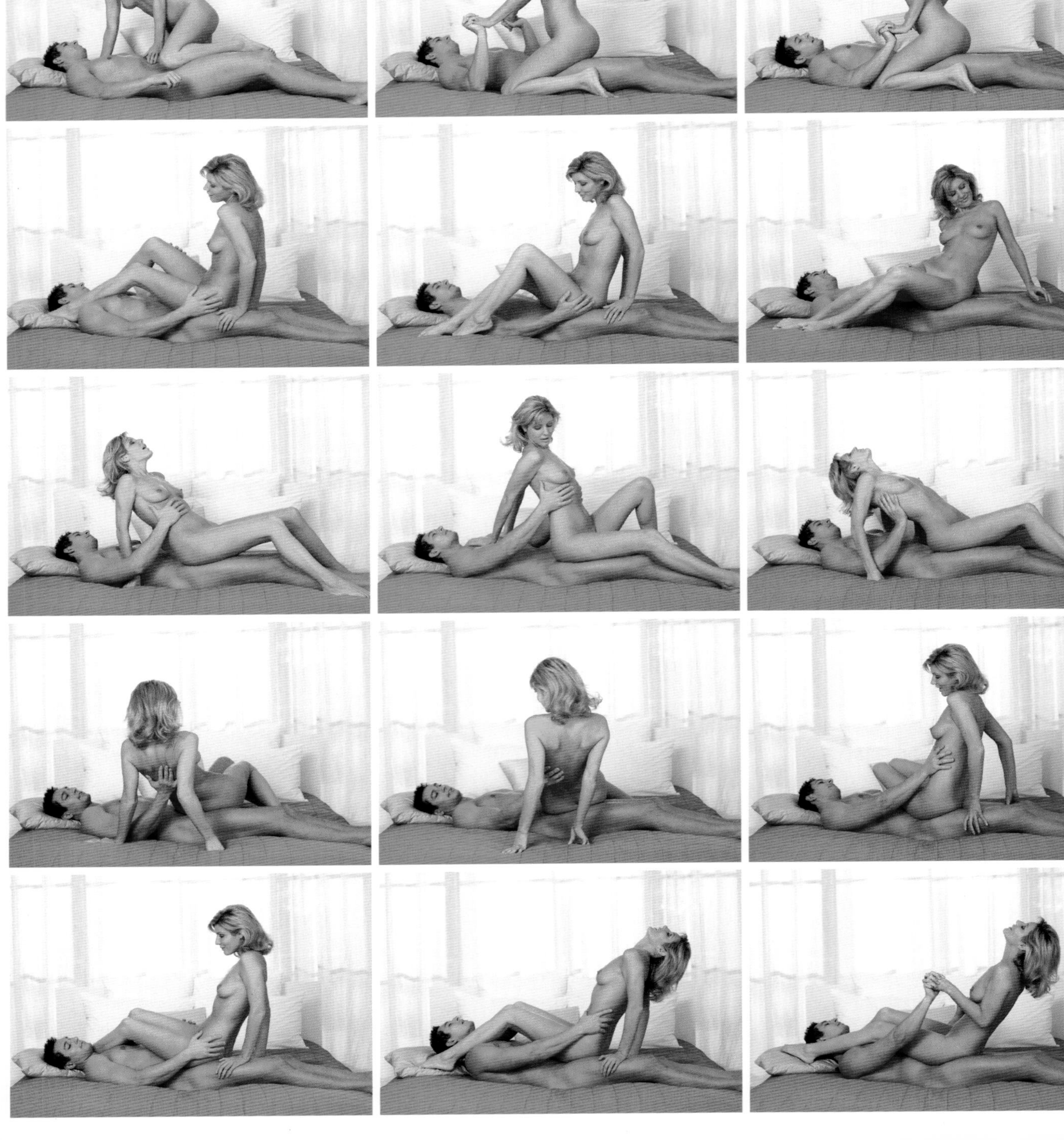

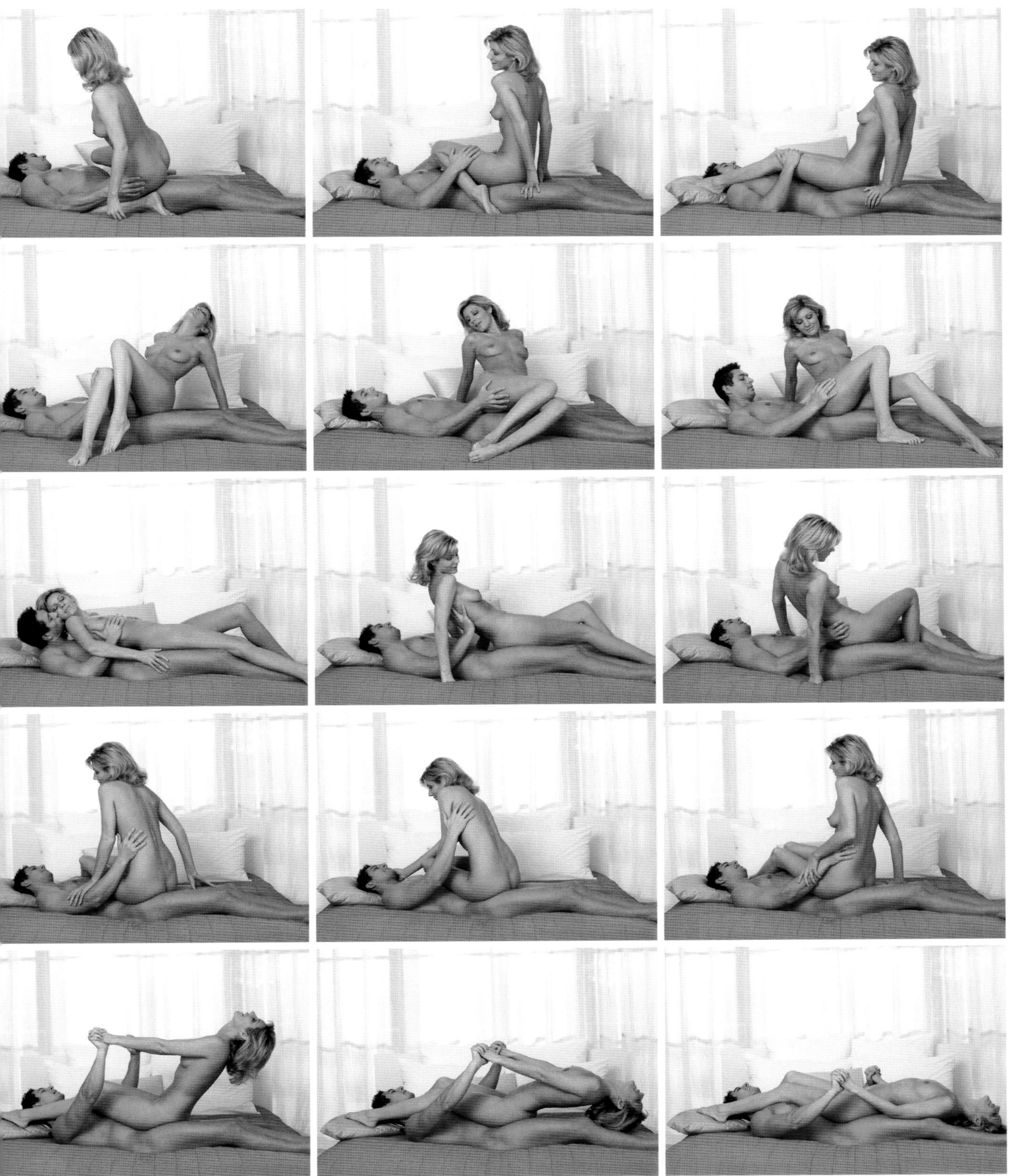

The second posture

☆☆☆☆☆ Kama sensation rating

Make this your grand finale to a long night of steamy passion. You're both taut with sexual tension and, at last, this is the point where you can let rip in full mattress-pounding glory before that explosive "yes… yes… yesssssss" moment.

Why it works

- The maximum depth of penetration is possible in this position, letting you express your lust as freely as you want.
- It's the ultimate invitation from her to him.
- It enhances sensation if he's smaller than average because her vagina is contracted.
- You'll both convulse with pleasure at the moment of entry.
- He can fire her passion by pulling out and popping down below to deliver some oral sex.
- Despite being separated by the barrier of her legs, you can make intense eye contact.

Turn on…

… Let yourself go. No one's watching, so you're free to moan, scream, thrash, and gyrate. If it feels cool, calm, and collected, you're not doing it right.

Turn off…

Neglecting to add additional clitoral friction if she needs it. You could take your penis out and rub it against her. Or you could bring her to orgasm with your hand or a vibrator postcoitally.

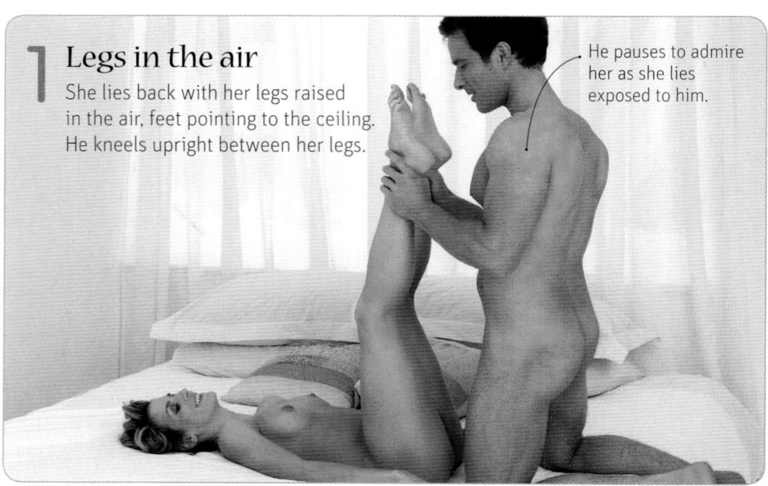

1 Legs in the air
She lies back with her legs raised in the air, feet pointing to the ceiling. He kneels upright between her legs.

He pauses to admire her as she lies exposed to him.

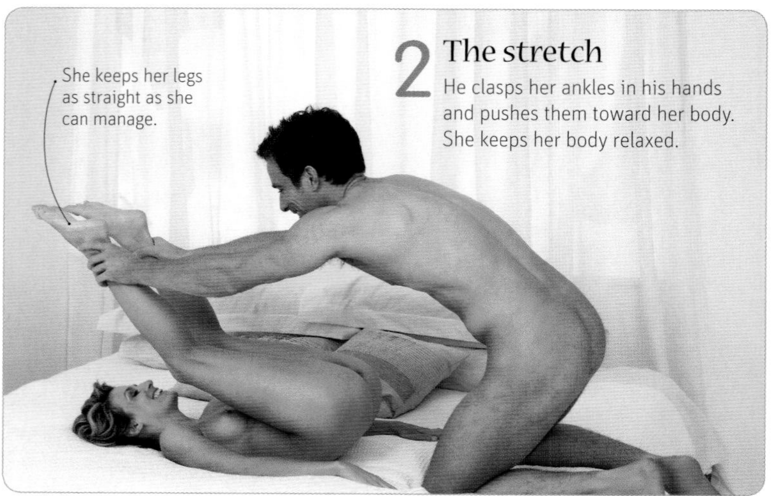

2 The stretch
He clasps her ankles in his hands and pushes them toward her body. She keeps her body relaxed.

She keeps her legs as straight as she can manage.

"Let the woman lie on her back, lift her legs into the air, so that her right leg be near her right ear, and the left one near her left ear." THE PERFUMED GARDEN

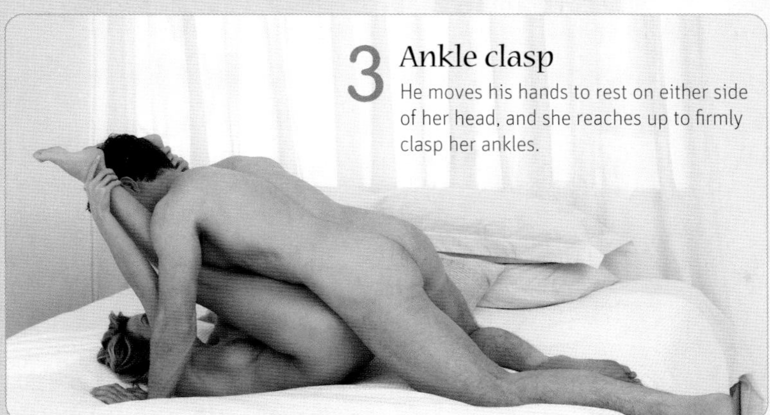

3 Ankle clasp

He moves his hands to rest on either side of her head, and she reaches up to firmly clasp her ankles.

Taking it further

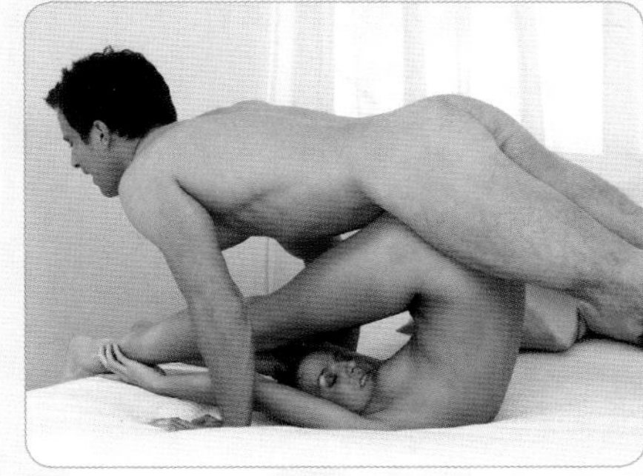

Flexible fun

If she's super-flexible, she takes this position to the next level by resting her toes on the bed behind her head (like the Plow in yoga).

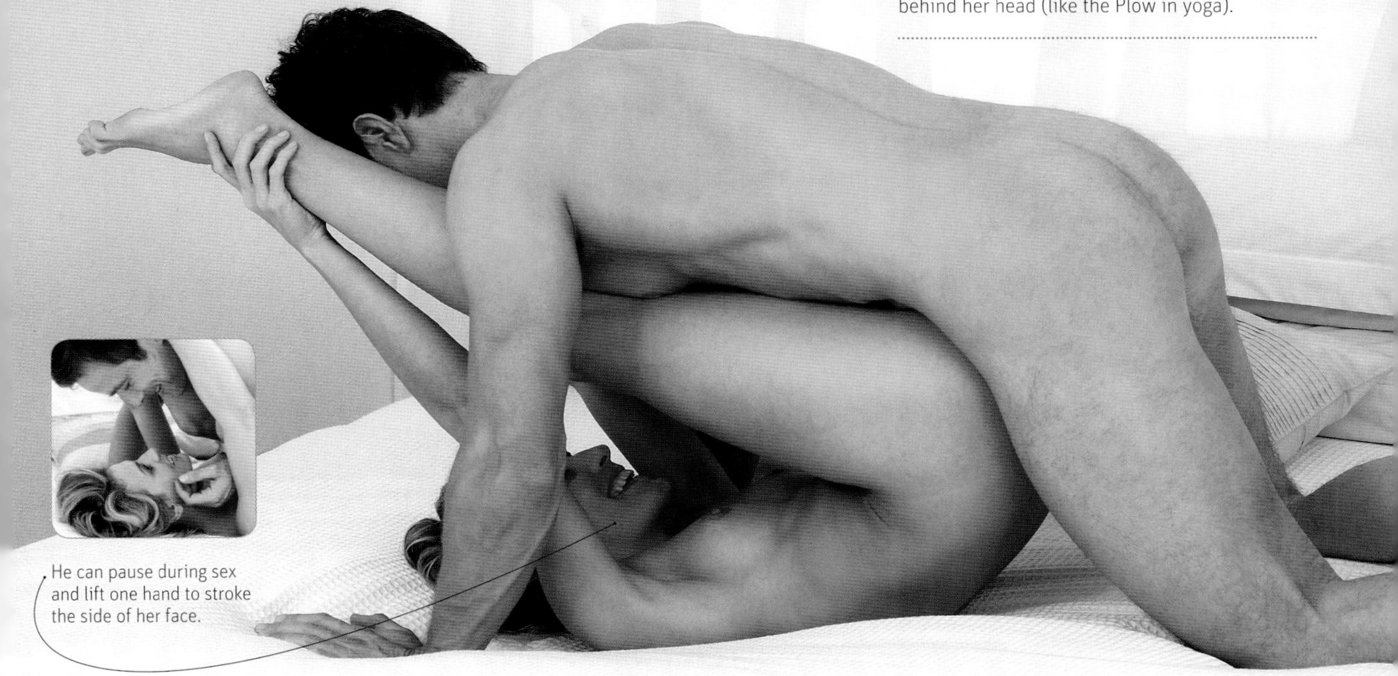

He can pause during sex and lift one hand to stroke the side of her face.

4 Ankles to head

She draws her ankles as close to her head as she can. He penetrates gently but deeply.

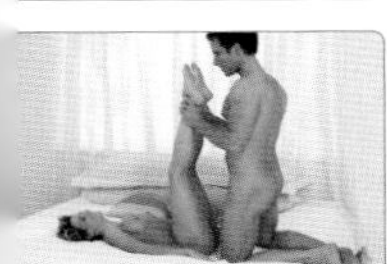
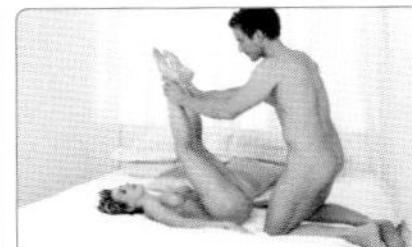
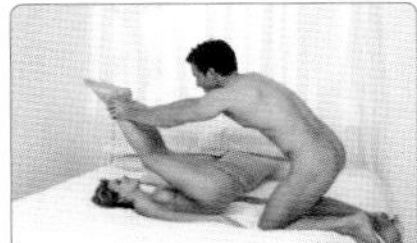
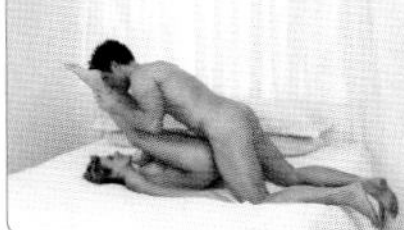
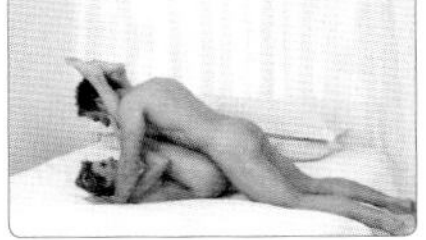
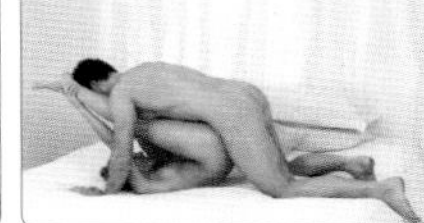

Happy endings

You've just completed a sex marathon, and you're lying limp and satisfied in each other's arms. The *Kama Sutra* at this point says: "go modestly to the bathing place without looking at each other." Feel free to disregard it on this occasion; post-orgasmic bliss is much better shared.

After sex you're awash with feel-good chemicals such as oxytocin and endorphins, which are the body's natural opiates. These combine to give you a natural high, which is why it's a good idea to bask in this state for as long it lasts.

Carnal comedown Cuddle up to each other and whisper softly. Hover in the delicious state between sleep and wakefulness, and zone in on all the warm, tingling post-sex sensations coursing through your bodies. Stroke each other. Take the chance to declare your tenderest feelings.

The *Ananga Ranga* had the right idea; Kalyana Malla's advice to men was: "When your amorous frolics are at an end, take care not to get up brusquely. Instead, gently withdraw your member and stay with your lover. Lie on your right side in the bed of pleasure. In this way you won't resemble a man who mounts a woman like a mule and pays no attention to the art of love."

Going around again The postcoital period can also be the time when she has her first/second/third orgasm. If she's still itching with desire and he's spent and flaccid, seek a compromise: you can both take turns to stimulate her, or he can provide some static vaginal penetration with his fingers while she goes to work on her clitoris. A vibrator is also an excellent postcoital orgasm provider.

Alternatively, she can hang on for round two. Depending on how old he is (and how tired and how motivated), the time it takes for him to get hard again may be anything from minutes to hours. The quickest way to get him back in the mood is a power nap, followed by liquid refreshments, a sexy massage, and her X-rated suggestions whispered in his ear.

Refueling Sharing a sensual postcoital snack is a great way to prolong the mood and stay in that intimate "we've-just-had-sex" bubble. This is especially true if you share the same tub of slightly melted ice cream, sip from the same glass of full-bodied red wine, or feed each other succulent grapes or strawberries with your fingers. Even Vatsyayana, who discouraged postcoital eye contact and sent lovers off to the bathroom for a brisk after-sex scrub, recommends postcoital bonding over a drink and a snack. You may want to skip the gruel, though:

"The man should embrace her with his left arm and encourage her to drink from a cup that he holds in his hand. The couple can eat sweetmeats, they can drink fresh juice, soup, gruel, extracts of meat, sherbet, the juice of mango fruit, or the extract of the juice of the citron tree."

Postcoital positions Find a position that lets you relax your whole body so that you can relish that just-melted feeling in comfort. Spoons position is good for staying close but, for the ultimate in intimacy, try rolling into Side-by-Side Clasping (see page 38) and pressing your foreheads together. Alternatively, there's something quirkily snug about ending up with your heads by each other's feet. And after strenuous, bed-breaking bouts of sex, nothing beats lying on your backs and holding hands while grinning at the ceiling.

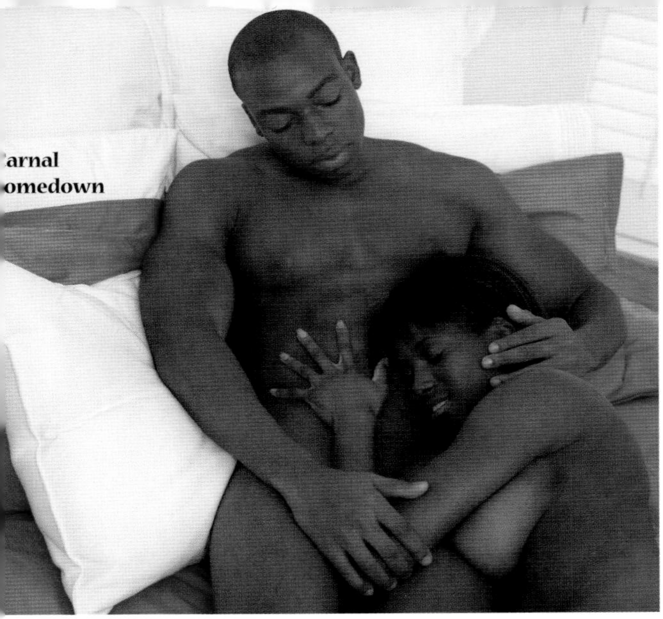

arnal omedown

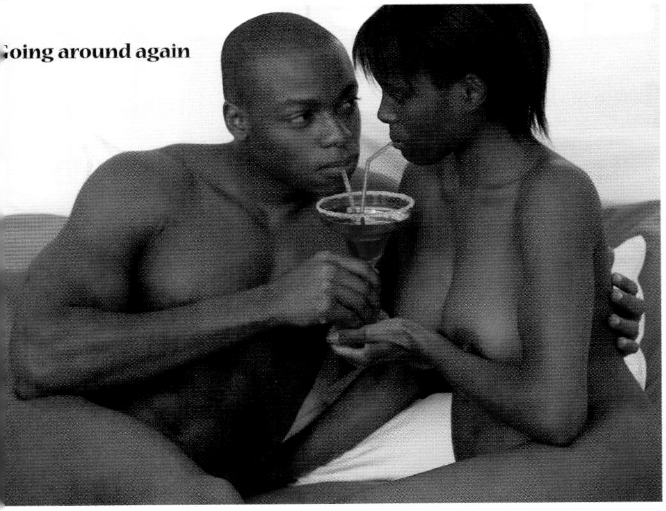

Postcoital positions

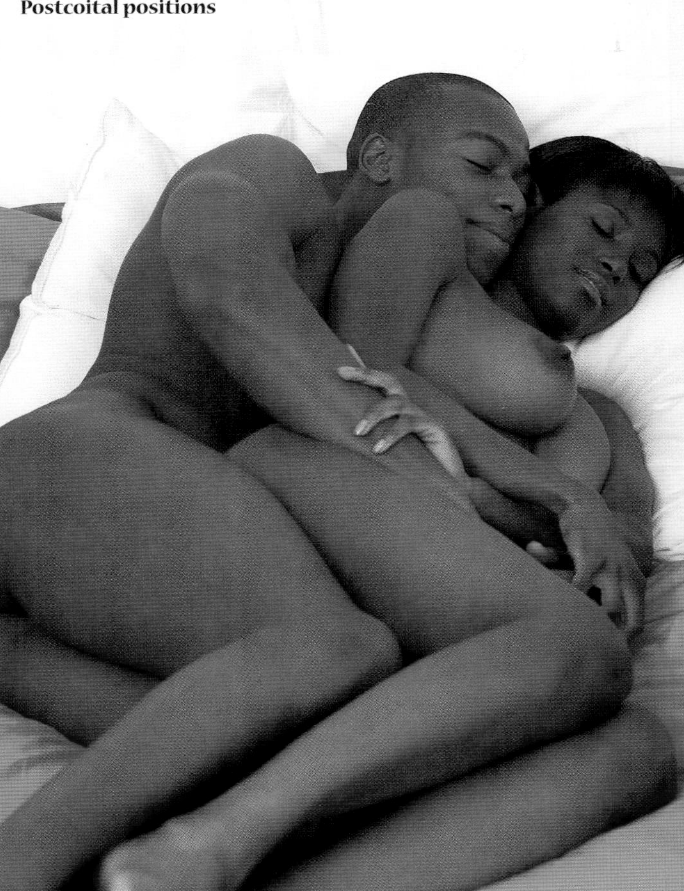

oing around again

efueling

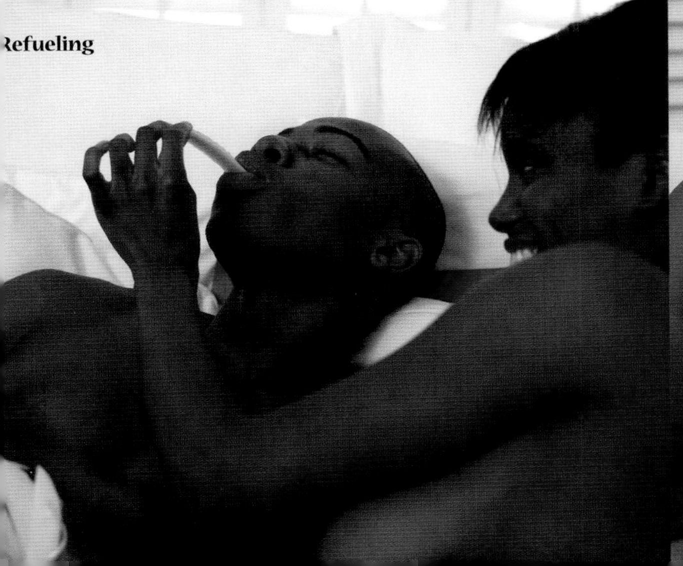

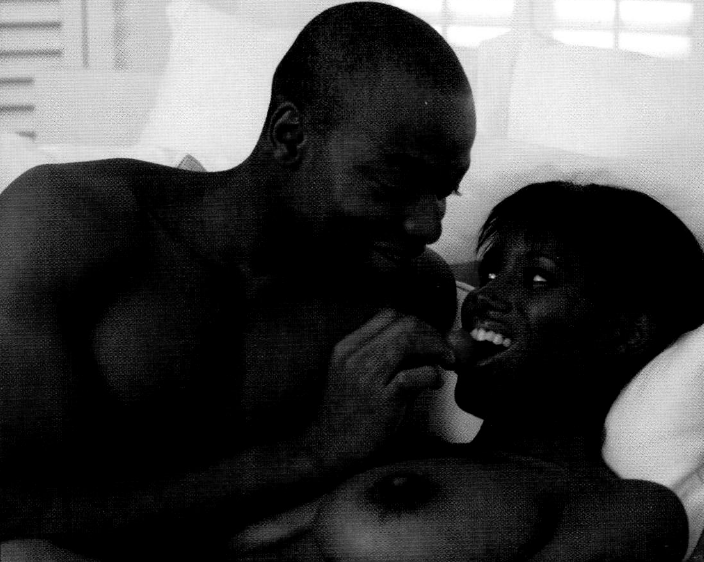

Index

e

f

g

h

i

k

l

t

uv

w

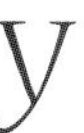

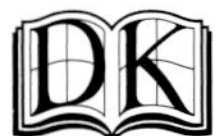

LONDON, NEW YORK, MELBOURNE, MUNICH, AND DELHI

US Editor: Chuck Wills
Project Editor: Daniel Mills
Senior Art Editor: Helen Spencer
Project Art Editor: Natasha Montgomery
Executive Managing Editor: Adèle Hayward
Managing Art Editor: Kat Mead
Senior Production Editor: Jennifer Murray
Production Controller: Bethan Blase
Creative Technical Support: Sonia Charbonnier
Art Director: Peter Luff
Publisher: Stephanie Jackson
Produced for DK by: Ruth Patrick (Editor) and Alison Fenton (designer).

Previously published in the United States as
Kama Sutra Step by Step, 2009
This edition first published in 2012 by
DK Publishing, 375 Hudson Street, New York, New York 10014

12 13 14 15 16 10 9 8 7 6
006—182626—Jan/2012

Published in Great Britain by Dorling Kindersley Limited.

A catalog record for this book is available from the Library of Congress.

ISBN: 978-0-7566-8961-2

Color reproduction by MDP, UK.
Printed and bound in China by South China Printing Co. Ltd

Discover more at
www.dk.com

ACKNOWLEDGMENTS
Jacket design: Charlotte Seymour and Wendy Bartlet
Photographer: John Rowley
Photographer's assistants: Jon Gorrigan and Russell Burton
Hair and make-up: Enzo Volpe
Photography production: Peter Mallory
Photographic direction and additional photography: Kat Mead
Proofreader: Siobhán O'Connor
Indexer: Laurence Errington
Additional design work: Katherine Raj and Collette Sadler
Retouching: Steve Crozier, Miranda Benzies, Jennifer Murray, and Jill Wooster

For kind permission to photograph sari cloths:
Punjab Textiles, London, UK
Anmol Fashion, London, UK.

DK encourages safe and responsible sex

- Use condoms to reduce your risk of sexually transmitted infections (STIs).
- Ensure that you and your new partner have been tested for STIs before any unprotected sexual activity.
- Speak to your doctor if you have any concerns about your sexual health.